Changes | An Insider's View

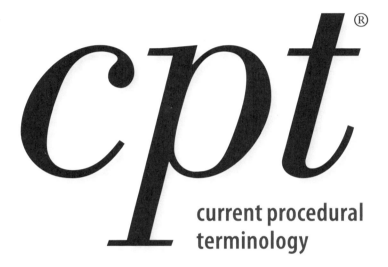

current procedural terminology

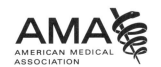

Executive Vice President, Chief Executive Officer: James L. Madara, MD
Senior Vice President, Health Solutions: Laurie A.S. McGraw
Vice President, Coding and Reimbursement Policy and Strategy: Jay Ahlman
Director, CPT Content Management and Development: Leslie W. Prellwitz
Director, CPT Editorial and Regulatory Services: Zachary Hochstetler
Manager, CPT Editorial Panel Processes: Desiree Rozell
Manager, CPT Content Management and Development: Karen E. O'Hara
Healthcare Coding Analysts/Senior Healthcare Coding Analysts: Thilani Attale; Jennifer Bell; Martha Espronceda; Desiree Evans; Dehandro Hayden; Lianne Stancik, Keisha Sutton
Program Manager, CPT Editorial Processes: Caitlin Dale
Vice President, Operations: Denise Foy
Manager, Publishing Operations: Elizabeth Goodman Duke
Senior Developmental Editor: Lisa Chin-Johnson
Production Specialist: Mary Ann Albanese
Business Operations Coordinator: Michael Pellegrino
Vice President, Sales: Lori Prestesater
Director, Channel Sales: Erin Kalitowski
Executive, Key Account Manager: Mark Daniels
Vice President, Product Development: Dave Sosnow
Product Manager, Print and Digital Products: Mark Ruthman
Marketing Manager: Vanessa Prieto

Copyright © 2019 by the American Medical Association. All rights reserved.
CPT® is a registered trademark of the American Medical Association

Printed in the United States of America. 19 20 21/ BD-WE / 9 8 7 6 5 4 3 2 1
Additional copies of this book may be ordered by calling 800-621-8335 or visit the AMA Store at **amastore.com**. Refer to product number OP512920.

No part of this publication may be reproduced, stored in a retrieval system, transmitted in any form, or by any means, electronic, mechanical, photocopying, recording, or otherwise, without prior written permission of the publisher.

Current Procedural Terminology (CPT®) is copyright 1966, 1970, 1973, 1977, 1981, 1983–2019 by the American Medical Association. All rights reserved.

The AMA does not directly or indirectly practice medicine or dispense medical services. This publication does not replace the AMA's *Current Procedural Terminology* codebook or other appropriate coding authority. The coding information in this publication should be used only as a guide.

Internet address: www.ama-assn.org

To request a license for distribution of products containing or reprinting CPT codes and/or guidelines, please see our website at www.ama-assn.org/go/cpt, or contact the American Medical Association CPT/DBP Intellectual Property Services, 330 North Wabash Avenue, Suite 39300, Chicago, IL 60611, 312 464-5022.

ISBN: 978-1-62202-900-6

Contents

Foreword...ix

Using This Book..xi
   The Symbols...xi
   The Rationale...xi
   Reading the Clinical Examples..xii
   Summary of Additions, Deletions, and Revisions and Indexes...........xii
   CPT Codebook Conventions and Styles..................................xii

Introduction..1
   Section Numbers and Their Sequences....................................1
      Add-on Codes...1
      Code Symbols...1

Evaluation and Management...3
   Summary of Additions, Deletions, and Revisions.........................3
   Domiciliary, Rest Home (eg, Assisted Living Facility), or Home Care Plan Oversight Services.....4
   Prolonged Services...4
      Prolonged Service Without Direct Patient Contact.................4
   Care Plan Oversight Services...5
   Preventive Medicine Services...5
      Counseling Risk Factor Reduction and Behavior Change Intervention.....5
   Non-Face-to-Face Services..6
      Telephone Services...6
      ►Online Digital Evaluation and Management Services◄..............6
      Interprofessional Telephone/Internet/Electronic Health Record Consultations.....9
      Digitally Stored Data Services/Remote Physiologic Monitoring.....10
      Remote Physiologic Monitoring Treatment Management Services.....12
   Special Evaluation and Management Services............................13
      Work Related or Medical Disability Evaluation Services..........13
   Inpatient Neonatal Intensive Care Services and Pediatric and Neonatal Critical Care Services...13
      Inpatient Neonatal and Pediatric Critical Care..................13
   Care Management Services..13
      Complex Chronic Care Management Services........................15
   Transitional Care Management Services.................................15

Surgery..17
   Summary of Additions, Deletions, and Revisions........................17
   Integumentary System..21
      Introduction..21
      Repair (Closure)..21
      Breast..25

►◄ = Contains new or revised text

Contents

Musculoskeletal System...29
    General...29
    Neck (Soft Tissues) and Thorax..34
    Spine (Vertebral Column)..34
    Femur (Thigh Region) and Knee Joint.....................................35
Respiratory System..35
    Nose...35
    Accessory Sinuses..35
    Larynx...37
    Lungs and Pleura...37
Cardiovascular System...39
    Heart and Pericardium..39
    Arteries and Veins...50
Hemic and Lymphatic Systems...62
    Lymph Nodes and Lymphatic Channels.......................................62
Digestive System..62
    Esophagus..62
    Anus...63
    Pancreas...65
    Abdomen, Peritoneum, and Omentum...65
Urinary System..67
    Urethra..67
Male Genital System...67
    Testis...67
Nervous System..67
    Skull, Meninges, and Brain...67
    Spine and Spinal Cord..68
    Extracranial Nerves, Peripheral Nerves, and Autonomic Nervous System.....70
Eye and Ocular Adnexa...80
    Anterior Segment...80
    Ocular Adnexa..84
    Conjunctiva..84
Auditory System...84
    Middle Ear...84
Operating Microscope..85

Radiology 87
Summary of Additions, Deletions, and Revisions......................................87
Diagnostic Radiology (Diagnostic Imaging)...89
    Chest..89
    Abdomen..89

Contents

      Gastrointestinal Tract 89
      Vascular Procedures 93
      Other Procedures 93
   Diagnostic Ultrasound 94
      Genitalia 94
      Ultrasonic Guidance Procedures 94
      Other Procedures 95
   Radiologic Guidance 95
      Fluoroscopic Guidance 95
      Computed Tomography Guidance 95
   Nuclear Medicine 96
      Diagnostic 96

Pathology and Laboratory 109
   Summary of Additions, Deletions, and Revisions 109
   Therapeutic Drug Assays 113
   Molecular Pathology 114
      Tier 1 Molecular Pathology Procedures 114
      Tier 2 Molecular Pathology Procedures 116
   Multianalyte Assays with Algorithmic Analyses 124
   Microbiology 125
   Reproductive Medicine Procedures 126
   Proprietary Laboratory Analyses 126

Medicine 145
   Summary of Additions, Deletions, and Revisions 145
   Vaccines, Toxoids 149
   Psychiatry 150
      Psychiatric Diagnostic Procedures 150
   Biofeedback 150
   Gastroenterology 151
   Ophthalmology 151
      Special Ophthalmological Services 151
   Special Otorhinolaryngologic Services 153
      Vestibular Function Tests, With Recording (eg, ENG) 153
      Evaluative and Therapeutic Services 153
   Cardiovascular 155
      Cardiography 155
      Cardiovascular Monitoring Services 155
      Implantable, Insertable, and Wearable Cardiac Device Evaluations 155
      Echocardiography 158
      Cardiac Catheterization 158

▶ ◀ = Contains new or revised text   American Medical Association   **v**

Contents

    Intracardiac Electrophysiological Procedures/Studies.................................. 160

    Noninvasive Physiologic Studies and Procedures 162

    Home and Outpatient International Normalized Ratio (INR) Monitoring Services 163

Noninvasive Vascular Diagnostic Studies 164

    Extremity Arterial Studies (Including Digits) 164

    Extremity Venous Studies (Including Digits) 164

    Extremity Arterial-Venous Studies... 164

Pulmonary 165

    Pulmonary Diagnostic Testing and Therapies 165

Neurology and Neuromuscular Procedures 166

    Sleep Medicine Testing 166

    Routine Electroencephalography (EEG) 166

    ▶Range of Motion Testing◀ 167

    Ischemic Muscle Testing and Guidance for Chemodenervation 167

    Special EEG Tests... 168

    Neurostimulators, Analysis-Programming 178

Adaptive Behavior Services 179

    Adaptive Behavior Assessments 179

    Adaptive Behavior Treatment.. 180

Central Nervous System Assessments/Tests (eg, Neuro-Cognitive, Mental Status,
Speech Testing) 180

▶Health Behavior Assessment and Intervention◀ 181

Physical Medicine and Rehabilitation 184

    Therapeutic Procedures 184

    Tests and Measurements... 185

Acupuncture 186

Education and Training for Patient Self-Management 186

Non-Face-to-Face Nonphysician Services 187

    Telephone Services.. 187

    ▶Qualified Nonphysician Health Care Professional Online Digital Evaluation
    and Management Service◀ 187

Category II Codes 191

Summary of Additions, Deletions, and Revisions 191

Physical Examination 192

Diagnostic/Screening Processes or Results... 192

Category III Codes.. 195

Summary of Additions, Deletions, and Revisions 195

Contents

Appendix A **233**
    Summary of Additions, Deletions, and Revisions 233
    Modifiers 234
        Modifiers Approved for Ambulatory Surgery Center (ASC) Hospital Outpatient Use 234

Appendix E **235**
    Summary of Additions, Deletions, and Revisions 235
    Summary of CPT Codes Exempt from Modifier 51 236

Appendix O **237**
    Summary of Additions, Deletions, and Revisions 237
    Multianalyte Assays with Algorithmic Analyses and Proprietary Laboratory Analyses 249

Indexes **271**
    Instructions for the Use of the Changes Indexes 271
        Index of Coding Changes 273
        Index of Modifiers 277

▶ ◀ = Contains new or revised text

Foreword

The American Medical Association (AMA) is pleased to offer *CPT® Changes 2020: An Insider's View (CPT Changes)*. Since this book was first published in 2000, it has served as the definitive text on additions, revisions, and deletions to the CPT code set.

In developing this book, it was our intention to provide CPT users with a glimpse of the logic, rationale, and proposed function of the changes in the CPT code set that resulted from the decisions of the CPT Editorial Panel and the yearly update process. The AMA staff members have the unique perspective of being both participants in the CPT editorial process and users of the CPT code set.

CPT Changes is intended to bridge understanding between clinical decisions made by the CPT Editorial Panel regarding appropriate service or procedure descriptions with functional interpretations of coding guidelines, code intent, and code combinations, which are necessary for users of the CPT code set. A new edition of this book, like the CPT codebook, is published annually.

To assist CPT users in applying the new and revised CPT codes, this book includes clinical examples that describe the typical patient who might undergo the procedure and detailed descriptions of the procedure. Both of these are required as a part of the CPT code change proposal process, which are used by the CPT Editorial Panel in crafting language, guidelines, and parenthetical notes associated with the new or revised codes. In addition, many of the clinical examples and descriptions of the procedures are used in the AMA/Specialty Society Relative Value Scale (RVS) Update (RUC) process to conduct surveys on physician work and to develop work relative value recommendations to the Centers for Medicare & Medicaid Services (CMS) as part of the Medicare physician fee schedule (MPFS).

We are confident that the information provided in *CPT Changes* will prove to be a valuable resource to CPT users, not only as they apply changes for the year of publication, but also as a resource for frequent reference as they continue their education in CPT coding. The AMA makes every effort to be a voice of clarity and consistency in an otherwise confusing system of health care claims and payment, and *CPT Changes 2020: An Insider's View* demonstrates our continued commitment to assist users of the CPT code set.

Using This Book

This book is designed to serve as a reference guide to understanding the changes contained in the Current Procedural Terminology (CPT®) 2020 code set and is not intended to replace the CPT codebook. Every effort is made to ensure accuracy, however, if differences exist, you should always defer to the information in the *CPT 2020* codebook.

The Symbols

This book uses the same coding conventions as those used in the CPT nomenclature.

- ● Indicates a new procedure number was added to the CPT nomenclature
- ▲ Indicates a code revision has resulted in a substantially altered procedure descriptor
- + Indicates a CPT add-on code
- ⊘ Indicates a code that is exempt from the use of modifier 51 but is not designated as a CPT add-on procedure or service
- ►◄ Indicates revised guidelines, cross-references, and/or explanatory text
- ⁄ Indicates a code for a vaccine that is pending FDA approval
- # Indicates a resequenced code. Note that rather than deleting and renumbering, resequencing allows existing codes to be relocated to an appropriate location for the code concept, regardless of the numeric sequence. Numerically placed references (ie, Code is out of numerical sequence. See…) are used as navigational alerts in the CPT codebook to direct the user to the location of an out-of-sequence code. Therefore, remember to refer to the CPT codebook for these references.
- ★ Indicates a telemedicine code
- ⋈ Indicates a duplicate PLA test
- ↑↓ Indicates a Category I PLA

Whenever possible, complete segments of text from the CPT codebook are provided; however, in some instances, only pertinent text is included.

The Rationale

After listing each change or series of changes from the CPT codebook, a rationale is provided. The rationale is intended to provide a brief clarification and explanation of the changes. Nevertheless, it is important to note that they may not address every question that may arise as a result of the changes.

►◄ = Contains new or revised text

Reading the Clinical Examples

The clinical examples and their procedural descriptions, which reflect typical clinical situations found in the health-care setting, are included in this text with many of the codes to provide practical situations for which the new and/or revised codes in the CPT 2020 code set would be appropriately reported. It is important to note that these examples do not suggest limiting the use of a code; instead, they are meant to represent the typical patient and service or procedure, as previously stated. In addition, they do not describe the universe of patients for whom the service or procedure would be appropriate. It is important to also note that third-party payer reporting policies may differ.

Summary of Additions, Deletions, and Revisions and Indexes

A **summary of additions, deletions, and revisions** for the section is presented in a tabular format at the beginning of each section. This table provides readers with the ability to quickly search and have an overview of all of the new, revised, and deleted codes for 2020. In addition to the tabular review of changes, the coding index individually lists all of the new, revised, and deleted codes with each code's status (new, revised, deleted) in parentheses. For more information about these indexes, please read the **Instructions for the Use of the Changes Indexes** on page 271.

CPT Codebook Conventions and Styles

Similar to the CPT codebook, the guidelines and revised and new CPT code descriptors and parenthetical notes in *CPT Changes 2020* are set in green type. Any revised text, guidelines, and/or headings are indicated with the ▶ ◀ symbols. To match the style used in the codebook, the revised or new text symbol is placed at the beginning and end of a paragraph or section that contains revisions, and the use of green text visually indicates new and/or revised content. Similarly, each section's and subsections' (Surgery) complete code range are listed in the tabs, regardless if these codes are discussed in this book. In addition, all of the different level of headings in the codebook are also picked up, as appropiate, and set in the same style and color. Besides matching the convention and style used in the CPT codebook, the Rationales are placed within a shaded box to distinguish them from the rest of the content for quick and easy reference.

Introduction

Current Procedural Terminology (CPT®), Fourth Edition, is a set of codes, descriptions, and guidelines intended to describe procedures and services performed by physicians and other health care professionals, or entities. Each procedure or service is identified with a five-digit code. The use of CPT codes simplifies the reporting of procedures and services. In the CPT code set, the term "procedure" is used to describe services, including diagnostic tests.

…

Section Numbers and Their Sequences

Evaluation and Management............99201-99499

…

Add-on Codes

Some of the listed procedures are commonly carried out in addition to the …

The add-on code concept in CPT 2020 applies …

▶Add-on codes are always performed in addition to the primary service or procedure and must never be reported as a stand-alone code. When the add-on procedure can be reported bilaterally and is performed bilaterally, the appropriate add-on code is reported twice, unless the code descriptor, guidelines, or parenthetical instructions for that particular add-on code instructs otherwise. Do not report modifier 50, Bilateral procedures, in conjunction with add-on codes. All add-on codes in the CPT code set are exempt from the multiple procedure concept. See the definitions of modifier 50 and 51 in **Appendix A.**◀

Rationale

In support of the revision to instructions for reporting add-on procedures when performed bilaterally, the Add-on Codes guidelines in the Introduction section have been revised. The guidelines state that unless the code descriptor, guidelines, or parenthetical instructions for that particular add-on code instructs otherwise, the add-on procedure that can be reported bilaterally and is performed bilaterally is reported twice.

Refer to the codebook and the Rationale for modifier 50, *Bilateral Procedure*, guideline revisions for a full discussion of these changes.

Code Symbols

A summary listing of additions, deletions, and revisions…

Resequenced codes that…

Duplicate proprietary laboratory analyses (PLA) tests are annotated by the ✶ symbol. PLA codes describe…

▶Unless specifically noted, even though the Proprietary Laboratory Analyses section of the code set is located at the end of the Pathology and Laboratory section of the code set, a PLA code does not fulfill Category I code criteria. A PLA code(s) that has Category I status is annotated by the ↑↓ symbol.◀

Rationale

The Code Symbols guidelines in the Introduction section have been revised to include the addition of the new PLA symbol ↑↓. Even though PLA codes are not required to fulfill the Category I criteria, any PLA coded test that satisfies Category I criteria and has been accepted by the CPT Editorial Panel will be designated with the ↑↓ symbol to the existing PLA code and will remain in the PLA section of the code set.

Refer to the codebook and the Rationale in the Pathology and Laboratory, Proprietary Laboratory Analyses subsection for a full discussion of these changes.

Notes

Evaluation and Management

Summary of Additions, Deletions, and Revisions

The summary of changes shows the actual changes that have been made to the code descriptors.

New codes appear with a bullet (●) and are indicated as "Code added." Revised codes are preceded with a triangle (▲). Within revised codes, or if a code symbol has been deleted, the deleted language and code symbol appear with a ~~strikethrough~~ (⊖), while new text appears underlined.

The ⁄ symbol is used to identify codes for vaccines that are pending FDA approval. The # symbol is used to identify codes that have been resequenced. CPT add-on codes are annotated by the ✚ symbol. The ⊘ symbol is used to identify codes that are exempt from the use of modifier 51. The ★ symbol is used to identify codes that may be used for reporting telemedicine services. The ✳ is used to identify proprietary laboratory analyses (PLA) test that has an identical descriptor as another PLA test. A PLA code that satisfies Category I code criteria and has been accepted by the CPT Editorial Panel is annotated with the ⇅ symbol.

Code	Description
#●99421	Code added
#●99422	Code added
#●99423	Code added
99444	~~Online evaluation and management service provided by a physician or other qualified health care professional who may report evaluation and management services provided to an established patient or guardian, not originating from a related E/M service provided within the previous 7 days, using the Internet or similar electronic communications network~~
#●99473	Code added
#●99474	Code added
#▲99457	Remote physiologic monitoring treatment management services, ~~20 minutes or more of~~ clinical staff/physician/other qualified health care professional time in a calendar month requiring interactive communication with the patient/caregiver during the month<u>; first 20 minutes</u>
#✚●99458	Code added

Evaluation and Management

Domiciliary, Rest Home (eg, Assisted Living Facility), or Home Care Plan Oversight Services

(For instructions on the use of 99339, 99340, see introductory notes for 99374-99380)

(For care plan oversight services for patients under the care of a home health agency, hospice, or nursing facility, see 99374-99380)

▶(Do not report 99339, 99340 for time reported with 98966, 98967, 98968, 99421, 99422, 99423, 99441, 99442, 99443)◀

99339 Individual physician supervision of a patient (patient not present) in home, domiciliary or rest home (eg, assisted living facility) requiring complex and multidisciplinary care modalities involving regular physician development and/or revision of care plans, review of subsequent reports of patient status, review of related laboratory and other studies, communication (including telephone calls) for purposes of assessment or care decisions with health care professional(s), family member(s), surrogate decision maker(s) (eg, legal guardian) and/or key caregiver(s) involved in patient's care, integration of new information into the medical treatment plan and/or adjustment of medical therapy, within a calendar month; 15-29 minutes

99340 30 minutes or more

(Do not report 99339, 99340 for patients under the care of a home health agency, enrolled in a hospice program, or for nursing facility residents)

(Do not report 99339, 99340 during the same month with 99487-99489)

(Do not report 99339, 99340 when performed during the service time of codes 99495 or 99496)

Rationale

In accordance with the deletion of codes 98969 and 99444 and the addition of codes 99421, 99422, and 99423, the parenthetical note in the Domiciliary, Rest Home (eg, Assisted Living Facility), or Home Care Plan Oversight Services subsection has been revised to reflect these changes.

Refer to the codebook and the Rationale for codes 98970, 98971, 98972, 99421, 99422, and 99423 for a full discussion of these changes.

Prolonged Services

Prolonged Service Without Direct Patient Contact

Codes 99358 and 99359 are used when a prolonged service is provided that is neither face-to-face time in the office or outpatient setting, nor additional unit/floor time in the hospital or nursing facility setting during the same session of an evaluation and management service and is beyond the usual physician or other qualified health care professional service time.

This service is to be reported in relation to other physician or other qualified health care professional services, including evaluation and management services at any level. This prolonged service may be reported on a different date than the primary service to which it is related. For example, extensive record review may relate to a previous evaluation and management service performed earlier and commences upon receipt of past records. However, it must relate to a service or patient where (face-to-face) patient care has occurred or will occur and relate to ongoing patient management. A typical time for the primary service need not be established within the CPT code set.

Codes 99358 and 99359 are used to report the total duration of non-face-to-face time spent by a physician or other qualified health care professional on a given date providing prolonged service, even if the time spent by the physician or other qualified health care professional on that date is not continuous. Code 99358 is used to report the first hour of prolonged service on a given date regardless of the place of service. It should be used only once per date.

Prolonged service of less than 30 minutes total duration on a given date is not separately reported because the work involved is included in the total work of the evaluation and management or psychotherapy codes.

Code 99359 is used to report each additional 30 minutes beyond the first hour regardless of the place of service. It may also be used to report the final 15 to 30 minutes of prolonged service on a given date.

Prolonged service of less than 15 minutes beyond the first hour or less than 15 minutes beyond the final 30 minutes is not reported separately.

▶Do not report 99358, 99359 for time spent in care plan oversight services (99339, 99340, 99374-99380), home and outpatient INR monitoring (93792, 93793), medical team conferences (99366-99368), or online digital evaluation and management services (99421, 99422, 99423).◀

99358 **Prolonged evaluation and management service** before and/or after direct patient care; first hour

+ 99359 each additional 30 minutes (List separately in addition to code for prolonged service)

Rationale

In accordance with the addition of codes 99421, 99422, and 99423, the guidelines for prolonged service without direct patient contact have been revised.

Refer to the codebook and the Rationale for codes 99421, 99422, and 99423 for a full discussion of these changes.

Care Plan Oversight Services

Care plan oversight services are reported separately from codes for office/outpatient, hospital, home, nursing facility or domiciliary, or non-face-to-face services. The complexity and approximate time of the care plan oversight services provided within a 30-day period determine code selection. Only one individual may report services for a given period of time, to reflect the sole or predominant supervisory role with a particular patient. These codes should not be reported for supervision of patients in nursing facilities or under the care of home health agencies unless they require recurrent supervision of therapy.

The work involved in providing very low intensity or infrequent supervision services is included in the pre- and post-encounter work for home, office/outpatient and nursing facility or domiciliary visit codes.

(For care plan oversight services of patients in the home, domiciliary, or rest home [eg, assisted living facility], see 99339, 99340, and for hospice agency, see 99377, 99378)

▶(Do not report 99374-99380 for time reported with 98966, 98967, 98968, 99421, 99422, 99423, 99441, 99442, 99443)◀

(Do not report 99374-99378 during the same month with 99487-99489)

(Do not report 99374-99380 when performed during the service time of codes 99495 or 99496)

99374 **Supervision** of a patient under care of home health agency (patient not present) in home, domiciliary or equivalent environment (eg, Alzheimer's facility) requiring complex and multidisciplinary care modalities involving regular development and/or revision of care plans by that individual, review of subsequent reports of patient status, review of related laboratory and other studies, communication (including telephone calls) for purposes of assessment or care decisions with health care professional(s), family member(s), surrogate decision maker(s) (eg, legal guardian) and/or key caregiver(s) involved in patient's care, integration of new information into the medical treatment plan and/or adjustment of medical therapy, within a calendar month; 15-29 minutes

99375 30 minutes or more

Rationale

In accordance with the deletion of codes 98969 and 99444 and the addition of codes 99421, 99422, and 99423, the parenthetical note in the Care Plan Oversight Services subsection has been revised to reflect these changes.

Refer to the codebook and the Rationale for codes 98970, 98971, 98972, 99421, 99422, and 99423 for a full discussion of these changes.

Preventive Medicine Services

Counseling Risk Factor Reduction and Behavior Change Intervention

New or Established Patient

These codes are used to report services provided face-to-face by a physician or other qualified health care professional for the purpose of promoting health and preventing illness or injury. They are distinct from evaluation and management (E/M) services that may be reported separately with modifier 25 when performed. Risk factor reduction services are used for persons without a specific illness for which the counseling might otherwise be used as part of treatment.

Preventive medicine counseling and risk factor reduction interventions will vary with age and should address such issues as family problems, diet and exercise, substance use, sexual practices, injury prevention, dental health, and diagnostic and laboratory test results available at the time of the encounter.

Behavior change interventions are for persons who have a behavior that is often considered an illness itself, such as tobacco use and addiction, substance abuse/misuse, or

Evaluation and Management

obesity. Behavior change services may be reported when performed as part of the treatment of condition(s) related to or potentially exacerbated by the behavior or when performed to change the harmful behavior that has not yet resulted in illness. Any E/M services reported on the same day must be distinct and reported with modifier 25, and time spent providing these services may not be used as a basis for the E/M code selection. Behavior change services involve specific validated interventions of assessing readiness for change and barriers to change, advising a change in behavior, assisting by providing specific suggested actions and motivational counseling, and arranging for services and follow-up.

For counseling groups of patients with symptoms or established illness, use 99078.

►Health behavior assessment and intervention services (96156, 96158, 96159, 96164, 96165, 96167, 96168, 96170, 96171) should not be reported on the same day as codes 99401-99412.◄

Rationale

In accordance with the deletion of codes 96150, 96151, 96152, 96153, 96154, and 96155, and the establishment of codes 96156, 96158, 96159, 96164, 96165, 96167, 96168, 96170, and 96171, a guideline within the Counseling Risk Factor Reduction and Behavior Change Intervention New or Established Patient subsection has been revised to reflect these changes.

Refer to the codebook and the Rationale for codes 96156, 96158, 96159, 96164, 96165, 96167, 96168, 96170, and 96171 for a full discussion of these changes.

Other Preventive Medicine Services

99421	Code is out of numerical sequence. See 99442-99447
99422	Code is out of numerical sequence. See 99442-99447
99423	Code is out of numerical sequence. See 99442-99447

Non-Face-to-Face Services

Telephone Services

►Telephone services are non-face-to-face evaluation and management (E/M) services provided to a patient using the telephone by a physician or other qualified health care professional, who may report evaluation and management services. These codes are used to report episodes of patient care initiated by an established patient or guardian of an established patient. If the telephone service ends with a decision to see the patient within 24 hours or next available urgent visit appointment, the code is not reported; rather the encounter is considered part of the preservice work of the subsequent E/M service, procedure, and visit. Likewise, if the telephone call refers to an E/M service performed and reported by that individual within the previous seven days (either requested or unsolicited patient follow-up) or within the postoperative period of the previously completed procedure, then the service(s) is considered part of that previous E/M service or procedure. (Do not report 99441-99443, if 99421, 99422, 99423 have been reported by the same provider in the previous seven days for the same problem.)◄

(For telephone services provided by a qualified nonphysician who may not report evaluation and management services [eg, speech-language pathologists, physical therapists, occupational therapists, social workers, dietitians], see 98966-98968)

99441 Telephone evaluation and management service by a physician or other qualified health care professional who may report evaluation and management services provided to an established patient, parent, or guardian not originating from a related E/M service provided within the previous 7 days nor leading to an E/M service or procedure within the next 24 hours or soonest available appointment; 5-10 minutes of medical discussion

99442 11-20 minutes of medical discussion

99443 21-30 minutes of medical discussion

Rationale

In accordance with the deletion of code 99444, and the addition of codes 99421, 99422, and 99423, the guidelines in the Non-Face-to-Face-Services Telephone Services subsection have been revised.

Refer to the codebook and the Rationale for codes 99421, 99422, and 99423 for a full discussion of these changes.

►Online Digital Evaluation and Management Services◄

►Online digital evaluation and management (E/M) services (99421, 99422, 99423) are patient-initiated services with physicians or other qualified health care professionals (QHPs). Online digital E/M services require physician or other QHP's evaluation, assessment, and management of the patient. These services are not for the nonevaluative electronic communication of test results, scheduling of appointments, or other communication that does not include E/M. While the patient's problem may be new to the physician or other QHP, the patient is an established patient. Patients initiate these services through Health Insurance Portability and Accountability Act (HIPAA)-compliant secure platforms, such as electronic health record (EHR) portals, secure email, or other digital applications, which allow digital communication with the physician or other QHP.

Online digital E/M services are reported once for the physician's or other QHP's cumulative time devoted to the service during a seven-day period. The seven-day period begins with the physician's or other QHP's initial, personal review of the patient-generated inquiry. Physician's or other QHP's cumulative service time includes review of the initial inquiry, review of patient records or data pertinent to assessment of the patient's problem, personal physician or other QHP interaction with clinical staff focused on the patient's problem, development of management plans, including physician- or other QHP generation of prescriptions or ordering of tests, and subsequent communication with the patient through online, telephone, email, or other digitally supported communication, which does not otherwise represent a separately reported E/M service. All professional decision making, assessment, and subsequent management by physicians or other QHPs in the same group practice contribute to the cumulative service time of the patient's online digital E/M service. Online digital E/M services require permanent documentation storage (electronic or hard copy) of the encounter.

If within seven days of the initiation of an online digital E/M service, a separately reported E/M visit occurs, then the physician or other QHP work devoted to the online digital E/M service is incorporated into the separately reported E/M visit (eg, additive of visit time for a time-based E/M visit or additive of decision-making complexity for a key component-based E/M visit). This includes E/M visits and procedures that are provided through synchronous telemedicine visits using interactive audio and video telecommunication equipment, which are reported with modifier 95 appended to the E/M service code. If the patient initiates an online digital inquiry for the same or a related problem within seven days of a previous E/M service, then the online digital visit is not reported. If the online digital inquiry is related to a surgical procedure and occurs during the postoperative period of a previously completed procedure, then the online digital E/M service is not reported separately. If the patient generates the initial online digital inquiry for a new problem within seven days of a previous E/M visit that addressed a different problem, then the online digital E/M service may be reported separately. If the patient presents a new, unrelated problem during the seven-day period of an online digital E/M service, then the physician's or other QHP's time spent on evaluation, assessment, and management of the additional problem is added to the cumulative service time of the online digital E/M service for that seven-day period.◄

▶(For online digital E/M services provided by a qualified nonphysician health care professional who may not report the physician or other qualified health care professional E/M services [eg, speech-language pathologists, physical therapists, occupational therapists, social workers, dietitians], see 98970, 98971, 98972)◄

#● **99421** Online digital evaluation and management service, for an established patient, for up to 7 days, cumulative time during the 7 days; 5-10 minutes

#● **99422** 11-20 minutes

#● **99423** 21 or more minutes

▶(Report 99421, 99422, 99423 once per 7-day period)◄

▶(Clinical staff time is not calculated as part of cumulative time for 99421, 99422, 99423)◄

▶(Do not report online digital E/M services for cumulative service time less than 5 minutes)◄

▶(Do not count 99421, 99422, 99423 time otherwise reported with other services)◄

▶(Do not report 99421, 99422, 99423 on a day when the physician or other qualified health care professional reports E/M services [99201, 99202, 99203, 99204, 99205, 99212, 99213, 99214, 99215, 99241, 99242, 99243, 99244, 99245])◄

▶(Do not report 99421, 99422, 99423 when using 99091, 99339, 99340, 99374, 99375, 99377, 99378, 99379, 99380, 99487, 99489, 99495, 99496 for the same communication[s])◄

▶(Do not report 99421, 99422, 99423 for home and outpatient INR monitoring when reporting 93792, 93793)◄

▶(99444 has been deleted. To report, see 99421, 99422, 99423)◄

Rationale

The On-Line Medical Evaluation subsection has been revised with the new heading, Online Digital Evaluation and Management Services, with new guidelines, and the addition of three new codes. In addition, existing code 99444 has been deleted.

The online digital evaluation and management (E/M) services are intended for patient-initiated digital communications that require a clinical decision that would otherwise have been typically provided in the office. These services provide a clinician the opportunity to gather information through, for example, review of patient records, and to develop a diagnosis and possible management plan. These services are not intended to

Evaluation and Management

represent the nonevaluative electronic communication that may be solely focused on dissemination of test results, processing of medication requests, or scheduling of appointments.

Online digital communication has been expanded to encompass multiple types and episodes of physician communication initiated by patient inquiries typically submitted via electronic health record (EHR) portals. Because the opportunities for patients to communicate digitally with their physicians have expanded, the cumulative work of addressing the patient's presenting problem may transpire over multiple encounters and over multiple consecutive days. With this accumulation of physician time, new codes were necessary to better reflect the extent of physician work required to complete the evaluation of the patient's inquiry.

Codes 99421, 99422, and 99423 are to be reported for online digital E/M services that are patient-initiated services with physicians or other qualified health care professionals (QHPs). These codes are reported for established patients and are time-based. Code 99421 is for the first 5-10 minutes, code 99422 is for 11-20 minutes, and code 99423 is for 21 or more minutes of service. Guidelines have been added to outline the components of these codes and their use.

A parenthetical note has been added to remind users that codes 99421, 99422, and 99423 may only be reported once per 7-day period. Exclusionary parenthetical notes have been added to indicate: if the online digital evaluation is less than 5 minutes, reporting of these codes is not appropriate; home INR monitoring codes 93792 and 93793 should be used if home INR is performed and not codes 99421, 99422, and 99423; and do not report codes 99421, 99422, and 99423 on a day when the physician or other QHP reports codes 99201, 99202, 99203, 99204, 99205, 99212, 99213, 99214, 99215, 99241, 99242, 99243, 99244, and 99245. In addition, an exclusionary note indicating that time otherwise reported with other services should not count for codes 99421, 99422, and 99423.

Code 99444 has been deleted as codes 99421, 99422, and 99423 have been established to report common practice.

Clinical Example (99421)

Patient 1: A mother submits an online query through her child's physician's electronic health record (EHR) portal about her six-year-old son, who developed itchy rash two days after an outdoor hike.

Patient 2: A 68-year-old patient submits an online query through his physician's EHR because he developed itchy rash two days after an outdoor hike.

Description of Procedure (99421)

Physician reviews the initial patient inquiry, medical history, documents sent by the patient and/or obtained by clinical staff, and checks online data registries or information exchanges. Assess medical condition described in the patient query. Formulate and send physician's response (eg, a diagnosis and treatment plan, and/or request for additional information). Review test results and other reports. Email prescriptions. Conduct follow-up communication with the patient. Interact with clinical staff to order diagnostic tests, coordinate care, and implement the care plan. Complete medical record documentation of all communications. Provide necessary care coordination, telephonic, or electronic communication assistance.

Clinical Example (99422)

Patient 1: A 16-year-old female asthmatic submits an online query through her physician's EHR portal about her increase in wheezing and cough.

Patient 2: A 75-year-old female with chronic obstructive pulmonary disease (COPD) and congestive heart failure (CHF) submits an online query through her physician's EHR portal about worsening shortness of breath and mild weight gain.

Description of Procedure (99422)

Physician reviews the initial patient inquiry, medical history, documents sent by the patient and/or obtained by clinical staff, and checks online data registries or information exchanges. Assess medical condition described in the patient query. Formulate and send physician's response (eg, a diagnosis and treatment plan, and/or request for additional information). Review test results and other reports. Email prescriptions. Conduct follow-up communication with the patient. Interact with clinical staff to order diagnostic tests, coordinate care, and implement the care plan. Complete medical record documentation of all communications. Provide necessary care coordination, telephonic, or electronic communication assistance.

Clinical Example (99423)

Patient 1: A mother submits an online query through her child's physician's EHR portal about her six-year-old son, who has attention-deficit/hyperactivity disorder (ADHD) with increased lability upon starting a new school.

Patient 2: An adult child of an 80-year-old parent submits through her parent's physician's EHR portal an online query about her parent, who has moderate dementia and has become increasingly confused.

Description of Procedure (99423)

Physician reviews the initial patient inquiry, medical history, documents sent by the patient and/or obtained by clinical staff, and checks online data registries or information exchanges. Assess medical condition described in the patient query. Formulate and send physician's response (eg, a diagnosis and treatment plan, and/or request for additional information). Review test results and other reports. Email prescriptions. Conduct follow-up communication with the patient. Interact with clinical staff to order diagnostic tests, coordinate care, and implement the care plan. Complete medical record documentation of all communications. Provide necessary care coordination, telephonic, or electronic communication assistance.

Interprofessional Telephone/Internet/Electronic Health Record Consultations

The consultant should use codes 99446, 99447, 99448, 99449, 99451 to report interprofessional telephone/Internet/electronic health record consultations. An interprofessional telephone/Internet/electronic health record consultation is an assessment and management service in which a patient's treating (eg, attending or primary) physician or other qualified health care professional requests the opinion and/or treatment advice of a physician with specific specialty expertise (the consultant) to assist the treating physician or other qualified health care professional in the diagnosis and/or management of the patient's problem without patient face-to-face contact with the consultant.

The patient for whom the interprofessional telephone/Internet/electronic health record consultation is requested may be either a new patient to the consultant or an established patient with a new problem or an exacerbation of an existing problem. However, the consultant should not have seen the patient in a face-to-face encounter within the last 14 days. When the telephone/Internet/electronic health record consultation leads to a transfer of care or other face-to-face service (eg, a surgery, a hospital visit, or a scheduled office evaluation of the patient) within the next 14 days or next available appointment date of the consultant, these codes are not reported.

Review of pertinent medical records, laboratory studies, imaging studies, medication profile, pathology specimens, etc is included in the telephone/Internet/electronic health record consultation service and should not be reported separately when reporting 99446, 99447, 99448, 99449, 99451. The majority of the service time reported (greater than 50%) must be devoted to the medical consultative verbal or Internet discussion. If greater than 50% of the time for the service is devoted to data review and/or analysis, 99446, 99447, 99448, 99449 should not be reported. However, the service time for 99451 is based on total review and interprofessional-communication time.

If more than one telephone/Internet/electronic health record contact(s) is required to complete the consultation request (eg, discussion of test results), the entirety of the service and the cumulative discussion and information review time should be reported with a single code. Codes 99446, 99447, 99448, 99449, 99451 should not be reported more than once within a seven-day interval.

The written or verbal request for telephone/Internet/electronic health record advice by the treating/requesting physician or other qualified health care professional should be documented in the patient's medical record, including the reason for the request. Codes 99446, 99447, 99448, 99449 conclude with a verbal opinion report and written report from the consultant to the treating/requesting physician or other qualified health care professional. Code 99451 concludes with only a written report.

▶Telephone/Internet/electronic health record consultations of less than five minutes should not be reported. Consultant communications with the patient and/or family may be reported using 98966, 98967, 98968, 99421, 99422, 99423, 99441, 99442, 99443, and the time related to these services is not used in reporting 99446, 99447, 99448, 99449. Do not report 99358, 99359 for any time within the service period, if reporting 99446, 99447, 99448, 99449, 99451.◀

When the sole purpose of the telephone/Internet/electronic health record communication is to arrange a transfer of care or other face-to-face service, these codes are not reported.

The treating/requesting physician or other qualified health care professional may report 99452 if spending 16-30 minutes in a service day preparing for the referral and/or communicating with the consultant. Do not report 99452 more than once in a 14-day period. The treating/requesting physician or other qualified health care professional may report the prolonged service codes 99354, 99355, 99356, 99357 for the time spent on the interprofessional telephone/Internet/electronic health record discussion with the consultant (eg, specialist) if the time **exceeds 30 minutes** beyond the typical time of the appropriate E/M service performed and the patient is present (on-site) and accessible to the treating/requesting physician or other qualified health care professional. If the interprofessional telephone/Internet/electronic health record assessment and management service occurs when the patient is not present and the time spent in a day **exceeds 30 minutes,** then the non-face-to-face prolonged service codes 99358, 99359 may be reported by the treating/requesting physician or other qualified health care professional.

(For telephone services provided by a physician to a patient, see 99441, 99442, 99443)

(For telephone services provided by a qualified health care professional to a patient, see 98966, 98967, 98968)

▶(For online digital E/M services provided by a physician or other qualified health care professional to a patient, see 99421, 99422, 99423)◀

Rationale

In accordance with the deletion of codes 98969 and 99444, and the addition of codes 98970, 98971, 98972, 99421, 99422, and 99423, the guidelines and parenthetical notes in the Interprofessional Telephone/Internet/Electronic Health Record Consultations subsection have been revised to reflect these changes.

Refer to the codebook and the Rationale for codes 98970, 98971, 98972, 99421, 99422, and 99423 for a full discussion of these changes.

Digitally Stored Data Services/Remote Physiologic Monitoring

Codes 99453 and 99454 are used to report remote physiologic monitoring services (eg, weight, blood pressure, pulse oximetry) during a 30-day period. To report 99453, 99454, the device used must be a medical device as defined by the FDA, and the service must be ordered by a physician or other qualified health care professional. Code 99453 may be used to report the set-up and patient education on use of the device(s). Code 99454 may be used to report supply of the device for daily recording or programmed alert transmissions. Codes 99453, 99454 are not reported if monitoring is less than 16 days. Do not report 99453, 99454 when these services are included in other codes for the duration of time of the physiologic monitoring service (eg, 95250 for continuous glucose monitoring requires a minimum of 72 hours of monitoring).

Code 99091 should be reported no more than once in a 30-day period to include the physician or other qualified health care professional time involved with data accession, review and interpretation, modification of care plan as necessary (including communication to patient and/or caregiver), and associated documentation.

▶If the services described by 99091 or 99474 are provided on the same day the patient presents for an evaluation and management (E/M) service to the same provider, these services should be considered part of the E/M service and not reported separately.◀

Do not report 99091 in the same calendar month as care plan oversight services (99374, 99375, 99377, 99378, 99379, 99380), home, domiciliary, or rest home care plan oversight services (99339, 99340), and remote physiologic monitoring services (99457). Do not report 99091 if other more specific codes exist (eg, 93227, 93272 for cardiographic services; 95250 for continuous glucose monitoring). Do not report 99091 for transfer and interpretation of data from hospital or clinical laboratory computers.

Code 99453 is reported for each episode of care. For coding remote monitoring of physiologic parameters, an episode of care is defined as beginning when the remote monitoring physiologic service is initiated, and ends with attainment of targeted treatment goals.

Rationale

In accordance with the addition of code 99474, the guidelines for Digitally Stored Data Services/Remote Physiologic Monitoring subsection have been revised to include code 99474 and to indicate that code 99474 should not be reported separately with an E/M service on the same day by the same provider when measured blood pressure (BP) monitoring is performed.

Refer to the codebook and the Rationale for code 99474 for a full discussion of these changes.

99453   Remote monitoring of physiologic parameter(s) (eg, weight, blood pressure, pulse oximetry, respiratory flow rate), initial; set-up and patient education on use of equipment

(Do not report 99453 more than once per episode of care)

(Do not report 99453 for monitoring of less than 16 days)

99454   device(s) supply with daily recording(s) or programmed alert(s) transmission, each 30 days

(For physiologic monitoring treatment management services, use 99457)

(Do not report 99454 for monitoring of less than 16 days)

(Do not report 99453, 99454 in conjunction with codes for more specific physiologic parameters [eg, 93296, 94760])

▶(For self-measured blood pressure monitoring, see 99473, 99474)◀

Rationale

In accordance with the addition of codes 99473 and 99474, a parenthetical note following code 99454 has been added to direct users to codes 99473 and 99474 when measured blood pressure monitoring is performed.

Refer to the codebook and the Rationale for codes 99473 and 99474 for a full discussion of these changes.

 # 99091 Collection and interpretation of physiologic data (eg, ECG, blood pressure, glucose monitoring) digitally stored and/or transmitted by the patient and/or caregiver to the physician or other qualified health care professional, qualified by education, training, licensure/regulation (when applicable) requiring a minimum of 30 minutes of time, each 30 days

(Do not report 99091 in conjunction with 99457)

(Do not report 99091 if it occurs within 30 days of 99339, 99340, 99374, 99375, 99377, 99378, 99379, 99380, 99457)

#● 99473 Self-measured blood pressure using a device validated for clinical accuracy; patient education/training and device calibration

▶(Do not report 99473 more than once per device)◀

▶(For ambulatory blood pressure monitoring, see 93784, 93786, 93788, 93790)◀

#● 99474 separate self-measurements of two readings one minute apart, twice daily over a 30-day period (minimum of 12 readings), collection of data reported by the patient and/or caregiver to the physician or other qualified health care professional, with report of average systolic and diastolic pressures and subsequent communication of a treatment plan to the patient

▶(Do not report 99473, 99474 in the same calendar month as 93784, 93786, 93788, 93790, 99091, 99453, 99454, 99457, 99487, 99489, 99490, 99491)◀

▶(Do not report 99474 more than once per calendar month)◀

Rationale

Codes 99473 and 99474 have been established to report self-measured BP monitoring using a device that has been validated for clinical accuracy. These codes enable the reporting of self-measured BP monitoring adequately and better describe current clinical practice.

The United States Preventive Services Task Force (USPSTF) released updated recommendations for screening of high BP and determined that reliance on measurement of BP in the clinical setting for diagnosis of hypertension can result in measurement errors, a smaller number of measurements, and white-coat hypertension. In addition, the USPSTF has confirmed that out-of-office BP monitoring is an effective method of confirming hypertension. While the USPSTF identifies ambulatory BP monitoring (ABPM) as the reference standard for evaluation of noninvasive BP measurements, the list of evidence is growing to confirm that self-measured BP may also be effective.

Code 99473 includes patient education and training on device calibration, which is typically performed by a care-team member and should only be reported once per device. An exclusionary parenthetical note has been added to preclude the reporting of code 99473 more than once for the same device.

Code 99474 is reported for reviewing individual readings, averaging the readings, and providing instructions to the clinical staff on what should be communicated to the patient. This code may only be reported once per calendar month, which is why an exclusionary parenthetical note that precludes the use of this code more than once per calendar month has been added after code 99474.

In addition, an exclusionary note has been added following code 99474 that precludes the reporting of codes 99473 and 99474 with codes 93784, 93786, 93788, 93790, 99091, 99453, 99454, 99457, 99487, 99489, 99490, and 99491 in the same calendar month.

Clinical Example (99473)

A 65-year-old male presents with repeated office visit measurements of blood pressure (BP) greater than normal or goal. Self-measured BP is ordered.

Description of Procedure (99473)

N/A

Clinical Example (99474)

A 65-year-old male presents with repeated office visit measurements of BP greater than normal or goal. Self-measured BP is ordered.

Description of Procedure (99474)

Physician reviews the clinical staff–developed data and report with individual and mean systolic and diastolic BPs from the recording period. Provide instructions to the clinical staff regarding care plan information to be communicated to the patient.

Evaluation and Management | CPT Changes 2020

Remote Physiologic Monitoring Treatment Management Services

▶Remote physiologic monitoring treatment management services are provided when clinical staff/physician/other qualified health care professional use the results of remote physiological monitoring to manage a patient under a specific treatment plan. To report remote physiological monitoring, the device used must be a medical device as defined by the FDA, and the service must be ordered by a physician or other qualified health care professional. Do not use 99457, 99458 for time that can be reported using more specific monitoring services (eg, for the patient that requires reevaluation of medication regimen and/or changes in treatment). Codes 99457, 99458 may be reported during the same service period as chronic care management services (99487, 99489, 99490), transitional care management services (99495, 99496), and behavioral health integration services (99484, 99492, 99493, 99494); however, time spent performing these services should remain separate and no time should be counted toward the required time for both services in a single month. Codes 99457, 99458 require a live, interactive communication with the patient/caregiver. For the first 20 minutes of clinical staff/physician/other qualified health care professional time in a calendar month report 99457, and report 99458 for each additional 20 minutes. Do not report services of less than 20 minutes. Report 99457 one time regardless of the number of physiologic monitoring modalities performed in a given calendar month.

Do not count any time on a day when the physician or other qualified health care professional reports an E/M service (office or other outpatient services 99201, 99202, 99203, 99204, 99205, 99211, 99212, 99213, 99214, 99215, domiciliary, rest home services 99324, 99325, 99326, 99327, 99328, 99334, 99335, 99336, 99337, home services 99341, 99342, 99343, 99344, 99345, 99347, 99348, 99349, 99350, inpatient services 99221, 99222, 99223, 99231, 99232, 99233, 99251, 99252, 99253, 99254, 99255). Do not count any time related to other reported services (eg, 93290, 93793, 99291, 99292).◀

#▲ **99457** Remote physiologic monitoring treatment management services, clinical staff/physician/other qualified health care professional time in a calendar month requiring interactive communication with the patient/caregiver during the month; first 20 minutes

(Report 99457 once each 30 days, regardless of the number of parameters monitored)

▶(Do not report 99457 for services of less than 20 minutes)◀

▶(Do not report 99457 in conjunction with 93264, 99091)◀

▶(Do not report 99457 in the same month as 99473, 99474)◀

#+● **99458** each additional 20 minutes (List separately in addition to code for primary procedure)

▶(Use 99458 in conjunction with 99457)◀

▶(Report only 99457 if you have not completed 20 minutes of additional treatment regardless of time spent)◀

▶(Do not report 99458 for services of less than 20 minutes)◀

Rationale

A new subsection (Remote Physiologic Monitoring Treatment Management Services) and guidelines were added in 2019 to the E/M Services section. For CPT 2020, the guidelines and code 99457 have been revised to report remote physiologic monitoring treatment management services for the first 20 minutes of service. Code 99457 requires interactive communication with the patient/caregiver during the month. As indicated in the guidelines, it is important to note that the device used to provide these services must be a medical device defined by the United States Food and Drug Administration (FDA), and it must be ordered by a physician or other QHP.

Code 99457 provides physicians and other QHPs the ability to report remote monitoring of conditions not currently reportable with existing CPT codes. Code 99457 was approved to report remote monitoring management for the first 20 minutes.

A new add-on code (99458) has also been established to report each additional 20 minutes of remote physiologic monitoring treatment management services. This code should be reported in addition to code 99457. Parenthetical notes have been added following codes 99457 and 99458 that preclude the reporting of these codes if the services are less than 20 minutes. If 20 minutes of additional treatment has not been completed, only code 99457 should be reported. In addition, the second exclusionary parenthetical note following code 99457 has been revised to include code 93264 as a code that should not be reported in conjunction with code 99457.

These revisions build on the remote physiologic monitoring treatment management code (99457) to allow for more intensive monitoring services needed for patients with physiologic monitors who require particularly intense remote management.

In accordance with the addition of codes 99473 and 99474, a parenthetical note following code 99457 has been added to direct users to codes 99473 and 99474 when self-measured BP monitoring is performed.

Refer to the codebook and the Rationale for codes 99473 and 99474 for a full discussion of these changes.

★=Telemedicine +=Add-on code ⦸=FDA approval pending #=Resequenced code ⊘=Modifier 51 exempt

Clinical Example (99458)

An 82-year-old female with systolic dysfunction heart failure is enrolled in a heart failure management program that uses remote physiologic monitoring services. During the course of monitoring, adjustments in therapy and continued monitoring and evaluation are required. [**Note:** This is an add-on code and represents the services performed after 20 minutes of time reported with code 99457.]

Description of Procedure (99458)

Based on interpreted data, the physician or other qualified health care professional (QHP) uses medical decision making to assess patient's clinical stability, communicates the results to the patient, and oversees the management and/or coordination of services, as needed, for all medical conditions.

Special Evaluation and Management Services

Work Related or Medical Disability Evaluation Services

99458 Code is out of numerical sequence. See 99448-99455

Inpatient Neonatal Intensive Care Services and Pediatric and Neonatal Critical Care Services

Inpatient Neonatal and Pediatric Critical Care

99473 Code is out of numerical sequence. See 99448-99455

99474 Code is out of numerical sequence. See 99448-99455

Care Management Services

Care management services are management and support services provided by clinical staff, under the direction of a physician or other qualified health care professional, or may be provided personally by a physician or other qualified health care professional to a patient residing at home or in a domiciliary, rest home, or assisted living facility. Services include establishing, implementing, revising, or monitoring the care plan, coordinating the care of other professionals and agencies, and educating the patient or caregiver about the patient's condition, care plan, and prognosis. The physician or other qualified health care professional provides or oversees the management and/or coordination of services, as needed, for all medical conditions, psychosocial needs, and activities of daily living.

A plan of care must be documented and shared with the patient and/or caregiver. A care plan is based on a physical, mental, cognitive, social, functional, and environmental assessment. It is a comprehensive plan of care for all health problems. It typically includes, but is not limited to, the following elements: problem list, expected outcome and prognosis, measurable treatment goals, symptom management, planned interventions, medication management, community/social services ordered, how the services of agencies and specialists unconnected to the practice will be directed/coordinated, identification of the individuals responsible for each intervention, requirements for periodic review, and, when applicable, revision of the care plan.

Codes 99487, 99489, 99490, 99491 are reported only once per calendar month and may only be reported by the single physician or other qualified health care professional who assumes the care management role with a particular patient for the calendar month.

For 99487, 99489, 99490 the face-to-face and non-face-to-face time spent by the clinical staff in communicating with the patient and/or family, caregivers, other professionals, and agencies; creating, revising, documenting, and implementing the care plan; or teaching self-management is used in determining the care management clinical staff time for the month. Only the time of the clinical staff of the reporting professional is counted. Only count the time of one clinical staff member when two or more clinical staff members are meeting about the patient. For 99491, only count the time personally spent by the physician or other qualified health care professional. Do not count any of the clinical staff time spent on the day of an initiating visit (the creation of the care plan, initial explanation to the patient and/or caregiver, and obtaining consent).

Care management activities performed by clinical staff, or personally by the physician or other qualified health care professional, typically include:

- communication and engagement with patient, family members, guardian or caretaker, surrogate decision makers, and/or other professionals regarding aspects of care;
- communication with home health agencies and other community services utilized by the patient;

- collection of health outcomes data and registry documentation;
- patient and/or family/caregiver education to support self-management, independent living, and activities of daily living;
- assessment and support for treatment regimen adherence and medication management;
- identification of available community and health resources;
- facilitating access to care and services needed by the patient and/or family;
- management of care transitions not reported as part of transitional care management (99495, 99496);
- ongoing review of patient status, including review of laboratory and other studies not reported as part of an E/M service, noted above;
- development, communication, and maintenance of a comprehensive care plan.

The care management office/practice must have the following capabilities:

- provide 24/7 access to physicians or other qualified health care professionals or clinical staff including providing patients/caregivers with a means to make contact with health care professionals in the practice to address urgent needs regardless of the time of day or day of week;
- provide continuity of care with a designated member of the care team with whom the patient is able to schedule successive routine appointments;
- provide timely access and management for follow-up after an emergency department visit or facility discharge;
- utilize an electronic health record system so that care providers have timely access to clinical information;
- use a standardized methodology to identify patients who require care management services;
- have an internal care management process/function whereby a patient identified as meeting the requirements for these services starts receiving them in a timely manner;
- use a form and format in the medical record that is standardized within the practice;
- be able to engage and educate patients and caregivers as well as coordinate care among all service professionals, as appropriate for each patient.

►E/M services may be reported separately by the same physician or other qualified health care professional during the same calendar month. A physician or other qualified health care professional who reports codes 99487, 99489, 99490, may not report care plan oversight services (99339, 99340, 99374-99380), prolonged services without direct patient contact (99358, 99359), home and outpatient INR monitoring (93792, 93793), medical team conferences (99366, 99367, 99368), education and training (98960, 98961, 98962, 99071, 99078), telephone services (99441, 99442, 99443), preparation of special reports (99080), analysis of data (99091), transitional care management services (99495, 99496), medication therapy management services (99605, 99606, 99607), and, if performed, these services may not be reported separately during the month for which 99487, 99489, 99490 are reported. All other services may be reported. Do not report 99487, 99489, 99490, 99491 if reporting ESRD services (90951-90970) during the same month. If the care management services are performed within the postoperative period of a reported surgery, the same individual may not report 99487, 99489, 99490, 99491. When reporting 99487, 99489, 99490, do not report 99421, 99422, 99423 during the same time.◄

Care management may be reported in any calendar month during which the clinical staff time or physician or other qualified health care professional personal time requirements are met. If care management resumes after a discharge during a new month, start a new period or report transitional care management services (99495, 99496) as appropriate. If discharge occurs in the same month, continue the reporting period or report Transitional Care Management Services. Do not report 99487, 99489, 99490 for any post-discharge care management services for any days within 30 days of discharge, if reporting 99495, 99496.

When behavioral or psychiatric collaborative care management services are also provided, 99484, 99492, 99493, 99494 may be reported in addition.

Rationale

In accordance with the deletion of codes 98969 and 99444, and the addition of codes 98970, 98971, 98972, 99421, 99422, and 99423, the guidelines for care management services have been revised to reflect these changes.

Refer to the codebook and the Rationale for codes 98970, 98971, 98972, 99421, 99422, and 99423 for a full discussion of these changes.

Complex Chronic Care Management Services

99487 Complex chronic care management services, with the following required elements:

- multiple (two or more) chronic conditions expected to last at least 12 months, or until the death of the patient,
- chronic conditions place the patient at significant risk of death, acute exacerbation/decompensation, or functional decline,
- establishment or substantial revision of a comprehensive care plan,
- moderate or high complexity medical decision making;
- 60 minutes of clinical staff time directed by a physician or other qualified health care professional, per calendar month.

(Complex chronic care management services of less than 60 minutes duration, in a calendar month, are not reported separately)

+ 99489 each additional 30 minutes of clinical staff time directed by a physician or other qualified health care professional, per calendar month (List separately in addition to code for primary procedure)

(Report 99489 in conjunction with 99487)

(Do not report 99489 for care management services of less than 30 minutes additional to the first 60 minutes of complex chronic care management services during a calendar month)

▶(Do not report 99487, 99489, 99490 during the same month with 90951-90970, 93792, 93793, 98960-98962, 98966, 98967, 98968, 99071, 99078, 99080, 99091, 99339, 99340, 99358, 99359, 99366-99368, 99374-99380, 99441, 99442, 99443, 99495, 99496, 99605-99607)◀

Rationale

In accordance with the deletion of codes 98969 and 99444, the parenthetical note following code 99489 has been revised to reflect these changes.

Refer to the codebook and the Rationale for codes 98969 and 99444 for a full discussion of these changes.

Transitional Care Management Services

Codes 99495 and 99496 are used to report transitional care management services (TCM). These services are for a new or established patient whose medical and/or psychosocial problems require moderate or high complexity medical decision making during transitions in care from an inpatient hospital setting (including acute hospital, rehabilitation hospital, long-term acute care hospital), partial hospital, observation status in a hospital, or skilled nursing facility/nursing facility to the patient's community setting (home, domiciliary, rest home, or assisted living). TCM commences upon the date of discharge and continues for the next 29 days.

TCM is comprised of one face-to-face visit within the specified timeframes, in combination with non-face-to-face services that may be performed by the physician or other qualified health care professional and/or licensed clinical staff under his/her direction.

Non-face-to-face services provided by clinical staff, under the direction of the physician or other qualified health care professional, may include:

- communication (with patient, family members, guardian or caretaker, surrogate decision makers, and/or other professionals) regarding aspects of care,
- communication with home health agencies and other community services utilized by the patient,
- patient and/or family/caretaker education to support self-management, independent living, and activities of daily living,
- assessment and support for treatment regimen adherence and medication management,
- identification of available community and health resources,
- facilitating access to care and services needed by the patient and/or family

Non-face-to-face services provided by the physician or other qualified health care provider may include:

- obtaining and reviewing the discharge information (eg, discharge summary, as available, or continuity of care documents);
- reviewing need for or follow-up on pending diagnostic tests and treatments;
- interaction with other qualified health care professionals who will assume or reassume care of the patient's system-specific problems;
- education of patient, family, guardian, and/or caregiver;
- establishment or reestablishment of referrals and arranging for needed community resources;
- assistance in scheduling any required follow-up with community providers and services.

TCM requires a face-to-face visit, initial patient contact, and medication reconciliation within specified time frames. The first face-to-face visit is part of the TCM service and not reported separately. Additional E/M services provided on subsequent dates after the first face-to-face visit may be reported separately. TCM requires an interactive contact with the patient or caregiver, as appropriate, within two business days of discharge. The contact may be direct (face-to-face), telephonic, or by electronic means. Medication reconciliation and management must occur no later than the date of the face-to-face visit.

These services address any needed coordination of care performed by multiple disciplines and community service agencies. The reporting individual provides or oversees the management and/or coordination of services, as needed, for all medical conditions, psychosocial needs and activity of daily living support by providing first contact and continuous access.

Medical decision making and the date of the first face-to-face visit are used to select and report the appropriate TCM code. For 99496, the face-to-face visit must occur within 7 calendar days of the date discharge and medical decision making must be of high complexity. For 99495, the face-to-face visit must occur within 14 calendar days of the date of discharge and medical decision making must be of at least moderate complexity.

Type of Medical Decision Making	Face-to-Face Visit Within 7 Days	Face-to-Face Visit Within 8 to 14 Days
Moderate Complexity	99495	99495
High Complexity	99496	99495

Medical decision making is defined by the E/M Services Guidelines. The medical decision making over the service period reported is used to define the medical decision making of TCM. Documentation includes the timing of the initial post discharge communication with the patient or caregivers, date of the face-to-face visit, and the complexity of medical decision making.

Only one individual may report these services and only once per patient within 30 days of discharge. Another TCM may not be reported by the same individual or group for any subsequent discharge(s) within the 30 days. The same individual may report hospital or observation discharge services and TCM. However, the discharge service may not constitute the required face-to-face visit. The same individual should not report TCM services provided in the postoperative period of a service that the individual reported.

▶A physician or other qualified health care professional who reports codes 99495, 99496 may not report care plan oversight services (99339, 99340, 99374-99380), prolonged services without direct patient contact (99358, 99359), home and outpatient INR monitoring (93792, 93793), medical team conferences (99366-99368), education and training (98960-98962, 99071, 99078), telephone services (98966-98968, 99441-99443), end stage renal disease services (90951-90970), preparation of special reports (99080), analysis of data (99091), complex chronic care coordination services (99487-99489), medication therapy management services (99605-99607), during the time period covered by the transitional care management services codes. When reporting 99495, 99496, do not report 99421, 99422, 99423 during the same time period.◀

Rationale

In accordance with the deletion of codes 98969 and 99444, and the addition of codes 98970, 98971, 98972, 99421, 99422, and 99423, the guidelines for transitional care management services have been revised to reflect these changes.

Refer to the codebook and the Rationale for codes 98970, 98971, 98972, 99421, 99422, and 99423 for a full discussion of these changes.

★ **99495** **Transitional Care Management Services** with the following required elements:

- Communication (direct contact, telephone, electronic) with the patient and/or caregiver within 2 business days of discharge
- Medical decision making of at least moderate complexity during the service period
- Face-to-face visit, within 14 calendar days of discharge

★ **99496** **Transitional Care Management Services** with the following required elements:

- Communication (direct contact, telephone, electronic) with the patient and/or caregiver within 2 business days of discharge
- Medical decision making of high complexity during the service period
- Face-to-face visit, within 7 calendar days of discharge

(Do not report 99495, 99496 in conjunction with 93792, 93793)

▶(Do not report 90951-90970, 98960-98962, 98966, 98967, 98968, 99071, 99078, 99080, 99091, 99339, 99340, 99358, 99359, 99366-99368, 99374-99380, 99441, 99442, 99443, 99487-99489, 99605-99607, when performed during the service time of code 99495 or 99496)◀

Rationale

In accordance with the deletion of codes 98969 and 99444, the parenthetical note following code 99496 has been revised to reflect these changes.

Refer to the codebook and the Rationale for codes 98969 and 99444 for a full discussion of these changes.

Surgery

Summary of Additions, Deletions, and Revisions

The summary of changes shows the actual changes that have been made to the code descriptors.

New codes appear with a bullet (●) and are indicated as "Code added." Revised codes are preceded with a triangle (▲). Within revised codes, or if a code symbol has been deleted, the deleted language and code symbol appear with a strikethrough (⊖), while new text appears underlined.

The ⚡ symbol is used to identify codes for vaccines that are pending FDA approval. The # symbol is used to identify codes that have been resequenced. CPT add-on codes are annotated by the ✚ symbol. The ⊘ symbol is used to identify codes that are exempt from the use of modifier 51. The ★ symbol is used to identify codes that may be used for reporting telemedicine services. The ✤ is used to identify proprietary laboratory analyses (PLA) test that has an identical descriptor as another PLA test. A PLA code that satisfies Category I code criteria and has been accepted by the CPT Editorial Panel is annotated with the ↑↓ symbol.

Code	Description
#●15769	Code added
●15771	Code added
✚●15772	Code added
●15773	Code added
✚●15774	Code added
19260	Excision of chest wall tumor including ribs
19271	Excision of chest wall tumor involving ribs, with plastic reconstruction; without mediastinal lymphadenectomy
19272	with mediastinal lymphadenectomy
19304	Mastectomy, subcutaneous
#●20560	Code added
#●20561	Code added
✚●20700	Code added
✚●20701	Code added
✚●20702	Code added
✚●20703	Code added
✚●20704	Code added
✚●20705	Code added
20926	Tissue grafts, other (eg, paratenon, fat, dermis)
●21601	Code added
●21602	Code added

▲ = Revised code ● = New code ▶ ◀ = Contains new or revised text ✤ = Duplicate PLA test ↑↓ = Category I PLA

Code	Description
●21603	Code added
▲31233	Nasal/sinus endoscopy, diagnostic with maxillary sinusoscopy (via inferior meatus or canine fossa puncture); with maxillary sinusoscopy (via inferior meatus or canine fossa puncture)
▲31235	with sphenoid sinusoscopy (via puncture of sphenoidal face or cannulation of ostium)
▲31292	Nasal/sinus endoscopy, surgical, with orbital decompression; with medial or inferior orbital wall decompression
▲31293	with medial orbital wall and inferior orbital wall decompression
▲31294	Nasal/sinus endoscopy, surgical, with optic nerve decompression; with optic nerve decompression
▲31295	Nasal/sinus endoscopy, surgical, with dilation (eg, balloon dilation); with dilation of maxillary sinus ostium (eg, balloon dilation), transnasal or via canine fossa
▲31296	with dilation of frontal sinus ostium (eg, balloon dilation)
▲31297	with dilation of sphenoid sinus ostium (eg, balloon dilation)
▲31298	with dilation of frontal and sphenoid sinus ostia (eg, balloon dilation)
33010	Pericardiocentesis; initial
33011	subsequent
33015	Tube pericardiostomy
●33016	Code added
●33017	Code added
●33018	Code added
●33019	Code added
#▲33275	Transcatheter removal of permanent leadless pacemaker, right ventricular, including imaging guidance (eg, fluoroscopy, venous ultrasound, ventriculography, femoral venography), when performed
●33858	Code added
●33859	Code added
33860	Ascending aorta graft, with cardiopulmonary bypass, includes valve suspension, when performed
33870	Transverse arch graft, with cardiopulmonary bypass
●33871	Code added
#+●34717	Code added
#●34718	Code added
▲35701	Exploration (not followed by surgical repair,), with or without lysis of artery; neck (eg, carotid artery, subclavian)
●35702	Code added
●35703	Code added
35721	femoral artery
35741	popliteal artery

Code	Description
35761	other vessels
43401	Transection of esophagus with repair, for esophageal varices
#▲46945	Hemorrhoidectomy, internal, by ligation other than rubber band; single hemorrhoid column/group, without imaging guidance
#▲46946	2 or more hemorrhoid columns/groups, without imaging guidance
#●46948	Code added
●49013	Code added
●49014	Code added
▲54640	Orchiopexy, inguinal approach, with or without hernia repair scrotal approach
▲62270	Spinal puncture, lumbar, diagnostic;
#●62328	Code added
▲62272	Spinal puncture, therapeutic, for drainage of cerebrospinal fluid (by needle or catheter);
#●62329	Code added
▲64400	Injection(s), anesthetic agent(s) and/or steroid; trigeminal nerve, any division or branch each branch (ie, ophthalmic, maxillary, mandibular)
64402	facial nerve
▲64405	greater occipital nerve
▲64408	vagus nerve
64410	phrenic nerve
64413	cervical plexus
▲64415	brachial plexus, single
▲64416	brachial plexus, continuous infusion by catheter (including catheter placement)
▲64417	axillary nerve
▲64418	suprascapular nerve
▲64420	intercostal nerve, single level
+▲64421	intercostal nerve, multiple, regional block each additional level (List separately in addition to code for primary procedure)
▲64425	ilioinguinal, iliohypogastric nerves
▲64430	pudendal nerve
▲64435	paracervical (uterine) nerve
▲64445	sciatic nerve, single
▲64446	sciatic nerve, continuous infusion by catheter (including catheter placement)
▲64447	femoral nerve, single

▲ = Revised code   ● = New code   ▶◀ = Contains new or revised text   ✕ = Duplicate PLA test   ↑↓ = Category I PLA

Code	Description
▲64448	femoral nerve, continuous infusion by catheter (including catheter placement)
▲64449	lumbar plexus, posterior approach, continuous infusion by catheter (including catheter placement)
▲64450	other peripheral nerve or branch
●64451	Code added
●64454	Code added
#●64624	Code added
#●64625	Code added
▲66711	cyclophotocoagulation, endoscopic, without concomitant removal of crystalline lens
▲66982	Extracapsular cataract removal with insertion of intraocular lens prosthesis (1-stage procedure), manual or mechanical technique (eg, irrigation and aspiration or phacoemulsification), complex, requiring devices or techniques not generally used in routine cataract surgery (eg, iris expansion device, suture support for intraocular lens, or primary posterior capsulorrhexis) or performed on patients in the amblyogenic developmental stage; without endoscopic cyclophotocoagulation
▲66984	Extracapsular cataract removal with insertion of intraocular lens prosthesis (1 stage procedure), manual or mechanical technique (eg, irrigation and aspiration or phacoemulsification); without endoscopic cyclophotocoagulation
#●66987	Code added
#●66988	Code added

Surgery

Integumentary System

Introduction

11981 Insertion, non-biodegradable drug delivery implant

▶(For manual preparation and insertion of deep [eg, subfascial], intramedullary, or intra-articular drug-delivery device, see 20700, 20702, 20704)◀

▶(Do not report 11981 in conjunction with 20700, 20702, 20704)◀

11982 Removal, non-biodegradable drug delivery implant

▶(For removal of deep [eg, subfascial], intramedullary, or intra-articular drug-delivery device, see 20701, 20703, 20705)◀

▶(Do not report 11982 in conjunction with 20701, 20703, 20705)◀

Rationale

In accordance with the addition of codes 20700, 20701, 20702, 20703, 20704, and 20705, new parenthetical notes have been added following codes 11981 and 11982 on the use of the new codes.

Refer to the codebook and the Rationale for codes 20700, 20701, 20702, 20703, 20704, and 20705 for a full discussion of these changes.

Repair (Closure)

Use the codes in this section to designate wound closure utilizing sutures, staples, or tissue adhesives (eg, 2-cyanoacrylate), either singly or in combination with each other, or in combination with adhesive strips. Wound closure utilizing adhesive strips as the sole repair material should be coded using the appropriate E/M code.

Definitions

The repair of wounds may be classified as Simple, Intermediate, or Complex.

Simple repair is used when the wound is superficial; eg, involving primarily epidermis or dermis, or subcutaneous tissues without significant involvement of deeper structures, and requires simple one layer closure. This includes local anesthesia and chemical or electrocauterization of wounds not closed.

▶*Intermediate repair* includes the repair of wounds that, in addition to the above, require layered closure of one or more of the deeper layers of subcutaneous tissue and superficial (non-muscle) fascia, in addition to the skin (epidermal and dermal) closure. It includes limited undermining (defined as a distance less than the maximum width of the defect, measured perpendicular to the closure line, along at least one entire edge of the defect). Single-layer closure of heavily contaminated wounds that have required extensive cleaning or removal of particulate matter also constitutes intermediate repair.

Complex repair includes the repair of wounds that, in addition to the requirements for intermediate repair, require at least one of the following: exposure of bone, cartilage, tendon, or named neurovascular structure; debridement of wound edges (eg, traumatic lacerations or avulsions); extensive undermining (defined as a distance greater than or equal to the maximum width of the defect, measured perpendicular to the closure line along at least one entire edge of the defect); involvement of free margins of helical rim, vermilion border, or nostril rim; placement of retention sutures. Necessary preparation includes creation of a limited defect for repairs or the debridement of complicated lacerations or avulsions. Complex repair does not include excision of benign (11400-11446) or malignant (11600-11646) lesions, excisional preparation of a wound bed (15002-15005) or debridement of an open fracture or open dislocation.◀

Extensive Undermining

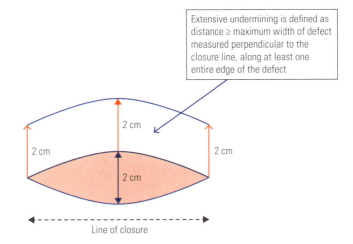

Surgery

CPT Changes 2020

Rationale

The guidelines for Integumentary/Repair (Closure) subsection have been revised to clarify the distinction between intermediate and complex repair. A new illustration of extensive undermining has been added to this subsection as well.

Prior to 2020, complex repair was distinguished from intermediate repair by the inclusion of layered closure that was part of intermediate repair plus scar revision, debridement, extensive undermining, use of stents or retention sutures, and preparation that included creation of a limited defect for repairs or the debridement of complicated lacerations or avulsions. It was determined that more descriptive language about the work involved in complex repair would make the distinction between complex and intermediate repairs clearer. This clarification would in turn ensure more accurate code selection.

For 2020, the guidelines have been revised to clarify that intermediate repair includes limited undermining and to provide a definition of limited undermining. The guidelines also clarify that complex repair includes the requirements listed for intermediate repair and at least one of the following: exposure of bone, cartilage, tendon, or named neurovascular structure; debridement of wound edges; extensive undermining; involvement of free margins of the helical rim, vermilion border, or nostril rim; placement of retention sutures. In addition, the guidelines include definitions with an illustration of extensive undermining. Reference to scar revision and stents has been removed from the complex repair guidelines. Necessary preparation including creation of a limited defect for repairs or the debridement of complicated lacerations or avulsions is still part of complex repair.

Other Flaps and Grafts

Code 15740 describes a cutaneous flap, transposed into a nearby but not immediately adjacent defect, with a pedicle that incorporates an anatomically named axial vessel into its design. The flap is typically transferred through a tunnel underneath the skin and sutured into its new position. The donor site is closed directly.

Neurovascular pedicle procedures are reported with 15750. This code includes not only skin but also a functional motor or sensory nerve(s). The flap serves to reinnervate a damaged portion of the body dependent on touch or movement (eg, thumb).

Repair of donor site requiring skin graft or local flaps should be reported as an additional procedure.

For random island flaps, V-Y subcutaneous flaps, advancement flaps, and other flaps from adjacent areas without clearly defined anatomically named axial vessels, see 14000-14302.

►Code 15769 may be used to report autologous soft tissue grafts, such as fat, dermis, fascia, or other soft tissues, which are harvested from the patient using an excisional technique. The autologous soft tissue grafts are then placed into a defect during the same operation. Autologous grafts that are already defined in the CPT code set, including skin, bone, nerve, tendon, fascia lata or vessels, should be reported with the specific codes for each tissue type. For harvesting, preparation or injection(s) of platelet-rich plasma, use 0232T.

Codes 15771, 15772, 15773, 15774 may be used to report autologous fat grafting when the adipose cells are harvested via a liposuction technique, prepared with minimal manipulation, and then injected via cannula in multiple small aliquots to the defect. The regions listed refer to the recipient area (not the donor site). Volumes are based on total injectate. For multiple sites of injection, sum the total volume of injectate to anatomic sites that are grouped together into the same code descriptor. Do not report 11950, 11951, 11952, 11954 in conjunction with 15771, 15772, 15773, 15774, for the same anatomic site.◄

15760   Graft; composite (eg, full thickness of external ear or nasal ala), including primary closure, donor area

15769   Code is out of numerical sequence. See 15760-15772

15770   derma-fat-fascia

#● 15769   Grafting of autologous soft tissue, other, harvested by direct excision (eg, fat, dermis, fascia)

►(For injection[s] of platelet-rich plasma, use 0232T)◄

● 15771   Grafting of autologous fat harvested by liposuction technique to trunk, breasts, scalp, arms, and/or legs; 50 cc or less injectate

►(Report 15771 only once per session)◄

+● 15772   each additional 50 cc injectate, or part thereof (List separately in addition to code for primary procedure)

►(Use 15772 in conjunction with 15771)◄

● 15773   Grafting of autologous fat harvested by liposuction technique to face, eyelids, mouth, neck, ears, orbits, genitalia, hands, and/or feet; 25 cc or less injectate

►(Report 15773 only once per session)◄

+● 15774   each additional 25 cc injectate, or part thereof (List separately in addition to code for primary procedure)

►(Use 15774 in conjunction with 15773)◄

►(Do not report 15769, 15771, 15772, 15773, 15774 in conjunction with 15876, 15877, 15878, 15879, 0232T, 0481T, 0489T, 0490T)◄

▶(For injection[s], autologous white blood cell concentrate [autologous protein solution], any site, including image guidance, harvesting and preparation, when performed, use 0481T)◀

Rationale

Five new codes (15769, 15771, 15772, 15773, 15774) have been established to report autologous soft tissue and fat grafting. New guidelines and parenthetical notes have also been added to provide instruction on the appropriate use of these five new codes. The grafts (or implants) guidelines in the Musculoskeletal System section have been revised, and code 20926 has been deleted.

Code 15769 has been established to report autologous soft tissue grafting, such as fat, dermis, fascia, or other soft tissues that are harvested from the patient using an excisional technique and placed into a defect for reconstructive purposes.

Codes 15771, 15772, 15773, and 15774 have been established to report autologous fat grafting (or lipofilling) when the adipose cells are harvested via a liposuction technique, prepared with minimal manipulation, and injected via cannula in multiple small aliquots to the defect. The defect can be secondary to surgical resection, trauma, radiation, developmental abnormalities, or aging.

Codes 15771 and 15772 are reported for 50 cc or less of injectate in the trunk, breasts, scalp, arms, and/or legs. Codes 15773 and 15774 are reported for 25 cc or less of injectate in the face, eyelids, mouth, neck, ears, orbits, genitalia, hands, and/or feet.

The guidelines for Grafts (or Implants) have been revised to direct users to the appropriate codes to report autologous soft-tissue grafts harvested by direct excision and for autologous fat grafting harvested by liposuction technique. In addition, code 20926, *Tissue grafts, other (eg, paratenon, fat, dermis),* has been deleted because it was identified as potentially misvalued by the AMA/Specialty Society Relative Value Scale (RVS) Update Committee (RUC) Relativity Assessment Workgroup (RAW). It was determined that this code was being used to represent more than one procedure. Therefore, these procedures are now more clearly described by codes 15769, 15771, 15772, 15773, and 15774.

Clinical Example (15769)

A 58-year-old male presents with a left-sided parotid mass. The mass is excised, leaving a defect in the parotid bed. An enbloc fat graft is planned to correct the soft-tissue deficiency.

Description of Procedure (15769)

Make an incision, followed by a meticulous dissection and preparation of the recipient bed and facial nerve identification. Re-excise the margins of the previous incision, debriding and removing fibrous and poorly vascularized tissue. Obtain hemostasis and pack the wound with wet sponges. Measure and plan the needed graft size. Carefully measure and re-mark the donor site. Make an elliptical abdominal incision, just through the epithelium. Fastidiously remove all of the epithelium from the dermis. Make the elliptical incision again, but through the dermis and subcutaneous tissues for the second time around. Perform a dissection deep to the subcutaneous tissues. Remove the graft and set aside in saline for later implantation. Undermine and close the wound, primarily in three separate layers. Remove the sponges from the recipient wound and reinspect the site. Trim the donor abdominal dermis and fat to fill the defect, and place en bloc into the defect to fill the soft-tissue void. Fix the graft in place with long-lasting absorbable sutures. Bring out a drain through a separate, stab incision and suture in place. Close the wound in a layered fashion.

Clinical Example (15771)

A 35-year-old female presents with a postlumpectomy defect in the superior medial pole of the breast and wishes to use her own tissue to repair the concavity. Examination documents a 40-ml volumetric defect in the area of the lumpectomy. Fat grafting to the breast is requested.

Description of Procedure (15771)

Infiltrate the graft donor sites (often thighs or abdomen) with a liposuction wetting (tumescent) solution. Wait for the hemostatic effects of the epinephrine and anesthetic effects of the lidocaine. Connect a liposuction cannula to gentle, subatmospheric pressure and use it to harvest the fat and associated aspirate from the soft tissues of the donor site, taking care to avoid the creation of soft-tissue deformities. Close the donor incisions in a layered fashion. Place the lipoaspirate into syringes and place in an operating room (OR) centrifuge. After completion of the centrifuge cycle, drain the separated blood and wick the oil away from the usable fat graft. Transfer the graft into small-volume syringes. Use small cannulas to subcutaneously inject the fat in small aliquots to fill the soft-tissue defect. This requires placement of the grafts in multiple planes and depths in order to ensure viability of the graft. Infiltrate the fat grafts into the soft tissues until the desired volumetric filling is achieved. Filling is often evaluated with the patient in an upright position on the OR table, which requires the patient to be sitting up. Close the small stab wounds primarily.

Clinical Example (15772)

A 35-year-old female presents with a postlumpectomy defect in the superior medial pole of the breast and wishes to use her own tissue to repair the concavity. Examination documents a 75-ml volumetric defect in the area of the lumpectomy. Fat grafting to the breast is requested.

Description of Procedure (15772)

Wait for hemostatic effects of the epinephrine and anesthetic effects of the lidocaine. Connect a liposuction cannula to gentle, subatmospheric pressure and use it to harvest the additional fat and associated aspirate from the soft tissues of donor site, taking care to avoid the creation of soft-tissue deformities. Close the donor incisions in a layered fashion. Place the lipoaspirate into syringes and place in an OR centrifuge. Each centrifuge is able to hold six syringes, which results in an average of 50 cc of additional usable fat graft. After completion of the centrifuge cycle, drain the separated blood and wick the oil away from the usable fat graft. Transfer the graft into small-volume syringes. Use small cannulas to subcutaneously inject the fat in small aliquots to fill the soft-tissue defect. This requires placement of the grafts in multiple planes and depths in order to ensure viability of the graft. Infiltrate the fat grafts into the soft tissues until the desired volumetric filling is achieved. Filling is often evaluated with the patient in an upright position on the OR table, which requires the patient to sit up.

Clinical Example (15773)

A 60-year-old male presents 15 years after radical, local excision of a rhabdomyosarcoma of his left masseter followed by irradiation. Examination shows a 20-ml volumetric soft-tissue defect on left jaw at the previous surgical site.

Description of Procedure (15773)

Bring the patient to the operating room. Prepare both the facial and the abdominal donor site. Infiltrate the abdominal donor site with a liposuction wetting (tumescent) solution. Connect a liposuction cannula to gentle, subatmospheric pressure and use it to harvest the fat and associated aspirate from the soft tissue of the abdomen. Close the donor incisions. Place the lipoaspirate into syringes and place in an OR centrifuge. Drain the separated blood and wick the oil away from the usable fat graft. Transfer the graft into small-volume syringes. Use small cannulas to subcutaneously inject the fat in small aliquots to fill the soft-tissue defect. This requires placement of the grafts in multiple planes and depths in order to ensure viability of the graft. Close the small stab wounds primarily.

Clinical Example (15774)

A 60-year-old male presents 15 years after radical local excision of a rhabdomyosarcoma of his left masseter followed by irradiation. Examination shows a 40-ml volumetric soft-tissue defect on left jaw at the previous surgical site.

Description of Procedure (15774)

Wait for hemostatic effects of the epinephrine and anesthetic effects of the lidocaine. Connect a liposuction cannula to gentle, subatmospheric pressure and use it to harvest the additional fat and associated aspirate from the soft tissues of the donor site, taking care to avoid the creation of soft-tissue deformities. Close the donor incisions in a layered fashion. Place the lipoaspirate into syringes and place in an OR centrifuge. Each centrifuge is able to hold six syringes, which results in an average of 50 cc of additional usable fat graft. After completion of the centrifuge cycle, drain the separated blood and wick the oil away from the usable fat graft. Transfer the graft into small-volume syringes. Use small cannulas to subcutaneously inject the fat in small aliquots to fill the soft-tissue defect. This requires placement of the grafts in multiple planes and depths in order to ensure viability of the graft. Infiltrate the fat grafts into the soft tissues until the desired volumetric filling is achieved. Filling is often evaluated with the patient in an upright position on the OR table.

+ 15777 Implantation of biologic implant (eg, acellular dermal matrix) for soft tissue reinforcement (ie, breast, trunk) (List separately in addition to code for primary procedure)

(For implantation of biologic implants for soft tissue reinforcement in tissues other than breast and trunk, use 17999)

▶(For bilateral breast procedure, report 15777 twice. Do not report modifier 50 in conjunction with 15777)◀

(For implantation of mesh or other prosthesis for open incisional or ventral hernia repair, use 49568 in conjunction with 49560-49566)

(For insertion of mesh or other prosthesis for closure of a necrotizing soft tissue infection wound, use 49568 in conjunction with 11004-11006)

(For topical application of skin substitute graft to a wound surface, see 15271-15278)

(For repair of anorectal fistula with plug (eg, porcine small intestine submucosa [SIS]), use 46707)

(For insertion of mesh or other prosthesis for repair of pelvic floor defect, use 57267)

(For implantation of non-biologic or synthetic implant for fascial reinforcement of the abdominal wall, use 0437T)

(The supply of biologic implant should be reported separately in conjunction with 15777)

Rationale

In accordance with the revision to instructions for reporting add-on procedures when performed bilaterally, the instructional parenthetical note for add-on code 15777 has been revised to instruct that code 15777 should be reported twice when the procedure is performed bilaterally.

Refer to the codebook and the Rationale for modifier 50, *Bilateral Procedure,* guideline revisions, for a full discussion of these changes.

Other Procedures

15876	Suction assisted lipectomy; head and neck
15877	trunk
15878	upper extremity
15879	lower extremity

▶(Do not report 15876, 15877, 15878, 15879 in conjunction with 15771, 15772, 15773, 15774, 0489T, 0490T)◀

(For harvesting of adipose tissue for autologous adipose-derived regenerative cell therapy, use 0489T)

▶(For autologous fat grafting harvested by liposuction technique, see 15771, 15772, 15773, 15774)◀

Rationale

In accordance with the addition of codes 15771, 15772, 15773, and 15774, the exclusionary parenthetical note following code 15879 has been revised to preclude the use of these codes with codes 15876-15879. In addition, a new parenthetical note has also been added referring users to new codes 15771, 15772, 15773, and 15774 for the reporting of autologous fat grafting harvested by liposuction technique.

Refer to the codebook and the Rationale for codes 15771, 15772, 15773, and 15774 for a full discussion of these changes.

Breast

19000	Puncture aspiration of cyst of breast;
+ 19001	each additional cyst (List separately in addition to code for primary procedure)

(Use 19001 in conjunction with 19000)

(If imaging guidance is performed, see 76942, 77021)

19020	Mastotomy with exploration or drainage of abscess, deep
19030	Injection procedure only for mammary ductogram or galactogram

(For radiological supervision and interpretation, see 77053, 77054)

▶Breast biopsy procedures may be performed via a percutaneous or open approach and with or without imaging guidance.

Percutaneous image-guided breast biopsies, including the placement of breast localization device(s), when performed, are reported with 19081, 19082, 19083, 19084, 19085, 19086. Imaging codes 76098, 76942, 77002, 77021 may not be separately reported for the same lesion. When more than one percutaneous breast biopsy with or without localization device placement is performed using the same imaging modality, use an add-on code whether the additional service(s) is on the same or contralateral breast. If additional percutaneous biopsies with or without localization device placements are performed using different imaging modalities, report another primary code for each additional biopsy with or without localization device placement performed using a different image guidance modality.

To report bilateral image-guided breast biopsies, report 19081, 19083, 19085 for the initial biopsy. The contralateral and each additional breast image-guided biopsy are then reported with 19082, 19084, 19086.

Percutaneous breast biopsies without imaging guidance are reported with 19100.

Open incisional breast biopsy (19101) does not include imaging guidance. However, if an open incisional biopsy is performed after image-guided placement of a localization device, the appropriate image-guided localization device placement code (19281, 19282, 19283, 19284, 19285, 19286, 19287, 19288) may also be reported.

Percutaneous cryosurgical ablation of a fibroadenoma (19105) includes ultrasound guidance and, therefore, 76940, 76942 may not be separately reported. Code 19105 may only be reported once per cryoprobe insertion site, even if several adjacent lesions are ablated.

Open excision of a breast lesion (eg, lesions of breast duct[s], cyst[s], benign or malignant tumor[s]), without specific attention to adequate surgical margins, with or without the preoperative placement of radiological markers are reported with 19110, 19112, 19120, 19125, 19126. If an open excision of a breast lesion is performed after image-guided placement of a localization device, the appropriate image-guided localization device placement code (19281, 19282, 19283, 19284, 19285, 19286, 19287, 19288) may also be reported.

To report bilateral procedures for 19100, 19101, 19105, 19110, 19112, 19120, report modifier 50 with the procedure code.◄

Rationale

Significant changes have been made to several subsections within the Integumentary System, Musculoskeletal System, and Respiratory System sections of the CPT code set. Notable changes include:

1. Deletion of the "Incision" and "Excision" subheadings from the Integumentary System/Breast subsection.

2. New guidelines for breast biopsy procedures.

3. Revised guidelines in the Breast/Introduction subsection.

4. New guidelines in the Mastectomy Procedures subsection.

5. Relocation (and renumbering) of chest wall tumor resection codes 19260, 19271, and 19272 to the Musculoskeletal subsection.

6. New, revised, and updated parenthetical notes throughout several code set subsections to reflect these changes.

7. Deletion of mastectomy code 19304.

8. New cross-reference parenthetical notes to clarify appropriate reporting for breast-size reduction for gynecomastia (19300) and for breast-size reduction for other than gynecomastia (19318).

These significant changes have been made to: (1) modernize the Integumentary/Breast/Introduction/Mastectomy Procedures, Musculoskeletal System, Respiratory System, and the Thoracoscopy (Video-assisted thoracic surgery [VATS]) subsections to reflect current clinical practice; and (2) clarify appropriate reporting regarding nipple and skin sparing services.

As part of the process of modernizing and updating these subsections, the "Incision" and "Excision" subheadings have been removed from the Breast subsection. In addition, new guidelines have been added to the Breast subsection to clarify breast biopsy procedures performed percutaneously or by open approach and with or without imaging. The guidelines also describe among other things how to report breast biopsies with breast localization device(s), imaging services, and bilateral procedures. Another step in modernizing to reflect current clinical practice, the chest wall tumor resection codes (19260, 19271, 19272) and all related parenthetical notes have been relocated to the Musculoskeletal subsection and renumbered. To support this change, three deletion parenthetical notes were added following code 19126 to direct users to report new codes 21601, 21602, and 21603. In addition, parenthetical notes following codes 21600, 21603, 32100, 32445, 32491, 32504, 32506, 32674, and 38746 have been updated to reflect all affected changes as appropriate.

The Introduction subsection guidelines have been revised to clarify the codes in this subsection and for consistency and in support of the changes in the guidelines for the breast biopsy procedures. In addition, the guidelines also provide instruction on how to report add-on services and placement of radiotherapy catheters (afterloading expandable or afterloading brachytherapy). The Mastectomy Procedures subsection guidelines have been updated to describe the codes and provide guidance on how to report bilateral procedures. In addition, code 19304 (subcutaneous mastectomy) has been deleted due to low utilization. A deletion parenthetical note has been added following code 19303. To clarify the appropriate reporting of breast-size reduction for gynecomastia (19300) and breast-size reduction for other than gynecomastia (19318), new cross-reference notes have been added following mastectomy codes (19300, 19303).

19081 Biopsy, breast, with placement of breast localization device(s) (eg, clip, metallic pellet), when performed, and imaging of the biopsy specimen, when performed, percutaneous; first lesion, including stereotactic guidance

+ **19082** each additional lesion, including stereotactic guidance (List separately in addition to code for primary procedure)

(Use 19082 in conjunction with 19081)

19083 Biopsy, breast, with placement of breast localization device(s) (eg, clip, metallic pellet), when performed, and imaging of the biopsy specimen, when performed, percutaneous; first lesion, including ultrasound guidance

+ **19084** each additional lesion, including ultrasound guidance (List separately in addition to code for primary procedure)

(Use 19084 in conjunction with 19083)

19085 Biopsy, breast, with placement of breast localization device(s) (eg, clip, metallic pellet), when performed, and imaging of the biopsy specimen, when performed, percutaneous; first lesion, including magnetic resonance guidance

+ **19086** each additional lesion, including magnetic resonance guidance (List separately in addition to code for primary procedure)

(Use 19086 in conjunction with 19085)

(Do not report 19081-19086 in conjunction with 19281-19288, 76098, 76942, 77002, 77021 for same lesion)

19100 Biopsy of breast; percutaneous, needle core, not using imaging guidance (separate procedure)

(For fine needle aspiration biopsy, see 10004, 10005, 10006, 10007, 10008, 10009, 10010, 10011, 10012, 10021)

19101 open, incisional

(For placement of percutaneous localization clip with imaging guidance, see 19281-19288)

19105 Ablation, cryosurgical, of fibroadenoma, including ultrasound guidance, each fibroadenoma

(Do not report 19105 in conjunction with 76940, 76942)

▶(For cryoablation of malignant breast tumor[s], use 0581T)◀

(For adjacent lesions treated with 1 cryoprobe insertion, report once)

Rationale

In support of the establishment of new Category III code 0581T, a cross-reference parenthetical note directing users to report code 0581T for cryoablation of malignant breast tumor[s] has been added in the Integumentary System section following code 19105.

Refer to the codebook and the Rationale for code 0581T for a full discussion of these changes.

19110 Nipple exploration, with or without excision of a solitary lactiferous duct or a papilloma lactiferous duct

19112 Excision of lactiferous duct fistula

19120 Excision of cyst, fibroadenoma, or other benign or malignant tumor, aberrant breast tissue, duct lesion, nipple or areolar lesion (except 19300), open, male or female, 1 or more lesions

19125 Excision of breast lesion identified by preoperative placement of radiological marker, open; single lesion

+ 19126 each additional lesion separately identified by a preoperative radiological marker (List separately in addition to code for primary procedure)

(Use 19126 in conjunction with 19125)

(Intraoperative placement of clip[s] is not separately reported)

▶(19260 has been deleted. To report, use 21601)◀

▶(19271 has been deleted. To report, use 21602)◀

▶(19272 has been deleted. To report, use 21603)◀

Rationale

In support of the relocation and renumbering of codes 19260, 19271, and 19272 to the Musculoskeletal subsection, parenthetical notes have been added directing users to codes 21601-21603 to report these services.

Refer to the codebook and the Rationale for breast biopsy procedure codes for a full discussion of these changes.

Introduction

▶Percutaneous image-guided placement of breast localization device(s) without image-guided breast biopsy(ies) is reported with 19281, 19282, 19283, 19284, 19285, 19286, 19287, 19288. When more than one localization device placement without image-guided biopsy is performed using the same imaging modality, report an add-on code whether the additional service(s) is on the same or contralateral breast. If additional localization device placements without image-guided biopsy(ies) are performed using different imaging modalities, report another primary code for each additional localization device placement without image-guided biopsy performed using a different image guidance modality.◀

To report bilateral image-guided placement of localization devices report 19281, 19283, 19285, or 19287 for the initial lesion localized. The contra-lateral and each additional breast image-guided localization device placement is reported with code 19282, 19284, 19286 or 19288.

▶When an open breast biopsy or open excision of a breast lesion is performed after image-guided percutaneous placement of a localization device, the appropriate image-guided localization device placement code (19281, 19282, 19283, 19284, 19285, 19286, 19287, 19288) may also be reported.◀

Code 19294 is used to report the preparation of the tumor cavity with placement of an intraoperative radiation therapy applicator concurrent with partial mastectomy (19301, 19302).

▶Codes 19296, 19297, 19298 describe placement of radiotherapy catheters (afterloading expandable or afterloading brachytherapy) into the breast for interstitial radioelement application either concurrent or on a separate date from a partial mastectomy procedure. Imaging guidance is included and may not be separately reported.◀

19281 Placement of breast localization device(s) (eg, clip, metallic pellet, wire/needle, radioactive seeds), percutaneous; first lesion, including mammographic guidance

Surgery																																																											CPT Changes 2020

+ 19282 each additional lesion, including mammographic guidance (List separately in addition to code for primary procedure)

(Use 19282 in conjunction with 19281)

Rationale

In the Integumentary System/Breast/Introduction subsection, the introductory guidelines have been revised to clarify correct reporting of the codes in this subsection, for consistency, and to support the changes in the guidelines for breast biopsy procedures. In addition, the guidelines also provide instruction on how to report add-on services and placement of radiotherapy catheters (afterloading expandable or afterloading brachytherapy).

Refer to the codebook and the Rationale for breast biopsy procedure codes for a full discussion of these changes.

Mastectomy Procedures

►Mastectomy procedures (with the exception of gynecomastia [19300]) are performed either for treatment or prevention of breast cancer.

Code 19301 describes a partial mastectomy where only a portion of the ipsilateral breast tissue is removed (eg, lumpectomy, tylectomy, quadrantectomy, segmentectomy). When a complete axillary lymphadenectomy is performed in addition to a partial mastectomy, report 19302. When breast tissue is removed for breast-size reduction and not for treatment or prevention of breast cancer, report 19318 (reduction mammaplasty).

Code 19303 describes total removal of ipsilateral breast tissue with or without removal of skin and/or nipples (eg, nipple-sparing), for treatment or prevention of breast cancer. Code 19303 does not include excision of pectoral muscle(s) and/or axillary and internal mammary lymph nodes. When a total mastectomy is performed for gynecomastia, report 19300.

Codes 19305, 19306, 19307 describe radical procedures that include total removal of the ipsilateral breast tissue, including the nipple for treatment of breast cancer and excision of pectoral muscle(s) and/or axillary lymph nodes and/or internal mammary lymph nodes.

To report bilateral procedures for 19300, 19301, 19302, 19303, 19305, 19306, 19307, report modifier 50 with the procedure code.◄

Rationale

New introductory guidelines have been added in the Mastectomy Procedures subsection. These guidelines describe the codes in this subsection, as well as provide guidance on how to report bilateral procedures.

Refer to the codebook and the Rationale for breast biopsy procedure codes for a full discussion of these changes.

19300 Mastectomy for gynecomastia

▶(For breast tissue removed for breast-size reduction for other than gynecomastia, use 19318)◄

Rationale

A parenthetical note has been added following code 19300 to clarify reporting of breast tissue removed for breast-size reduction for other than gynecomastia.

Refer to the codebook and the Rationale for breast biopsy procedure codes for a full discussion of these changes.

19301 Mastectomy, partial (eg, lumpectomy, tylectomy, quadrantectomy, segmentectomy);

19302   with axillary lymphadenectomy

(For placement of radiotherapy afterloading balloon/brachytherapy catheters, see 19296-19298)

(Intraoperative placement of clip[s] is not separately reported)

(For the preparation of tumor cavity with placement of an intraoperative radiation therapy applicator concurrent with partial mastectomy, use 19294)

▶(For radiofrequency spectroscopy, real time, intraoperative margin assessment, at the time of partial mastectomy, with report, use 0546T)◄

Rationale

In support of the establishment of Category III code 0546T, a parenthetical note directing users to the new code for radiofrequency spectroscopy performed during mastectomy to assess the surgical margins has been added following codes 19301 and 19302 (partial mastectomy).

Refer to the codebook and the Rationale for code 0546T for a full discussion of these changes.

19303 Mastectomy, simple, complete

(Intraoperative placement of clip[s] is not separately reported)

(For immediate or delayed insertion of implant, see 19340, 19342)

(For gynecomastia, use 19300)

▶(19304 has been deleted)◀

▶(For breast tissue removed for breast-size reduction for gynecomastia, use 19300)◀

▶(For breast tissue removed for breast-size reduction for other than gynecomastia, use 19318)◀

Rationale

Code 19304 has been deleted because of low utilization, and as such, a deletion parenthetical note has been added following code 19303. In addition, two parenthetical notes to clarify the appropriate reporting of breast-size reduction for gynecomastia (19300) and for breast-size reduction for other than gynecomastia (19318) have been added following code 19303.

Refer to the codebook and the Rationale for breast biopsy procedure codes for a full discussion of these changes.

Musculoskeletal System

General

Introduction or Removal

20552 Injection(s); single or multiple trigger point(s), 1 or 2 muscle(s)

20553 single or multiple trigger point(s), 3 or more muscles

▶(Do not report 20552, 20553 in conjunction with 20560, 20561 for the same muscle[s])◀

(If imaging guidance is performed, see 76942, 77002, 77021)

#● **20560** Needle insertion(s) without injection(s); 1 or 2 muscle(s)

#● **20561** 3 or more muscles

20555 Placement of needles or catheters into muscle and/or soft tissue for subsequent interstitial radioelement application (at the time of or subsequent to the procedure)

20560 Code is out of numerical sequence. See 20552-20600

20561 Code is out of numerical sequence. See 20552-20600

Rationale

Two new codes have been established to identify needle insertion(s) without injection(s) for 1 or 2 muscle(s) (20560) and for 3 or more muscles (20561). In addition, following code 20553, a new exclusionary parenthetical note has been added to restrict reporting existing codes 20552 and 20553 with these two new codes for the same muscle(s).

Codes 20560 and 20561 have been added to identify services that are not specifically identified as acupuncture or injections (due to the absence of an injectate). Instead, these services are known by other names including "dry needling" and "trigger point acupuncture." To reduce confusion regarding what these codes are and how they may be reported, the new codes (20560, 20561) have been placed in the Musculoskeletal System/Introduction or Removal subsection to recognize the differences between these services and acupuncture services. The descriptors specify that a needle is inserted without injection and the number of muscles treated.

To assist users in reporting these services, parenthetical instructions have been placed within this subsection and in other subsections in the codebook directing users to the appropriate codes to report depending on the type of services rendered. Parenthetical notes and guidelines that restrict the use of codes that may be mutually excluded because of services overlap and/or alternative reporting instructions have been provided, which includes: (1) an exclusionary parenthetical note following code 20553 restricting reporting of trigger point injections (20552, 20553) in conjunction with needle insertions without injection codes 20560 and 20561 for the same muscle(s); (2) adding an instructional parenthetical note following code 97140 (manual therapy techniques) directing users to codes 20560 and 20561; (3) adding guideline in the Acupuncture subsection directing users to codes 20560 and 20561 for needle insertion(s) without injection(s); and (4) adding a parenthetical note following code 97814 restricting the use of acupuncture services (ie, 97810, 97811, 97813, 97814) in conjunction with codes 20560 and 20561 and providing guidance to report only the time-based acupuncture codes when both time-based acupuncture services and needle insertion(s) without injection(s) are performed.

Refer to the codebook and the Rationale for acupuncture codes for a full discussion of these changes.

Clinical Example (20560)

A 38-year-old female presents with diffuse right-shoulder myofascial pain.

Description of Procedure (20560)

Physician palpates and locates the trigger points to be needled. Secure the first muscle between the fingers of the nonneedling hand. Insert sterile, single-use, solid filament needles, varying from 32 to 38 gauge and 25 to 100 mm in length, at various depths and angles to achieve the desired result of releasing tight tissue, improving microcirculation, and removing neuronoxious chemicals. Make interactive reassessments throughout the procedure, noting needle fibrillation, local twitch response, and/or reproduction of symptoms, including but not limited to achiness, burning, and electricity. Repeat this process for each additional muscle to be treated. Withdraw the needles and apply pressure (hemostasis) directly to the skin over the needle-insertion site.

Clinical Example (20561)

A 38-year-old female presents with neck pain, muscle-tension headaches, and diffuse right-shoulder myofascial pain.

Description of Procedure (20561)

Physician palpates and locates the trigger points to be needled. Secure the first muscle between the fingers of the nonneedling hand. Insert sterile, single-use, solid filament needles, varying from 32 to 38 gauge and 25 to 100 mm in length, at various depths and angles to achieve the desired result of releasing tight tissue, improving microcirculation, and removing neuronoxious chemicals. Make interactive reassessments throughout the procedure, noting needle fibrillation, local twitch response, and/or reproduction of symptoms, including but not limited to achiness, burning, and electricity. Repeat this process for each additional muscle to be treated. Withdraw the needles and apply pressure (hemostasis) directly to the skin over the needle-insertion site.

20696 Application of multiplane (pins or wires in more than 1 plane), unilateral, external fixation with stereotactic computer-assisted adjustment (eg, spatial frame), including imaging; initial and subsequent alignment(s), assessment(s), and computation(s) of adjustment schedule(s)

(Do not report 20696 in conjunction with 20692, 20697)

⊘ **20697** exchange (ie, removal and replacement) of strut, each

(Do not report 20697 in conjunction with 20692, 20696)

▶Manual preparation involves the mixing and preparation of antibiotics or other therapeutic agent(s) with a carrier substance by the physician or other qualified health care professional during the surgical procedure and then shaping the mixture into a drug-delivery device(s) (eg, beads, nails, spacers) for placement in the deep (eg, subfascial) intramedullary or intra-articular space(s). Codes 20700, 20702, 20704 are add-on codes for the manual preparation and insertion of the drug-delivery device during the associated primary surgical procedure listed with each add-on code. Codes 20701, 20703, 20705 are add-on codes for the removal of drug-delivery device(s) during the associated primary surgical procedures listed in the parenthetical codes associated with each add-on code. Insertion of a prefabricated drug device(s) may not be reported with 20700, 20702, 20704. Report 20680, if removal of drug-delivery device(s) is performed alone. Report 20700, 20701, 20702, 20703, 20704, 20705 once per anatomic location.◀

+● **20700** Manual preparation and insertion of drug-delivery device(s), deep (eg, subfascial) (List separately in addition to code for primary procedure)

▶(Use 20700 in conjunction with 11010, 11011, 11012, 11043, 11044, 11046, 11047, 20240, 20245, 20250, 20251, 21010, 21025, 21026, 21501, 21502, 21510, 21627, 21630, 22010, 22015, 23030, 23031, 23035, 23040, 23044, 23170, 23172, 23174, 23180, 23182, 23184, 23334, 23335, 23930, 23931, 23935, 24000, 24134, 24136, 24138, 24140, 24147, 24160, 25031, 25035, 25040, 25145, 25150, 25151, 26070, 26230, 26235, 26236, 26990, 26991, 26992, 27030, 27070, 27071, 27090, 27301, 27303, 27310, 27360, 27603, 27604, 27610, 27640, 27641, 28001, 28002, 28003, 28020, 28120, 28122)◀

▶(Do not report 20700 in conjunction with 11981)◀

+● **20701** Removal of drug-delivery device(s), deep (eg, subfascial) (List separately in addition to code for primary procedure)

▶(Use 20701 in conjunction with 11010, 11011, 11012, 11043, 11044, 11046, 11047, 20240, 20245, 20250, 20251, 21010, 21025, 21026, 21501, 21502, 21510, 21627, 21630, 22010, 22015, 23030, 23031, 23035, 23040, 23044, 23170, 23172, 23174, 23180, 23182, 23184, 23334, 23335, 23930, 23931, 23935, 24000, 24134, 24136, 24138, 24140, 24147, 24160, 25031, 25035, 25040, 25145, 25150, 25151, 26070, 26230, 26235, 26236, 26990, 26991, 26992, 27030, 27070, 27071, 27090, 27301, 27303, 27310, 27360, 27603, 27604, 27610, 27640, 27641, 28001, 28002, 28003, 28020, 28120, 28122)◀

▶(Do not report 20701 in conjunction with 11982)◀

+● 20702   Manual preparation and insertion of drug-delivery device(s), intramedullary (List separately in addition to code for primary procedure)

▶(Use 20702 in conjunction with 20680, 20690, 20692, 20694, 20802, 20805, 20838, 21510, 23035, 23170, 23180, 23184, 23515, 23615, 23935, 24134, 24138, 24140, 24147, 24430, 24516, 25035, 25145, 25150, 25151, 25400, 25515, 25525, 25526, 25545, 25574, 25575, 27245, 27259, 27360, 27470, 27506, 27640, 27720)◀

▶(Do not report 20702 in conjunction with 11981)◀

+● 20703   Removal of drug-delivery device(s), intramedullary (List separately in addition to code for primary procedure)

▶(Use 20703 in conjunction with 20690, 20692, 20694, 20802, 20805, 20838, 21510, 23035, 23170, 23180, 23184, 23515, 23615, 23935, 24134, 24138, 24140, 24147, 24430, 24516, 25035, 25145, 25150, 25151, 25400, 25515, 25525, 25526, 25545, 25574, 25575, 27245, 27259, 27360, 27470, 27506, 27640, 27720)◀

▶(Do not report 20703 in conjunction with 11982)◀

+● 20704   Manual preparation and insertion of drug-delivery device(s), intra-articular (List separately in addition to code for primary procedure)

▶(Use 20704 in conjunction with 22864, 22865, 23040, 23044, 23334, 24000, 24160, 25040, 25250, 25251, 26070, 26075, 26080, 26990, 27030, 27090, 27301, 27310, 27603, 27610, 28020)◀

▶(Do not report 20704 in conjunction with 11981, 27091, 27488)◀

+● 20705   Removal of drug-delivery device(s), intra-articular (List separately in addition to code for primary procedure)

▶(Use 20705 in conjunction with 22864, 22865, 23040, 23044, 23334, 24000, 24160, 25040, 25250, 25251, 26070, 26075, 26080, 26990, 27030, 27090, 27301, 27310, 27603, 27610, 28020)◀

▶(Do not report 20705 in conjunction with 11982, 23335, 27091, 27125, 27130, 27134, 27137, 27138, 27236, 27438, 27446, 27486, 27487, 27488)◀

Rationale

Six new add-on codes (20700-20705) have been established along with new guidelines to describe insertion and removal of drug-delivery devices. These codes should only be reported once per anatomic location.

Codes 20700, 20702, and 20704 should be used to report manual preparation and insertion of the drug-delivery device(s) during the associated primary surgical procedures, which have been listed in instructional parenthetical notes following each of these codes.

Codes 20701, 20703, and 20705 should be used to report removal of the drug-delivery device(s) during the associated primary surgical procedures, which have been listed in instructional parenthetical notes following each of these codes.

If only the removal of drug-delivery device(s) is performed, ie, without an associated primary procedure, then code 20680 should be reported.

New guidelines that define manual preparation with instructions for correct reporting of these new codes have been added.

Exclusionary parenthetical notes have been added following each code precluding their use with other codes, including codes 11981 and 11982. The Integumentary System subsection codes 11981 and 11982 may be reported for insertion and removal of non-biodegradable drug-delivery implants. However, they do not include manual fabrication and insertion of devices and removal of these specific devices, which are included in the new codes.

Clinical Example (20700)

A 19-year-old male undergoes surgical treatment of infected bone and soft tissues (reported separately). The surgeon fabricates an antibiotic cement device that is placed deep (subfascial) in the affected area. [**Note:** This is an add-on code. Only consider the additional work for manual preparation and insertion of the antibiotic-delivery device.]

Description of Procedure (20700)

Following thorough debridement of the infected bone and soft tissue (report separately), estimate the size of the dead space or defect. On the back table, make the device. Mix polymethylmethacrylate (PMMA) powder with antibiotic powder; most commonly, 3.6 g of tobramycin and 1 g of vancomycin are used for each 40-g package of cement. Add liquid monomer and mix the materials in a vacuum-mixing system. As the cement begins to harden but is still soft, roll it into long rods 1.5 to 2.0 cm in diameter. Cut these into small segments of 1.0 to 2.0 cm in length. Roll each into 1.5- to 2.0-cm–diameter round beads. Thread the beads on the suture, maintaining reasonably equal spacing. After the cement has hardened, check each bead to make sure it is securely centered on the suture. Tie a large knot on one end, incorporating a metallic marker for imaging (eg, vessel clip). Provisionally set the string of beads in the defect until adequate fill is obtained; remove beads from the suture as needed. Tie a large knot on the other end of the suture with a metallic marker. Remove, count, then re-insert the entire string of beads.

Clinical Example (20701)

A 19-year-old male undergoes removal of a deep (subfascial) antibiotic-delivery device during surgical treatment of a deep infection. [**Note:** This is an add-on code. Only consider the additional work for removal of the antibiotic-delivery device.]

Description of Procedure (20701)

Use prior incision(s), in part or in total. Complete exposure and dissection until the device is identified. Carefully strip soft tissues from the device and remove it manually. Count the number of beads and use fluoroscopy to confirm that the entire device has been removed.

Clinical Example (20702)

A 19-year-old male undergoes surgical treatment of infected bone and soft tissues (reported separately). The surgeon fabricates an antibiotic-cement device that is placed within the intramedullary canal of the tibia. [**Note:** This is an add-on code. Only consider the additional work for manual preparation and insertion of the antibiotic-delivery device.]

Description of Procedure (20702)

Following thorough debridement of the infected bone and soft tissue (report separately), finalize the length and diameter of the drug-delivery nail device. Remove the instruments that were used for the dirty portion of the procedure; open and set up new instruments. Prepare and redrape the patient's limb. Begin the clean portion of the procedure. On the back table, make the device. Select an appropriate diameter silicone tubing or chest tube and cut to the correct length. Use sterile mineral oil to lubricate the inner portion. Mix PMMA powder with antibiotic powder; most commonly 3.6 g of tobramycin and 1 g of vancomycin are used with each 40-g package of cement. Add liquid monomer and mix the materials in a vacuum-mixing system. Transfer container with the liquid cement to a pressurized insertion gun. Clamp one end of the tube and inject the liquid cement to completely fill the tube. While the cement is still soft, pass a small-diameter rod or wire (eg, 5.0-mm threaded Harrington rod, 4.5-mm Ender nail, 4.0-mm ball-tipped guidewire) down the tube, remove the clamp, and advance the wire until it exits the other end. After the cement has hardened, cut the tube and strip off the PMMA antibiotic nail. At the distal end of the nail, bend the wire and/or thread a nut onto the rod. Under fluoroscopic control, advance the device down the medullary canal and confirm the position. Cut the proximal end of the wire or rod at the appropriate length to allow subsequent removal, when performed.

Clinical Example (20703)

A 19-year-old male undergoes removal of an intramedullary antibiotic-cement device during surgical treatment of a deep infection. [**Note:** This is an add-on code. Only consider the additional work for removal of the antibiotic-delivery device.]

Description of Procedure (20703)

Use the prior incision(s), in part or in total. Complete exposure and dissection until the device is identified. Use thin osteotomes to loosen the device at the bone-cement interface, taking care to minimize bone loss. Attach an extraction tool and remove the device. However, not infrequently, the cement fractures and multiple fragments must be removed individually. Remove supplemental anchoring components and/or cement in the medullary canal with osteotomes, curettes, and grasping instruments; fluoroscopic control may be utilized for this portion. Use fluoroscopy to confirm that the entire device has been removed.

Clinical Example (20704)

A 70-year-old male undergoes surgical treatment of a native joint infection (reported separately). The surgeon fabricates an antibiotic-cement device that is placed intra-articularly. [**Note:** This is an add-on code. Only consider the additional work for manual preparation and insertion of the antibiotic-delivery device.]

Description of Procedure (20704)

Following thorough debridement of the infected bone and soft tissue (separately reported), select the type of drug-delivery device and size of the components. Remove the instruments that were used for the dirty portion of the procedure; open and set up new instruments. Prepare and redrape the patient's limb. Change gown and gloves. Begin the clean portion of the procedure. On the back table, make the device. Select an appropriately sized mold. Use sterile mineral oil or ultrasound gel to lubricate the inner portion of the mold. Mix PMMA powder with antibiotic powder; most commonly 3.6 g of tobramycin and 1 g of vancomycin are used with each 40-g package of cement. Add liquid monomer and mix the materials in a vacuum-mixing system. Transfer container with liquid cement to a pressurized insertion gun. Inject the liquid cement to completely fill the mold. After the cement has hardened, remove the device from the mold. Determine the size and fit of the device by temporary application to the bone ends; assess range of motion and joint stability. Remove the device, prepare and dry the bone ends with pulse irrigation. Prepare another batch of antibiotic cement in similar fashion. Apply the liquid cement to the bone ends plus or minus the medullary canal, insert the device and stabilize until the cement is hard. Remove the excess cement. A commercially available nail, rod, or wire may be used to supplement the cement fixation. Confirm stability and mobility.

Clinical Example (20705)

A 70-year-old male undergoes removal of an intra-articular antibiotic-cement device during surgical treatment of an intra-articular infection. [**Note:** This is an add-on code. Only consider the additional work for removal of the antibiotic-delivery device.]

Description of Procedure (20705)

Use the prior incision(s), in part or in total. Complete exposure and dissection until the device is identified, typically at the insertion site, but frequently also at the site of the infection and/or fracture. Carefully strip soft tissues and use a semicircular osteotome to loosen the bone-device interface. Attach an extraction tool to the nail, rod, or wire and make attempts to remove the device under fluoroscopic control. However, not infrequently, the cement fractures and multiple fragments must be removed individually via the medullary canal and/or via the infection or fracture site. Use fluoroscopy to confirm that the entire device has been removed.

Grafts (or Implants)

►Codes for obtaining autogenous bone, cartilage, tendon, fascia lata grafts, bone marrow, or other tissues through separate skin/fascial incisions should be reported separately, unless the code descriptor references the harvesting of the graft or implant (eg, includes obtaining graft). Autologous grafts that are already defined in the CPT code set, including skin, bone, nerve, tendon, fascia lata, or vessels, should be reported with the more specific codes for each tissue type. Code 15769 may be used for other autologous soft tissue grafts harvested by direct excision. See 15771, 15772, 15773, 15774 for autologous fat grafting harvested by liposuction technique.◄

Do not append modifier 62 to bone graft codes 20900-20938.

(For spinal surgery bone graft[s] see codes 20930-20938)

20900 Bone graft, any donor area; minor or small (eg, dowel or button)

20902 major or large

Rationale

Grafts (or Implants) guidelines have been revised instructing users that autologous grafts should be reported with the more specific codes for each tissue type already defined in the code set. In addition, reporting of autologous soft tissue grafts harvested by direct excision and for autologous fat grafting harvested by liposuction technique should be reported with new codes 15769, 15771, 15772, 15773, and 15774.

Refer to the codebook and the Rationale for codes 15769, 15771, 15772, 15773, and 15774 for a full discussion of these changes.

20920 Fascia lata graft; by stripper

20922 by incision and area exposure, complex or sheet

20924 Tendon graft, from a distance (eg, palmaris, toe extensor, plantaris)

►(20926 has been deleted)◄

►(To report autologous soft tissue grafts harvested by direct excision, use 15769)◄

►(To report autologous fat grafting harvested by liposuction technique, see 15771, 15772, 15773, 15774)◄

+ 20930 Allograft, morselized, or placement of osteopromotive material, for spine surgery only (List separately in addition to code for primary procedure)

(Use 20930 in conjunction with 22319, 22532, 22533, 22548-22558, 22590-22612, 22630, 22633, 22634, 22800-22812)

Rationale

Code 20926, *Tissue grafts, other (eg, paratenon, fat, dermis),* has been deleted because it was identified as potentially misvalued by RAW. It was determined that this code was being used to report significantly different procedures, including:

1. Harvesting small autologous soft tissue grafts via a direct excision technique;

2. Placing autologous soft tissue grafts into a defect for reconstructive purposes including utilization in skull base surgery; and

3. Placing autologous soft tissue grafts for minor contour deformities from trauma/surgery.

Therefore, five new codes (15769, 15771, 15772, 15773, 15774) have been established to more clearly differentiate these procedures.

Parenthetical notes have been added referring users to the new codes to report autologous soft tissue grafts harvested by direct excision and for autologous fat grafting harvested by liposuction technique.

Refer to the codebook and the Rationale for codes 15769, 15771, 15772, 15773, and 15774 for a full discussion of these changes.

+ 20939 Bone marrow aspiration for bone grafting, spine surgery only, through separate skin or fascial incision (List separately in addition to code for primary procedure)

(Use 20939 in conjunction with 22319, 22532, 22533, 22534, 22548, 22551, 22552, 22554, 22556, 22558, 22590, 22595, 22600, 22610, 22612, 22630, 22633, 22634, 22800, 22802, 22804, 22808, 22810, 22812)

▶(For bilateral procedure, report 20939 twice. Do not report modifier 50 in conjunction with 20939)◀

(For aspiration of bone marrow for the purpose of bone grafting, other than spine surgery and other therapeutic musculoskeletal applications, use 20999)

(For bone marrow aspiration[s] for platelet-rich stem cell injection, use 0232T)

(For diagnostic bone marrow aspiration[s], see 38220, 38222)

Rationale

In support of the revision to instructions for reporting add-on procedures when performed bilaterally, the instructional parenthetical note for add-on code 20939 has been revised to indicate that code 20939 should be reported twice when the procedure is performed bilaterally.

Refer to the codebook and the Rationale for modifier 50, *Bilateral Procedure,* guideline revisions for a full discussion of these changes.

Neck (Soft Tissues) and Thorax

Excision

21600 Excision of rib, partial

▶(For radical resection of chest wall and rib cage for tumor, use 21601)◀

(For radical debridement of chest wall and rib cage for injury, see 11044, 11047)

Rationale

In support of the deletion of code 19260, the existing parenthetical note following code 21600 has been revised by replacing code 19260 with code 21601. This parenthetical note directs users to report code 21601 for radical resection of chest wall and rib cage for tumor.

Refer to the codebook and the Rationale for breast biopsy procedure codes for a full discussion of these changes.

● 21601 Excision of chest wall tumor including rib(s)
● 21602 Excision of chest wall tumor involving rib(s), with plastic reconstruction; without mediastinal lymphadenectomy
● 21603   with mediastinal lymphadenectomy

▶(Do not report 21601, 21602, 21603 in conjunction with 32100, 32503, 32504, 32551, 32554, 32555)◀

21610 Costotransversectomy (separate procedure)

Rationale

In support of the significant changes made in the Breast, Musculoskeletal, and Respiratory System sections, the chest wall tumor excision procedures described by codes 19260, 19271, and 19272 have been renumbered and relocated to the Musculoskeletal System subsection. In addition, the existing exclusionary parenthetical note that originally followed code 19272 has been relocated to the Musculoskeletal System subsection to follow new code 21603 and has been revised by replacing the deleted codes with new codes 21601, 21602, and 21603. This revised parenthetical note restricts reporting codes 21601, 21602, and 21603 in conjunction with codes 32100, 32503, 32504, 32551, 32554, and 32555.

Refer to the codebook and the Rationale for breast biopsy procedure codes for a full discussion of these changes.

Spine (Vertebral Column)

Spinal Instrumentation

22856 Total disc arthroplasty (artificial disc), anterior approach, including discectomy with end plate preparation (includes osteophytectomy for nerve root or spinal cord decompression and microdissection); single interspace, cervical

▶(Do not report 22856 in conjunction with 22554, 22845, 22853, 22854, 22859, 63075, when performed at the same level)◀

(Do not report 22856 in conjunction with 69990)

▶(For additional interspace cervical total disc arthroplasty, use 22858)◀

#+ 22858   second level, cervical (List separately in addition to code for primary procedure)

(Use 22858 in conjunction with 22856)

Rationale

In support of the deletion of Category III code 0375T, two parenthetical notes following code 22856 have been revised with the removal of this code.

Refer to the codebook and the Rationale for code 0375T for a full discussion of these changes.

Femur (Thigh Region) and Knee Joint

Repair, Revision, and/or Reconstruction

27412   Autologous chondrocyte implantation, knee

▶(Do not report 27412 in conjunction with 15769, 15771, 15772, 15773, 15774, 27331, 27570)◀

(For harvesting of chondrocytes, use 29870)

Rationale

In accordance with the deletion of code 20926 and addition of codes 15769, 15771, 15772, 15773, and 15774, the parenthetical note following code 27412 has been revised to remove the deleted code from its listing.

Refer to the codebook and the Rationale for codes 15769, 15771, 15772, 15773, 15774, and 20926 for a full discussion of these changes.

Respiratory System

Nose

Repair

▶(For obtaining tissues for graft, see 15769, 20900, 20902, 20910, 20912, 20920, 20922, 20924, 21210)◀

▶(For correction of nasal defects using fat harvested via liposuction technique, see 15773, 15774)◀

30400   Rhinoplasty, primary; lateral and alar cartilages and/or elevation of nasal tip

(For columellar reconstruction, see 13151 et seq)

30410   complete, external parts including bony pyramid, lateral and alar cartilages, and/or elevation of nasal tip

30420   including major septal repair

30465   Repair of nasal vestibular stenosis (eg, spreader grafting, lateral nasal wall reconstruction)

▶(30465 excludes obtaining graft. For graft procedure, see 15769, 20900, 20902, 20910, 20912, 20920, 20922, 20924, 21210)◀

(30465 is used to report a bilateral procedure. For unilateral procedure, use modifier 52)

Rationale

In support of the deletion of code 20926 and addition of autologous grafting codes, parenthetical notes in the Nose/Repair subsection of the Respiratory section have been affected. The parenthetical notes following the Repair heading and code 30465 have been revised by removing the deleted code and replacing it with new code 15769 for autologous soft tissue grafting. In addition, a new parenthetical note has been added directing users to new codes 15773 and 15774 for correction of nasal defects using fat harvested via liposuction technique.

Refer to the codebook and the Rationale for codes 15769, 15773, 15774, and 20926 for a full discussion of these changes.

Accessory Sinuses

Endoscopy

31231   Nasal endoscopy, diagnostic, unilateral or bilateral (separate procedure)

▲ 31233   Nasal/sinus endoscopy, diagnostic; with maxillary sinusoscopy (via inferior meatus or canine fossa puncture)

▶(Do not report 31233 in conjunction with 31256, 31267, 31295, when performed on the ipsilateral side)◀

▲ 31235   with sphenoid sinusoscopy (via puncture of sphenoidal face or cannulation of ostium)

▶(Do not report 31235 in conjunction with 31257, 31259, 31287, 31288, 31297, 31298, when performed on the ipsilateral side)◀

(To report endoscopic placement of a drug-eluting implant in the ethmoid sinus without any other nasal/sinus endoscopic surgical service, use 31299. To report endoscopic placement of a drug-eluting implant in the ethmoid sinus in conjunction with biopsy, polypectomy, or debridement, use 31237)

Surgery | CPT Changes 2020

31237 Nasal/sinus endoscopy, surgical; with biopsy, polypectomy or debridement (separate procedure)

▶(Do not report 31237 in conjunction with 31238, 31253, 31254, 31255, 31256, 31257, 31259, 31267, 31276, 31287, 31288, 31290, 31291, 31292, 31293, 31294, when performed on the ipsilateral side)◀

31238 with control of nasal hemorrhage

▶(Do not report 31238 in conjunction with 31237, 31241, when performed on the ipsilateral side)◀

31239 with dacryocystorhinostomy

31240 with concha bullosa resection

31241 with ligation of sphenopalatine artery

(Do not report 31241 in conjunction with 31238, when performed on the ipsilateral side)

31253 Code is out of numerical sequence. See 31254-31267

31254 Nasal/sinus endoscopy, surgical with ethmoidectomy; partial (anterior)

▶(Do not report 31254 in conjunction with 31237, 31253, 31255, 31257, 31259, 31290, 31291, 31292, 31293, 31294, when performed on the ipsilateral side)◀

31255 total (anterior and posterior)

▶(Do not report 31255 in conjunction with 31237, 31253, 31254, 31257, 31259, 31276, 31287, 31288, 31290, 31291, 31292, 31293, 31294, when performed on the ipsilateral side)◀

 # 31253 total (anterior and posterior), including frontal sinus exploration, with removal of tissue from frontal sinus, when performed

▶(Do not report 31253 in conjunction with 31237, 31254, 31255, 31276, 31290, 31291, 31292, 31293, 31294, 31296, 31298, when performed on the ipsilateral side)◀

 # 31257 total (anterior and posterior), including sphenoidotomy

▶(Do not report 31257 in conjunction with 31235, 31237, 31254, 31255, 31259, 31287, 31288, 31290, 31291, 31292, 31293, 31294, 31297, 31298, when performed on the ipsilateral side)◀

 # 31259 total (anterior and posterior), including sphenoidotomy, with removal of tissue from the sphenoid sinus

▶(Do not report 31259 in conjunction with 31235, 31237, 31254, 31255, 31257, 31287, 31288, 31290, 31291, 31292, 31293, 31294, 31297, 31298, when performed on the ipsilateral side)◀

31256 Nasal/sinus endoscopy, surgical, with maxillary antrostomy;

▶(Do not report 31256 in conjunction with 31233, 31237, 31267, 31295, when performed on the ipsilateral side)◀

31257 Code is out of numerical sequence. See 31254-31267

31259 Code is out of numerical sequence. See 31254-31267

31267 with removal of tissue from maxillary sinus

▶(Do not report 31267 in conjunction with 31233, 31237, 31256, 31295, when performed on the ipsilateral side)◀

31276 Nasal/sinus endoscopy, surgical, with frontal sinus exploration, including removal of tissue from frontal sinus, when performed

▶(Do not report 31276 in conjunction with 31237, 31253, 31255, 31296, 31298, when performed on the ipsilateral side)◀

31287 Nasal/sinus endoscopy, surgical, with sphenoidotomy;

▶(Do not report 31287 in conjunction with 31235, 31237, 31255, 31257, 31259, 31288, 31291, 31294, 31297, 31298, when performed on the ipsilateral side)◀

31288 with removal of tissue from the sphenoid sinus

▶(Do not report 31288 in conjunction with 31235, 31237, 31255, 31257, 31259, 31287, 31291, 31294, 31297, 31298, when performed on the ipsilateral side)◀

31290 Nasal/sinus endoscopy, surgical, with repair of cerebrospinal fluid leak; ethmoid region

▶(Do not report 31290 in conjunction with 31237, 31253, 31254, 31255, 31257, 31259, when performed on the ipsilateral side)◀

31291 sphenoid region

▶(Do not report 31291 in conjunction with 31237, 31253, 31254, 31255, 31257, 31259, 31287, 31288, when performed on the ipsilateral side)◀

▲ **31292** Nasal/sinus endoscopy, surgical, with orbital decompression; medial or inferior wall

▶(Do not report 31292 in conjunction with 31237, 31253, 31254, 31255, 31257, 31259, 31293, 31296, when performed on the ipsilateral side)◀

▲ **31293** medial and inferior wall

▶(Do not report 31293 in conjunction with 31237, 31253, 31254, 31255, 31257, 31259, 31292, when performed on the ipsilateral side)◀

▲ **31294** Nasal/sinus endoscopy, surgical, with optic nerve decompression

▶(Do not report 31294 in conjunction with 31237, 31253, 31254, 31255, 31257, 31259, 31287, 31288, when performed on the ipsilateral side)◀

▲ **31295** Nasal/sinus endoscopy, surgical, with dilation (eg, balloon dilation); maxillary sinus ostium, transnasal or via canine fossa

(Do not report 31295 in conjunction with 31233, 31256, 31267, when performed on the ipsilateral side)

▲ **31296** frontal sinus ostium

(Do not report 31296 in conjunction with 31253, 31276, 31297, 31298, when performed on the ipsilateral side)

▲ **31297** sphenoid sinus ostium

(Do not report 31297 in conjunction with 31235, 31257, 31259, 31287, 31288, 31296, 31298, when performed on the ipsilateral side)

▲ **31298** frontal and sphenoid sinus ostia

▶(Do not report 31298 in conjunction with 31235, 31253, 31257, 31259, 31276, 31287, 31288, 31296, 31297, when performed on the ipsilateral side)◀

Rationale

Existing codes and exclusionary parenthetical notes have been revised, new parenthetical notes have been added, and a number of parenthetical notes have been deleted to simplify and clarify the intended use of the nasal endoscopy codes.

The changes made to this section are editorial in nature because they do not change the intent of these codes. Instead, the changes have been made to simplify the use of this large section of codes, ie, to enable language conformity within the code descriptors and parenthetical notes, and to facilitate differentiation of services included in the subsection. The specific changes include:

1. Consolidation of common language within code descriptors in the same family. In these instances, common language has been moved from the descriptors of the individual codes to the parent code to precede the semicolon. This change occurred in codes 31292 and 31293, with the terms "orbital" and "decompression" relocated to precede the semicolon of parent code 31292. Because code 31294 did not share this verbiage, it has been revised as a stand-alone code. Similarly, in the code family 31295-31298, the shared language "with dilation" and "(eg, balloon dilation)" have been moved to the parent code 31295, preceding the semicolon. For codes 31233 and 31235, a parent/child code relationship was created upon consolidation of language. Code 31235 is now a child code to code 31233 as they both share the common language "Nasal/sinus endoscopy, diagnostic."

2. Editorial revision of the exclusionary parenthetical notes that follow codes 31233, 31235, 31238, 31253, 31254, 31255, 31257, 31259, 31267, 31276, 31287, 31288, and 31298 to reflect inherent inclusion of nasal endoscopy services codes. In addition, in several of the parenthetical notes, the term "same sinus" has been editorially revised to conform with other codes in the section to state "ipsilateral side."

3. Addition of exclusionary parenthetical notes following codes 31237, 31256, 31290, 31291, 31292, 31293, and 31294 to mirror other exclusionary parenthetical notes included in this subsection by prohibiting reporting of other nasal endoscopic services performed on the ipsilateral side.

4. Removal of redundant instructional parenthetical notes because the exclusionary parenthetical notes provide ample direction regarding use of codes that would be inappropriately reported together.

Larynx

Endoscopy

31545 Laryngoscopy, direct, operative, with operating microscope or telescope, with submucosal removal of non-neoplastic lesion(s) of vocal cord; reconstruction with local tissue flap(s)

31546 reconstruction with graft(s) (includes obtaining autograft)

▶(Do not report 31546 in conjunction with 15769, 15771, 15772, 15773, 15774 for graft harvest)◀

(For reconstruction of vocal cord with allograft, use 31599)

(Do not report 31545 or 31546 in conjunction with 31540, 31541, 69990)

Rationale

In support of the deletion of code 20926 and addition of codes 15769, 15771, 15772, 15773, and 15774, the parenthetical note following code 31546 has been revised by replacing the deleted code with the new grafting codes.

Refer to the codebook and the Rationale for codes 15769, 15771, 15772, 15773, 15774, and 20926 for a full discussion of these changes.

Lungs and Pleura

Incision

32100 Thoracotomy; with exploration

▶(Do not report 32100 in conjunction with 21601, 21602, 21603, 32503, 32504, 33955, 33956, 33957, 33963, 33964)◀

Rationale

In support of the relocation and renumbering of the chest wall tumor excision codes 19260, 19271, and 19272 to the Musculoskeletal System subsection, the existing parenthetical note following code 32100 has been revised with the new codes 21601, 21602, and 21603.

Refer to the codebook and the Rationale for breast biopsy procedure codes for a full discussion of these changes.

Removal

32440 Removal of lung, pneumonectomy;

32442 with resection of segment of trachea followed by broncho-tracheal anastomosis (sleeve pneumonectomy)

32445 extrapleural

(For extrapleural pneumonectomy, with empyemectomy, use 32445 and 32540)

▶(If lung resection is performed with chest wall tumor resection, report the appropriate chest wall tumor resection code [21601, 21602, 21603], in addition to lung resection code [32440-32445])◀

32480 Removal of lung, other than pneumonectomy; single lobe (lobectomy)

32482 2 lobes (bilobectomy)

32484 single segment (segmentectomy)

(For removal of lung with bronchoplasty, use 32501)

32486 with circumferential resection of segment of bronchus followed by broncho-bronchial anastomosis (sleeve lobectomy)

32488 with all remaining lung following previous removal of a portion of lung (completion pneumonectomy)

(For lobectomy or segmentectomy, with concomitant decortication, use 32320 and the appropriate removal of lung code)

32491 with resection-plication of emphysematous lung(s) (bullous or non-bullous) for lung volume reduction, sternal split or transthoracic approach, includes any pleural procedure, when performed

▶(If lung resection is performed with chest wall tumor resection, report the appropriate chest wall tumor resection code [21601, 21602, 21603] in addition to lung resection code [32480, 32482, 32484, 32486, 32488, 32505, 32506, 32507])◀

+ **32501** Resection and repair of portion of bronchus (bronchoplasty) when performed at time of lobectomy or segmentectomy (List separately in addition to code for primary procedure)

(Use 32501 in conjunction with 32480, 32482, 32484)

(32501 is to be used when a portion of the bronchus to preserved lung is removed and requires plastic closure to preserve function of that preserved lung. It is not to be used for closure for the proximal end of a resected bronchus)

32503 Resection of apical lung tumor (eg, Pancoast tumor), including chest wall resection, rib(s) resection(s), neurovascular dissection, when performed; without chest wall reconstruction(s)

32504 with chest wall reconstruction

▶(Do not report 32503, 32504 in conjunction with 21601, 21602, 21603, 32100, 32551, 32554, 32555)◀

32505 Thoracotomy; with therapeutic wedge resection (eg, mass, nodule), initial

(Do not report 32505 in conjunction with 32440, 32442, 32445, 32488)

+ **32506** with therapeutic wedge resection (eg, mass or nodule), each additional resection, ipsilateral (List separately in addition to code for primary procedure)

(Report 32506 only in conjunction with 32505)

▶(If lung resection is performed with chest wall tumor resection, report the appropriate chest wall tumor resection code [21601, 21602, 21603], in addition to lung resection code [32480, 32482, 32484, 32486, 32488, 32505, 32506, 32507])◀

+ **32507** with diagnostic wedge resection followed by anatomic lung resection (List separately in addition to code for primary procedure)

(Report 32507 in conjunction with 32440, 32442, 32445, 32480, 32482, 32484, 32486, 32488, 32503, 32504)

Rationale

In support of the relocation and renumbering of the chest wall tumor excision codes 19260, 19271, and 19272 to the Musculoskeletal System subsection, the existing parenthetical notes following codes 32445, 32491, 32504, and 32506 have been revised with the new codes 21601, 21602, and 21603.

Refer to the codebook and the Rationale for breast biopsy procedure codes for a full discussion of these changes.

Thoracoscopy (Video-assisted thoracic surgery [VATS])

32650 Thoracoscopy, surgical; with pleurodesis (eg, mechanical or chemical)

32651 with partial pulmonary decortication

+ 32674   with mediastinal and regional lymphadenectomy (List separately in addition to code for primary procedure)

(On the right, mediastinal lymph nodes include the paratracheal, subcarinal, paraesophageal, and inferior pulmonary ligament)

(On the left, mediastinal lymph nodes include the aortopulmonary window, subcarinal, paraesophageal, and inferior pulmonary ligament)

▶(Report 32674 in conjunction with 21601, 31760, 31766, 31786, 32096-32200, 32220-32320, 32440-32491, 32503-32505, 32601-32663, 32666, 32669-32673, 32815, 33025, 33030, 33050-33130, 39200-39220, 39560, 39561, 43101, 43112, 43117, 43118, 43122, 43123, 43287, 43288, 43351, 60270, 60505)◀

(To report mediastinal and regional lymphadenectomy via thoracotomy, use 38746)

Rationale

In support of the relocation and renumbering of the chest wall tumor excision codes 19260, 19271, and 19272 to the Musculoskeletal System, the existing parenthetical note following code 32674 has been revised with new code 21601.

Refer to the codebook and the Rationale for breast biopsy procedure codes for a full discussion of these changes.

Cardiovascular System

Heart and Pericardium

Pericardium

▶In order to report pericardial drainage with insertion of indwelling catheter (33017, 33018, 33019), the catheter needs to remain in place when the procedure is completed. Codes 33017, 33018, 33019 should not be reported when a catheter is placed to aspirate fluid and then removed at the conclusion of the procedure.

Congenital cardiac anomaly for reporting percutaneous pericardial drainage with insertion of indwelling catheter is defined as abnormal situs (heterotaxy, dextrocardia, mesocardia), single ventricle anomaly/physiology, or any patient in the first 90-day postoperative period after repair of a congenital cardiac anomaly.◀

(For thoracoscopic (VATS) pericardial procedures, see 32601, 32604, 32658, 32659, 32661)

▶(33010, 33011 have been deleted. To report, see 33016, 33017, 33018, 33019)◀

▶(33015 has been deleted. To report, see 33017, 33018, 33019)◀

● **33016**   Pericardiocentesis, including imaging guidance, when performed

▶(Do not report 33016 in conjunction with 76942, 77002, 77012, 77021)◀

● **33017**   Pericardial drainage with insertion of indwelling catheter, percutaneous, including fluoroscopy and/or ultrasound guidance, when performed; 6 years and older without congenital cardiac anomaly

● **33018**   birth through 5 years of age or any age with congenital cardiac anomaly

▶(Do not report 33017, 33018 in conjunction with 75989, 76942, 77002, 77012, 77021)◀

▶(Do not report 33016, 33017, 33018 in conjunction with 93303-93325 when echocardiography is performed solely for the purpose of pericardiocentesis guidance)◀

▶(For CT-guided pericardial drainage, use 33019)◀

● **33019**   Pericardial drainage with insertion of indwelling catheter, percutaneous, including CT guidance

▶(Do not report 33019 in conjunction with 75989, 76942, 77002, 77012, 77021)◀

33020   Pericardiotomy for removal of clot or foreign body (primary procedure)

Rationale

To reflect current clinical practice, changes have been made to pericardium procedures reporting. Codes 33010 and 33011 (pericardiocentesis) and code 33015 (tube pericardiostomy) have been deleted because they no longer reflect current clinical practice. Instead, new codes 33016 (pericardiocentesis) and 33017, 33018, and 33019 (pericardial drainage) have been created. Guidelines and parenthetical notes have also been added to provide instruction on the correct reporting of codes 33017, 33018, and 33019.

Prior to 2020, codes 33010 and 33011 were distinguished as initial and subsequent, respectively, and did not include imaging guidance with instruction given to separately report code 76930, *Ultrasonic guidance for pericardiocentesis, imaging supervision and interpretation,* if performed. However, in current clinical practice, it is not necessary to distinguish between initial and subsequent pericardiocentesis; imaging guidance is performed with the procedure frequently enough to warrant inclusion in the code; and ultrasound is not the only type of imaging guidance that is performed with the procedure. Therefore, new codes 33016-33019 were created. Code 33016 describes pericardiocentesis with imaging guidance, when performed, and does not distinguish between initial or subsequent procedure. Pericardiocentesis as described by code 33016 may require insertion of a small catheter in order to complete the procedure. If a catheter is used, it is removed at the end of the procedure and not reported separately.

Codes 33017, 33018, and 33019 describe percutaneous pericardial drainage with insertion of an indwelling catheter (previously reported with code 33015, which used the outdated term "tube pericardiostomy"). These codes differ from code 33016 (pericardiocentesis) in that a catheter is always inserted during the procedure and is left in place at the end of the procedure. The work and resources used in pericardial drainage performed on children from birth through age five or on patients of any age who have a congenital cardiac anomaly varies significantly enough from those used when the procedure is performed on patients age six and older with no congenital cardiac anomaly to require separate codes.

Code 33017 is reported for patients age six or older who do not have a congenital cardiac anomaly. Report code 33018 for two types of patients: (1) patients from birth through five years of age; and (2) patients of any age who have a congenital cardiac anomaly. The new guidelines provide a definition of "congenital cardiac anomaly" relative to codes 33017 and 33018. Similar to pericardiocentesis, imaging guidance is performed with percutaneous pericardial drainage frequently enough to warrant inclusion in the new codes. Codes 33017 and 33018 include fluoroscopy and/or ultrasound guidance, when performed. Code 33019 has been added for percutaneous pericardial drainage with insertion of indwelling catheter when performed with computed tomography (CT) guidance because the work involved in using CT guidance differs from that involved in other modes of imaging guidance. Code 33019 is reported for patients of any age. In order to report code 33019, CT guidance must be performed.

Clinical Example (33016)

A 52-year-old male with lung cancer presents with a large pericardial effusion, slowly accumulating over the past several weeks. Chest X ray (CXR) shows an enlarged cardiac silhouette and ultrasound confirms presence of a large pericardial effusion. Fluid sample is requested for purpose of assisting with establishing etiology and staging.

Description of Procedure (33016)

Use moderate sedation or general anesthesia, as applicable given the patient's clinical status and/or age. Depending on the clinical stability of the patient's condition, the procedure may be performed either at the bedside, often emergently, or in the cardiac catheterization laboratory. Carefully inject local anesthetic along the insertion site. With use of a sterile sleeve, continuous echocardiographic guidance is provided, typically by a second physician but not separately reportable. Identify the optimal pocket of fluid. Use percutaneous technique to pass a needle through the skin and soft tissue into the pericardial space until fluid is aspirated. Pass a thin guidewire through the needle into the pericardial space. This is often performed from the subxiphoid approach; however, it can vary significantly to almost anywhere along the costal margin, as appropriate. Fluoroscopy may or may not be used, depending on where the procedure is performed (not additionally reportable). Take care to ensure the needle and wire are in the pericardial space. Confirm this placement with direct echocardiography and/or fluoroscopy and an injection of agitated saline/blood mixture into the space. The needle can also be attached briefly to a pressure transducer to demonstrate absence of a ventricular waveform. Once absolutely certain of proper positioning, remove the needle. Make a small incision in the skin, dilate the tract with a dilator, and place the larger bore wire. Place a multisided-hole drain over that wire, within the pericardial sac, and manually aspirate fluid to expedite stabilizing the patient. Continue to withdraw fluid, with frequent reassessment by ultrasound and adjustment of the catheter position to ensure complete and thorough drainage. Reconnect the catheter to a pressure transducer to ensure the pericardial pressure has returned close to zero. Remove the drain. Divide the collected fluid into multiple tubes for cell counts, chemistries, bacterial cultures, cytology, and whatever else may be appropriate. Apply a sterile, occlusive dressing. Complete the extensive laboratory forms and associate them with the samples.

Clinical Example (33017)

A 62-year-old male presents with chronic heart failure (CHF) and acute hemodynamic instability. CXR shows an enlarged cardiac silhouette, and ultrasound confirms presence of a large pericardial effusion. The patient is transported to the cardiac catheterization laboratory for pericardial-drain placement.

Description of Procedure (33017)

Use moderate sedation or general anesthesia, as applicable given the patient's clinical status and/or age. Depending on the clinical stability of the patient's condition, the procedure may be performed either at the bedside, often emergently, or transferred to the cardiac catheterization laboratory. Complete injection of local anesthetic along the insertion site. With use of a sterile sleeve, continuous echocardiographic guidance is provided, typically by a second physician but not separately reportable. Identify the optimal pocket of fluid. Use percutaneous technique to pass a needle through the skin and soft tissue into the pericardial space until fluid is aspirated. Pass a thin guidewire through the needle into the pericardial space. This is often performed from the subxiphoid approach; however, it can vary significantly to almost anywhere along the costal margin, as appropriate. Fluoroscopy may or may not be used, depending on where the procedure is performed (not additionally reportable). Take care to ensure the needle and wire are in the pericardial space. Confirm this placement with direct echocardiography and/or fluoroscopy and an injection of agitated saline/blood mixture into the space. The needle can also be attached briefly to a pressure transducer to demonstrate absence of a ventricular waveform. Once absolutely certain of proper positioning, remove the needle. Make a small incision in the skin, dilate the tract with a dilator, and place the larger bore wire. Place a multisided-hole drain over that wire, within the pericardial sac, and manually aspirate fluid to expedite stabilizing the patient. Continue to withdraw fluid, with frequent reassessment by ultrasound and adjustment of the catheter position to ensure complete and thorough drainage. Reconnect the catheter to a pressure transducer to ensure the pericardial pressure has returned close to zero. Secure the drain either with sutures or other approved device and attach to suction. Divide collected fluid into multiple tubes for cell counts, chemistries, bacterial cultures, cytology, and whatever else may be appropriate and send for laboratory analysis. Apply a sterile, occlusive dressing. Complete the extensive laboratory forms and associate them with the samples. Secure the drain further against disruption by transit of the patient back to the intensive care unit.

Clinical Example (33018)

A three-month-old, 6-kg infant male presents status postopen-heart surgery for repair of coarctation of the aorta and an atrial septal defect. Postoperative day two, the infant has rapid deterioration and hemodynamic instability. The intensive care unit (ICU) staff obtains a stat transthoracic echocardiogram, which confirms the presence of a large pericardial effusion and evidence of tamponade physiology.

Description of Procedure (33018)

A second cardiologist typically provides continuous echocardiographic guidance with use of a sterile sleeve (report separately). Identify the optimal pocket of fluid. Use percutaneous technique to pass a needle through the skin and soft tissue into the pericardial space until fluid is aspirated. Pass a thin guidewire through the needle into the pericardial space. This is often performed from the subxiphoid approach; however, it can vary significantly to almost anywhere along the costal margin, as well as occasionally over the right chest for patients with dextrocardia. Fluoroscopy may or may not be used, depending on where the procedure is performed (not additionally reportable). Due to the extremely small size of the patient's heart and pericardial sac, take great care to ensure the needle and wire are in the pericardial space. Confirm placement with direct echocardiography and/or fluoroscopy. Occasionally, an injection of agitated saline/blood mixture into the space for confirmation is also performed. The needle can also be attached briefly to a pressure transducer to demonstrate absence of a ventricular waveform. Once absolutely certain of proper positioning, remove the needle. Make a small incision in the skin, dilate the tract with a dilator, and remove. Place a multisided-hole drain over the wire, within the pericardial sac, and manually aspirate fluid to expedite stabilizing the patient. Secure the drain either with sutures or other approved device and attach to suction. Send collected fluid for lab analysis. Apply a sterile, occlusive dressing.

Clinical Example (33019)

A 65-year-old male with a history of lymphoma, mediastinal radiation, and coronary artery bypass presents with an enlarged cardiac silhouette on CXR, tamponade physiology, and a loculated posteriorly located pericardial effusion demonstrated by echocardiography.

Description of Procedure (33019)

Supervise and interpret scout views of area to be imaged to select appropriate field of view. Obtain and interpret preliminary computed tomography (CT) images acquired to assess appropriate approach to the target(s); evaluate for unexpected findings and interval changes in target area(s); and adjust patient positioning or protocol as needed. Mark and prepare the skin entry site in sterile fashion. Perform intermittent or continuous CT guidance to direct needle to the pericardial space and reposition as necessary. Confirm satisfactory needle placement in the pericardial fluid collection. Aspirate fluid and send for appropriate laboratory analysis (eg, microbiology, chemistry, cell count) as needed. Pass a guidewire into the collection and perform repeat imaging. Serially dilate the tract to the necessary size. Advance a drainage catheter into the collection and perform imaging (may involve contrast injection) to verify proper catheter position within the collection. Secure the catheter in place and connect it to a drainage system (eg, suction, gravity). Obtain and interpret postprocedural CT images to evaluate for complications. Interpret all images resulting from the study, including dedicated review of the target(s), as well as all visualized viscera, fascial planes, vasculature, soft tissues, and osseous structures. Assess for complications or other unexpected findings.

Pacemaker or Implantable Defibrillator

A pacemaker system with lead(s) includes a pulse generator containing electronics, a battery, and one or more leads. A lead consists of one or more electrodes, as well as conductor wires, insulation, and a fixation mechanism. Pulse generators are placed in a subcutaneous "pocket" created in either a subclavicular site or just above the abdominal muscles just below the ribcage. Leads may be inserted through a vein (transvenous) or they may be placed on the surface of the heart (epicardial). The epicardial location of leads requires a thoracotomy for insertion.

A single chamber pacemaker system with lead includes a pulse generator and one electrode inserted in either the atrium or ventricle. A dual chamber pacemaker system with two leads includes a pulse generator and one lead inserted in the right atrium and one lead inserted in the right ventricle. In certain circumstances, an additional lead may be required to achieve pacing of the left ventricle (bi-ventricular pacing). In this event, transvenous (cardiac vein) placement of the lead should be separately reported using code 33224 or 33225. Epicardial placement of the lead should be separately reported using 33202, 33203.

A leadless cardiac pacemaker system includes a pulse generator with built-in battery and electrode for implantation in a cardiac chamber via a transcatheter approach. For implantation of a leadless pacemaker system, use 33274. Insertion, replacement, or removal of a leadless pacemaker system includes insertion of a catheter into the right ventricle.

Right heart catheterization (93451, 93453, 93456, 93457, 93460, 93461, 93530, 93531, 93532, 93533) may not be reported in conjunction with leadless pacemaker insertion and removal codes 33274, 33275 unless complete right heart catheterization is performed for an indication distinct from the leadless pacemaker procedure.

▶Like a pacemaker system, an implantable defibrillator system includes a pulse generator and electrodes. Three general categories of implantable defibrillators exist: transvenous implantable pacing cardioverter-defibrillator (ICD), subcutaneous implantable defibrillator (S-ICD), and substernal implantable cardioverter-defibrillator. Implantable pacing cardioverter-defibrillator devices use a combination of antitachycardia pacing, low-energy cardioversion or defibrillating shocks to treat ventricular tachycardia or ventricular fibrillation. The subcutaneous implantable defibrillator uses a single subcutaneous electrode to treat ventricular tachyarrhythmias. The substernal implantable cardioverter-defibrillator uses at least one substernal electrode to perform defibrillation, cardioversion, and antitachycardia pacing. Subcutaneous implantable defibrillators differ from transvenous implantable pacing cardioverter-defibrillators in that subcutaneous defibrillators do not provide antitachycardia pacing or chronic pacing. Substernal implantable defibrillators differ from both subcutaneous and transvenous implantable pacing cardioverter-defibrillators in that they provide antitachycardia pacing, but not chronic pacing.◀

Implantable defibrillator pulse generators may be implanted in a subcutaneous infraclavicular, axillary, or abdominal pocket. Removal of an implantable defibrillator pulse generator requires opening of the existing subcutaneous pocket and disconnection of the pulse generator from its electrode(s). A thoracotomy (or laparotomy in the case of abdominally placed pulse generators) is not required to remove the pulse generator.

▶The electrodes (leads) of an implantable defibrillator system may be positioned within the atrial and/or ventricular chambers of the heart via the venous system (transvenously), or placed on the surface of the heart (epicardial), or positioned under the skin overlying the heart (subcutaneous). Electrode positioning on the epicardial surface of the heart requires a thoracotomy or thoracoscopic placement of the leads. Epicardial placement of electrode(s) may be separately reported using 33202, 33203. The electrode (lead) of a subcutaneous implantable defibrillator system is tunneled under the skin to the left parasternal margin. Subcutaneous placement of electrode may be reported using 33270 or 33271. The electrode (lead) of a substernal implantable defibrillator system is tunneled subcutaneously and placed into the substernal anterior mediastinum without entering the pericardial cavity and may be reported using 0571T, 0572T. In certain circumstances, an additional electrode may be required to achieve pacing of the left ventricle (bi-ventricular pacing). In this event, transvenous (cardiac vein) placement of the electrode may be separately reported using 33224 or 33225.◀

Rationale

In support of the establishment of new Category III codes 0571T, 0572T, 0573T, 0574T, 0575T, 0576T, 0577T, 0578T, 0579T, and 0580T to report implantable cardioverter-defibrillator system with substernal electrode, the introductory guidelines have been updated and parenthetical notes added in the Cardiovascular System/Heart and Pericardium/Pacemaker or Implantable Defibrillator subsection to provide guidance and direct users to the new codes.

Refer to the codebook and the Rationale for Category III codes 0571T-0580T for full discussion of these changes.

Removal of a transvenous electrode(s) may first be attempted by transvenous extraction (33234, 33235, or 33244). However, if transvenous extraction is unsuccessful, a thoracotomy may be required to remove the electrodes (33238 or 33243). Use 33212, 33213, 33221, 33230, 33231, 33240 as appropriate, in addition to the thoracotomy or endoscopic epicardial lead placement codes (33202 or 33203) to report the insertion of the generator if done by the same physician during the same session. Removal of a subcutaneous implantable defibrillator electrode may be separately reported using 33272. For removal of a leadless pacemaker system without replacement, use 33275. For removal and replacement of a leadless pacemaker system during the same session, use 33274.

When the "battery" of a pacemaker system with lead(s) or implantable defibrillator is changed, it is actually the pulse generator that is changed. Removal of only the pacemaker or implantable defibrillator pulse generator is reported with 33233 or 33241. If only a pulse generator is inserted or replaced without any right atrial and/or right ventricular lead(s) inserted or replaced, report the appropriate code for only pulse generator insertion or replacement based on the number of final existing lead(s) (33227, 33228, 33229 and 33262, 33263, 33264). Do not report removal of a pulse generator (33233 or 33241) separately for this service. Insertion of a new pulse generator, when existing lead(s) are already in place and when no prior pulse generator is removed, is reported with 33212, 33213, 33221, 33230, 33231, 33240. When a pulse generator insertion involves the insertion or replacement of one or more right atrial and/or right ventricular lead(s) or subcutaneous lead(s), use system codes 33206, 33207, 33208 for pacemaker, 33249 for implantable pacing cardioverter-defibrillator, or 33270 for subcutaneous implantable defibrillator. When reporting the system insertion or replacement codes, removal of a pulse generator (33233 or 33241) may be reported separately, when performed. In addition, extraction of leads 33234, 33235 or 33244 for transvenous or 33272 for subcutaneous may be reported separately, when performed. An exception involves a pacemaker upgrade from single to dual system that includes removal of pulse generator, replacement of new pulse generator, and insertion of new lead, reported with 33214.

Revision of a skin pocket is included in 33206-33249, 33262, 33263, 33264, 33270, 33271, 33272, 33273. When revision of a skin pocket involves incision and drainage of a hematoma or complex wound infection, see 10140, 10180, 11042, 11043, 11044, 11045, 11046, 11047, as appropriate.

Relocation of a skin pocket for a pacemaker (33222) or implantable defibrillator (33223) is necessary for various clinical situations such as infection or erosion. Relocation of an existing pulse generator may be performed as a stand-alone procedure or at the time of a pulse generator or electrode insertion, replacement, or repositioning. When skin pocket relocation is performed as part of an explant of an existing generator followed by replacement with a new generator, the pocket relocation is reported separately. Skin pocket relocation includes all work associated with the initial pocket (eg, opening the pocket, incision and drainage of hematoma or abscess if performed, and any closure performed), in addition to the creation of a new pocket for the new generator to be placed.

Repositioning of a pacemaker electrode, implantable defibrillator electrode(s), or a left ventricular pacing electrode is reported using 33215, 33226, or 33273, as appropriate.

▶Device evaluation codes 93260, 93261, 93279-93298 for pacemaker system with lead(s) may not be reported in conjunction with pulse generator and lead insertion or revision codes 33206-33249, 33262, 33263, 33264, 33270, 33271, 33272, 33273. For leadless pacemaker systems, device evaluation codes 93279, 93286, 93288, 93294, 93296 may not be reported in conjunction with leadless pacemaker insertion and removal codes 33274, 33275. Defibrillator threshold testing (DFT) during transvenous implantable defibrillator insertion or replacement may be separately reported using 93640, 93641. DFT testing during subcutaneous implantable defibrillator system insertion is not separately reportable. DFT testing for transvenous or subcutaneous implantable defibrillator in follow-up or at the time of replacement may be separately reported using 93642 or 93644.◀

Radiological supervision and interpretation related to the pacemaker or implantable defibrillator procedure is included in 33206-33249, 33262, 33263, 33264, 33270, 33271, 33272, 33273, 33274, 33275. Fluoroscopy (76000, 77002), ultrasound guidance for vascular access (76937), right ventriculography (93566), and femoral venography (75820) are included in 33274, 33275, when performed). To report fluoroscopic guidance for diagnostic lead evaluation without lead insertion, replacement, or revision procedures, use 76000.

Rationale

In support of the deletion of code 93299, a paragraph in the guidelines of the Pacemaker or Implantable Defibrillator subsection has been revised by replacing the deleted code with code 93298.

Refer to the codebook and the Rationale for code 93299 for a full discussion of these changes.

33241 Removal of implantable defibrillator pulse generator only

(Do not report 33241 in conjunction with 93260, 93261)

(Do not report 33241 in conjunction with 33230, 33231, 33240 for removal and replacement of the implantable defibrillator pulse generator. Use 33262, 33263, 33264, as appropriate, when pulse generator replacement is indicated)

(For removal and replacement of an implantable defibrillator pulse generator and electrode[s], use 33241 in conjunction with either 33243 or 33244 and 33249 for transvenous electrode[s] or 33270 and 33272 for subcutaneous electrode)

▶(For removal of implantable defibrillator with substernal lead, generator only, use 0580T)◀

 # 33270 Insertion or replacement of permanent subcutaneous implantable defibrillator system, with subcutaneous electrode, including defibrillation threshold evaluation, induction of arrhythmia, evaluation of sensing for arrhythmia termination, and programming or reprogramming of sensing or therapeutic parameters, when performed

(Do not report 33270 in conjunction with 33271, 93260, 93261, 93644)

(For removal and replacement of an implantable defibrillator pulse generator and subcutaneous electrode, use 33241 in conjunction with 33270 and 33272)

(For insertion of subcutaneous implantable defibrillator lead[s], use 33271)

▶(For insertion or replacement of permanent implantable defibrillator system with substernal electrode, use 0571T)◀

 # 33271 Insertion of subcutaneous implantable defibrillator electrode

(Do not report 33271 in conjunction with 33240, 33262, 33270, 93260, 93261)

(For insertion or replacement of a cardiac venous system lead, see 33224, 33225)

▶(For insertion of substernal defibrillator electrode, use 0572T)◀

 # 33272 Removal of subcutaneous implantable defibrillator electrode

▶(For removal of substernal defibrillator electrode, use 0573T)◀

 # 33273 Repositioning of previously implanted subcutaneous implantable defibrillator electrode

(Do not report 33272, 33273 in conjunction with 93260, 93261)

▶(For repositioning of substernal defibrillator electrode, use 0574T)◀

Rationale

In support of the establishment of new Category III codes 0571T, 0572T, 0573T, 0574T, 0575T, 0576T, 0577T, 0578T, 0579T, and 0580T to report implantable cardioverter-defibrillator system with substernal electrode, parenthetical notes have been added following codes 33241, 33270, 33271, 33272, and 33273 directing users to the new codes.

Refer to the codebook and the Rationale for Category III codes 0571T-0580T for full discussion of these changes.

 # 33274 Transcatheter insertion or replacement of permanent leadless pacemaker, right ventricular, including imaging guidance (eg, fluoroscopy, venous ultrasound, ventriculography, femoral venography) and device evaluation (eg, interrogation or programming), when performed

 # ▲ 33275 Transcatheter removal of permanent leadless pacemaker, right ventricular, including imaging guidance (eg, fluoroscopy, venous ultrasound, ventriculography, femoral venography), when performed

(Do not report 33275 in conjunction with 33274)

(Do not report 33274, 33275 in conjunction with femoral venography [75820], fluoroscopy [76000, 77002], ultrasound guidance for vascular access [76937], right ventriculography [93566])

(Do not report 33274, 33275 in conjunction with 93451, 93453, 93456, 93457, 93460, 93461, 93530, 93531, 93532, 93533, unless complete right heart catheterization is performed for indications distinct from the leadless pacemaker procedure)

(For subsequent leadless pacemaker device evaluation, see 93279, 93286, 93288, 93294, 93296)

(For insertion, replacement, repositioning, and removal of pacemaker systems with leads, see 33202, 33203, 33206, 33207, 33208, 33212, 33213, 33214, 33215, 33216, 33217, 33218, 33220, 33221, 33227, 33228, 33229, 33233, 33234, 33235, 33236, 33237)

Rationale

Code 33275 has been revised to include imaging guidance when performed. In 2019, codes 33274 and 33275 were established for reporting transcatheter insertion or replacement of leadless pacemaker (33274) and transcatheter removal of leadless pacemaker (33275). An exclusionary parenthetical note was added at the time instructing users not to report codes 33274 and 33275 with femoral venography (75820); fluoroscopy (76000, 77002); ultrasound guidance for vascular access (76937); or right ventriculography (93566). The descriptor of code 33274 included fluoroscopy, venous ultrasound, ventriculography, and femoral venography, when performed. For 2020, code 33275 has been revised to include this language to be consistent with code 33274 and the exclusionary parenthetical note following code 33275.

Electrophysiologic Operative Procedures

Incision

33255 Operative tissue ablation and reconstruction of atria, extensive (eg, maze procedure); without cardiopulmonary bypass

33256 with cardiopulmonary bypass

▶(Do not report 33254-33256 in conjunction with 32100, 32551, 33120, 33130, 33210, 33211, 33390, 33391, 33404-33507, 33510-33523, 33533-33548, 33600-33853, 33858, 33859, 33863, 33864, 33910-33920)◀

+ 33257 Operative tissue ablation and reconstruction of atria, performed at the time of other cardiac procedure(s), limited (eg, modified maze procedure) (List separately in addition to code for primary procedure)

▶(Use 33257 in conjunction with 33120-33130, 33250, 33251, 33261, 33300-33335, 33365, 33390, 33391, 33404-33417, 33420-33476, 33478, 33496, 33500-33507, 33510-33516, 33533-33548, 33600-33619, 33641-33697, 33702-33732, 33735-33767, 33770, 33877, 33910-33922, 33925, 33926, 33975, 33976, 33977, 33978, 33979, 33980, 33981, 33982, 33983)◀

+ 33258 Operative tissue ablation and reconstruction of atria, performed at the time of other cardiac procedure(s), extensive (eg, maze procedure), without cardiopulmonary bypass (List separately in addition to code for primary procedure)

▶(Use 33258 in conjunction with 33130, 33250, 33300, 33310, 33320, 33321, 33330, 33365, 33420, 33470, 33471, 33501-33503, 33510-33516, 33533-33536, 33690, 33735, 33737, 33750, 33755, 33762, 33764, 33766, 33800-33813, 33820, 33822, 33824, 33840, 33845, 33851, 33852, 33875, 33877, 33915, 33925, 33981, 33982, when the procedure is performed without cardiopulmonary bypass)◀

+ 33259 Operative tissue ablation and reconstruction of atria, performed at the time of other cardiac procedure(s), extensive (eg, maze procedure), with cardiopulmonary bypass (List separately in addition to code for primary procedure)

▶(Use 33259 in conjunction with 33120, 33251, 33261, 33305, 33315, 33322, 33335, 33390, 33391, 33404, 33405, 33406, 33410, 33411, 33412, 33413, 33414, 33415, 33416, 33417, 33422-33468, 33474, 33475, 33476, 33478, 33496, 33500, 33504-33507, 33510-33516, 33533-33548, 33600-33688, 33692-33726, 33730, 33732, 33736, 33767, 33770, 33783, 33786-33788, 33814, 33853, 33858-33877, 33910, 33916-33922, 33926, 33975-33980, 33983, when the procedure is performed with cardiopulmonary bypass)◀

(Do not report 33257, 33258 and 33259 in conjunction with 32551, 33210, 33211, 33254-33256, 33265, 33266)

Rationale

In support of the deletion of code 33860 (ascending aortic graft) and addition of codes 33858 and 33859, the exclusionary parenthetical note following code 33256 and the inclusionary parenthetical note following code 33259 have been revised to reflect these changes.

The parenthetical notes for add-on codes 33257, 33258, and 33259 (operative tissue ablation [Maze]) have been updated to reflect CPT codes that have been added and deleted from the code set over the past few years.

Refer to the codebook and the Rationale for codes 33858, 33859, and 33860 for a full discussion of these changes.

Subcutaneous Cardiac Rhythm Monitor

33285 Insertion, subcutaneous cardiac rhythm monitor, including programming

33286 Removal, subcutaneous cardiac rhythm monitor

▶(Initial insertion includes programming. For subsequent electronic analysis and/or reprogramming, see 93285, 93291, 93298)◀

Rationale

In accordance with the deletion of code 93299, the existing parenthetical note following code 33286 has been revised with the removal of this code.

Refer to the codebook and the Rationale for code 93299 for a full discussion of these changes.

Surgery   CPT Changes 2020

Cardiac Valves

Aortic Valve

33361 Transcatheter aortic valve replacement (TAVR/TAVI) with prosthetic valve; percutaneous femoral artery approach

33362   open femoral artery approach

33363   open axillary artery approach

33364   open iliac artery approach

33365   transaortic approach (eg, median sternotomy, mediastinotomy)

33366   transapical exposure (eg, left thoracotomy)

+ 33367   cardiopulmonary bypass support with percutaneous peripheral arterial and venous cannulation (eg, femoral vessels) (List separately in addition to code for primary procedure)

▶(Use 33367 in conjunction with 33361, 33362, 33363, 33364, 33365, 33366, 33418, 33477, 0483T, 0484T, 0544T, 0545T, 0569T, 0570T)◀

(Do not report 33367 in conjunction with 33368, 33369)

+ 33368   cardiopulmonary bypass support with open peripheral arterial and venous cannulation (eg, femoral, iliac, axillary vessels) (List separately in addition to code for primary procedure)

▶(Use 33368 in conjunction with 33361, 33362, 33363, 33364, 33365, 33366, 33418, 33477, 0483T, 0484T, 0544T, 0545T, 0569T, 0570T)◀

(Do not report 33368 in conjunction with 33367, 33369)

+ 33369   cardiopulmonary bypass support with central arterial and venous cannulation (eg, aorta, right atrium, pulmonary artery) (List separately in addition to code for primary procedure)

▶(Use 33369 in conjunction with 33361, 33362, 33363, 33364, 33365, 33366, 33418, 33477, 0483T, 0484T, 0544T, 0545T, 0569T, 0570T)◀

(Do not report 33369 in conjunction with 33367, 33368)

Rationale

In support of the establishment of Category III codes 0544T and 0545T (mitral and tricuspid valve annulus reconstruction) and 0569T and 0570T (tricuspid valve repair), the inclusionary parenthetical notes following codes 33367, 33368, and 33369 have been revised to include the new codes.

Refer to the codebook and the Rationale for codes 0544T, 0545T, 0569T, and 0570T for a full discussion of these changes.

Mitral Valve

33418 Transcatheter mitral valve repair, percutaneous approach, including transseptal puncture when performed; initial prosthesis

(Do not report 33418 in conjunction with 93462 unless transapical puncture is performed)

+ 33419   additional prosthesis(es) during same session (List separately in addition to code for primary procedure)

(Use 33419 in conjunction with 33418)

(For transcatheter mitral valve repair, percutaneous approach via the coronary sinus, use 0345T)

(For transcatheter mitral valve implantation/replacement [TMVI], see 0483T, 0484T)

▶(For transcatheter mitral valve annulus reconstruction, use 0544T)◀

Rationale

In support of the establishment of Category III code 0544T, a new parenthetical note has been added following code 33419 directing users to the appropriate code to report transcatheter mitral valve annulus reconstruction.

Refer to the codebook and the Rationale for codes 0544T and 0545T for a full discussion of these changes.

Tricuspid Valve

▶(For transcatheter tricuspid valve repair [TTVr], see 0569T, 0570T)◀

Rationale

In support of the establishment of Category III codes 0569T and 0570T (transcatheter tricuspid valve repair), a cross-reference parenthetical note directing users to the new codes has been added above code 33460.

Refer to the codebook and the Rationale for codes 0569T and 0570T for a full discussion of these changes.

33460 Valvectomy, tricuspid valve, with cardiopulmonary bypass

33468 Tricuspid valve repositioning and plication for Ebstein anomaly

▶(For transcatheter tricuspid valve annulus reconstruction, use 0545T)◀

Rationale

In support of the establishment of Category III code 0545T, a new parenthetical note has been added following code 33468 to direct users to the appropriate code to report transcatheter tricuspid valve annulus reconstruction.

Refer to the codebook and the Rationale for codes 0544T and 0545T for a full discussion of these changes.

Thoracic Aortic Aneurysm

▶When ascending aortic disease involves the aortic arch, an aortic hemiarch graft may be necessary in conjunction with the ascending aortic graft and may be reported with add-on code 33866 in conjunction with the appropriate ascending aortic graft code (33858, 33859, 33863, 33864). Aortic hemiarch graft requires all of the following components:

1. Either total circulatory arrest or isolated cerebral perfusion (retrograde or antegrade);
2. Incision into the transverse arch extending under one or more of the arch vessels (eg, innominate, left common carotid, or left subclavian arteries); and
3. Extension of the ascending aortic graft under the aortic arch by construction of a beveled anastomosis to the distal ascending aorta and aortic arch without a cross-clamp (an open anastomosis).

An ascending aortic repair with a beveled anastomosis into the arch with a cross-clamp cannot be reported separately as a hemiarch graft using 33866. Use 33866 for aortic hemiarch graft when performed in conjunction with the ascending aortic graft codes 33858, 33859, 33863, 33864. Code 33871 describes a complete transverse arch graft placement, and is not used to report an aortic hemiarch graft procedure.◀

● **33858** Ascending aorta graft, with cardiopulmonary bypass, includes valve suspension, when performed; for aortic dissection

● **33859** for aortic disease other than dissection (eg, aneurysm)

▶(33860 has been deleted. To report, see 33858, 33859)◀

33863 Ascending aorta graft, with cardiopulmonary bypass, with aortic root replacement using valved conduit and coronary reconstruction (eg, Bentall)

▶(Do not report 33863 in conjunction with 33405, 33406, 33410, 33411, 33412, 33413, 33858, 33859)◀

33864 Ascending aorta graft, with cardiopulmonary bypass with valve suspension, with coronary reconstruction and valve-sparing aortic root remodeling (eg, David Procedure, Yacoub Procedure)

▶(Do not report 33864 in conjunction with 33858, 33859, 33863)◀

+ **33866** Aortic hemiarch graft including isolation and control of the arch vessels, beveled open distal aortic anastomosis extending under one or more of the arch vessels, and total circulatory arrest or isolated cerebral perfusion (List separately in addition to code for primary procedure)

▶(Use 33866 for aortic hemiarch graft performed in conjunction with ascending aortic graft [33858, 33859, 33863, 33864])◀

▶(Do not report 33866 in conjunction with 33871)◀

▶(33870 has been deleted. To report, use 33871)◀

● **33871** Transverse aortic arch graft, with cardiopulmonary bypass, with profound hypothermia, total circulatory arrest and isolated cerebral perfusion with reimplantation of arch vessel(s) (eg, island pedicle or individual arch vessel reimplantation)

▶(Do not report 33871 for aortic hemiarch graft)◀

▶(Do not report 33871 in conjunction with 33866)◀

▶(For aortic hemiarch graft performed in conjunction with ascending aortic graft [33858, 33859, 33863, 33864], use 33866)◀

Rationale

Code 33860, *Ascending aorta graft, with cardiopulmonary bypass, includes valve suspension, when performed*, has been deleted, and two new codes (33858 and 33859) have been established for this procedure. The new codes distinguish use of a graft for aortic dissection (33858) and for aortic disease other than dissection (33859). Like code 33860, codes 33858 and 33859 include valve suspension, when performed, and cardiopulmonary bypass. Code 33870, *Transverse arch graft, with cardiopulmonary bypass*, has been deleted, and code 33871 has been created to report this procedure with cardiopulmonary bypass, profound hypothermia, total circulatory arrest, and isolated cerebral perfusion with reimplantation of arch vessel(s). The thoracic aortic aneurysm guidelines have been revised and several parenthetical notes have been revised and added to provide instructions on the correct reporting of these codes.

Repair of aortic aneurysm using an ascending aortic graft (33859) involves resecting the aneurysm and suturing the graft to healthy aortic tissue proximally and distally. In the case of aortic dissection (33858), the remaining proximal and/or distal tissue may still be thin and lack sufficient tensile strength, such that a buttressing material (eg, using a circumferential felt strip) is added to the suture lines to reinforce the proximal and/or distal anastomoses.

> Code 33870 (transverse arch graft) has been deleted instead of being revised because the original concept of the code has changed extensively. The concept of permanence principle was applied, and a new code, 33871, has been added to describe where the arch vessels are reimplanted into the graft and clarifies the distinction between this procedure and the hemiarch graft procedure described by add-on code 33866. Code 33866 describes repair of a portion of the aortic arch and may only be performed in conjunction with other ascending aortic graft procedures. Repair of the entire transverse aortic arch is described in code 33871. Cardiopulmonary bypass with profound hypothermia, total circulatory arrest, and isolated cerebral perfusion with reimplantation of arch vessel(s) are included in code 33871. When an ascending aortic aneurysm or dissection extends into the aortic arch, it may be necessary to repair the entire transverse aortic arch in addition to the ascending aortic repair. In this case, the transverse arch grafting code (33871) would be reported in addition to the appropriate ascending aortic repair code (33858-33864).

Clinical Example (33858)

A 62-year-old male presents to the emergency room (ER) with severe tearing pain in the chest. Transesophageal echocardiogram confirms an aortic dissection, and the patient is taken to the OR for ascending aortic graft repair.

Description of Procedure (33858)

Following a standard median sternotomy incision, divide the sternum with a saw. Determine which artery to use for arterial access while on cardiopulmonary bypass following median sternotomy and exposure of the heart and great vessels. This may require exposure and use of the aortic arch, innominate artery, subclavian artery, brachial artery, or even femoral artery, depending on the extent of the dissection and the condition of the ascending aorta. If necessary, anastomose an 8-mm graft to a peripheral artery to facilitate cardiopulmonary bypass (reported separately). Place a venous cannula directly into the right atrium. Heparinize the patient and initiate cardiopulmonary bypass with immediate systemic cooling. Because the ascending aorta is dissected to a variable and unpredictable degree, use of a standard antegrade cannula for cardioplegia solution delivery is not possible. Insert a retrograde cardioplegia cannula into the coronary sinus to administer cardioplegia and induce cardiac arrest. Continually assess the heart for distention, myocardial cooling, and sustained cardioplegic arrest. Cross-clamp the aorta just below the innominate artery. Arrest the heart with retrograde cardioplegia. Transect the dissected aorta.

Identify the two coronary ostia. Direct cannulation allows for delivery of additional cardioplegia in antegrade fashion as necessary. Determine the location and complete extent of the aortic intimal entry tear and include in the resection specimen. Following resection of the ascending aorta, size the remaining aorta for an appropriate tube graft. Assess the integrity of the aortic valve and, if necessary, resuspend the valve within the proximal ascending aorta. Reinforce the cut end of the proximal ascending aorta with a circumferential felt strip. Suture the tube graft to this reinforced proximal aorta with a running 5-0 polypropylene stitch. Measure the tube graft to length distally and suture to the distal aorta below the aortic cross-clamp using running 5-0 polypropylene stitch. In some cases, reinforce the distal suture line with felt before performing the anastomosis. In some cases the distal anastomosis may not be possible with the cross-clamp in place due to the extent of dissection and/or quality of the aortic tissue. In these situations, cool the patient to a nasopharyngeal or bladder temperature to the range of 15° to 20°C. Once the patient is cooled to the desired temperature, turn the cardiopulmonary bypass machine circuit off and interrupt circulation to the entire body. Retrograde and/or antegrade cerebral perfusion is established in some cases. Upon achieving total circulatory arrest, remove any cross-clamp, if present, allowing unobstructed view of the intimal integrity of the ascending aorta and transverse arch within a bloodless aorta. Confirm and resect the entire extent of the entry aortic tear. Cut the aorta and prepare with felt reinforcement before performing the distal anastomosis to the tube graft. Start rewarming the patient during this anastomosis. Upon completion of the distal aortic anastomosis, place the patient in the Trendelenburg position. Evacuate air from the graft as cardiopulmonary bypass is slowly re-established. Once full cardiopulmonary bypass is re-established, re-apply an aortic cross-clamp to the prosthetic graft, and re-administer antegrade or retrograde cardioplegia as needed during the rewarming period. When the patient has been rewarmed to an acceptable temperature, remove the cross-clamp, discontinue cardioplegia, and allow the heart to resume normal electrical activity. Vent the aortic root until left ventricle (LV) ejection has been present for 5 to 10 minutes. Use transesophageal echocardiogram to confirm air evaluation from the left side of heart, as well as from the tube graft, and to assess for any aortic valve insufficiency (reported separately). Accomplish continued resuscitation of the heart by allowing it to beat while unloaded on cardiopulmonary bypass. Establishing meticulous hemostasis is critical because patients are most often profoundly coagulopathic following profound hypothermia and total circulatory arrest. Place temporary pacing wires and initiate electrical pacing if necessary. Carefully wean the patient from cardiopulmonary bypass. Remove arterial, venous, and cardioplegia cannulas and secure or repair cannulation sites. Place chest tubes, and re-approximate the sternum. Close the sternal wound.

Clinical Example (33859)

A 60-year-old male is followed with serial echocardiograms looking for increasing aortic dimensions. Echocardiogram shows a 5.5-cm ascending aorta that has increased in size by 1 cm in one year. The patient is referred for surgical repair.

Description of Procedure (33859)

Perform standard median sternotomy skin incision, divide the sternum in the midline with a saw, and place arterial cardiopulmonary bypass cannula above the aneurysmal portion of the aorta. Place a venous cannula directly into the right atrium. Assess ascending aorta. Administer heparin and determine level of heparinization, establish cardiopulmonary bypass, initiate systemic cooling, and place antegrade and retrograde cardioplegia cannulas. Cross-clamp the aorta just below the innominate artery. Arrest the heart with antegrade and retrograde cardioplegia and assess heart for distention, cooling, and efficacy of cardioplegic arrest. Transect the aorta where the ascending aortic dilatation begins, most commonly at the sinotubular junction. Size the cut end of the aorta for the appropriate tube graft. Suture the tube graft to the proximal aorta with a running 5-0 polypropylene stitch. Measure the tube graft to length distally and suture to the distal ascending aorta below the aortic cross-clamp using running 5-0 polypropylene stitch, thereby excluding the entire aneurysmal portion of the ascending aorta. Place the patient in the Trendelenburg position. Evacuate air from the LV and ascending tube graft. Remove the cross-clamp and vent the aortic root until LV ejection has been present for 5 to 10 minutes. Use transesophageal echocardiography (TEE) to confirm and evaluate air in left side of heart and to assess for any aortic valve insufficiency using TEE (reported separately). Resuscitate the heart by allowing it to beat while unloaded on cardiopulmonary bypass. Ensure hemostasis, place temporary pacing wires, and begin pacing if necessary. Discontinue cardiopulmonary bypass, remove cannulas, and repair cannulation sites. Ensure hemostasis, place chest tubes, re-approximate the sternum, and close chest wound.

Clinical Example (33871)

Upon routine CXR, a 60-year-old male is found to have an enlarged aortic arch with an aortic aneurysm and is referred for additional workup. Echocardiogram, CT, magnetic resonance imaging (MRI), and angiogram are obtained. Although the patient is asymptomatic, the findings show that the aneurysm involves the entire aortic arch. The patient is scheduled for a transverse aortic arch graft placement.

Description of Procedure (33871)

Perform standard median sternotomy skin incision, and divide the sternum in the midline with a saw. Determine which artery will be used for arterial access while on cardiopulmonary bypass following median sternotomy and exposure of the heart and great vessels. This may require exposure and use of the innominate artery, right subclavian artery, brachial artery, or even femoral artery. If necessary, anastomose an 8-mm graft to a peripheral artery to facilitate cardiopulmonary bypass (reported separately). Insert a venous cannula. Dissect free the entire transverse arch, including the innominate artery, left carotid artery, and left subclavian artery, and isolate with vascular tapes. Identify and protect the recurrent laryngeal nerve as it crosses under the distal aortic arch. Heparinize the patient systemically and determine the level of heparinization. Establish cardiopulmonary bypass and initiate systemic cooling to establish deep hypothermia. Establish retrograde and/or antegrade cerebral perfusion with appropriate cannulae for delivery of cardioplegia when appropriate. Apply an aortic cross-clamp to the ascending aorta and transect the aorta above the cross-clamp. Anastomose an appropriately sized tube graft to the cut end of the ascending aorta. Once the patient is cooled to the desired temperature, turn off the cardiopulmonary bypass machine circuit and interrupt circulation to the entire body. Transect the arch vessels at the base, open and resect the transverse arch. Anastomose an appropriately sized tubular arch graft to the cut end of the proximal descending aorta. The remaining arch vessels (innominate artery, left carotid artery, and left subclavian artery) may be individually anastomosed to the arch tube graft, or the three arch vessels can be left attached to a remnant of the resected arch (configured as an island), which is then anastomosed to the newly constructed arch tube graft. Start a prolonged period of systemic warming as the anastomoses are being completed. This includes the final graft-to-graft (ascending aortic graft and transverse arch graft) anastomosis. As the patient approaches normothermia and bleeding has been sufficiently controlled, place the patient in Trendelenburg position and re-establish cardiopulmonary bypass slowly in order to evacuate air from the ascending aortic and transverse arch grafts. Vent the aortic root until LV ejection has been present for 5 to 10 minutes. Assess residual air (if any) in the left side of heart as well as myocardial contractility using transesophageal echocardiogram (reported separately). Resuscitate the heart by allowing it to beat while unloaded on cardiopulmonary bypass. Establishing meticulous hemostasis is critical because the patients are most often profoundly coagulopathic following profound hypothermia and total circulatory arrest. Place temporary pacing wires and initiate electrical pacing if necessary. Carefully wean the patient from cardiopulmonary bypass. Remove arterial, venous, and cardioplegia cannulas and secure or repair cannulation sites. Place chest tubes and re-approximate the sternum. Close the sternal wound.

Arteries and Veins

Endovascular Repair of Abdominal Aorta and/or Iliac Arteries

Codes 34701, 34702, 34703, 34704, 34705, 34706 describe introduction, positioning, and deployment of an endograft for treatment of abdominal aortic pathology (with or without rupture), such as aneurysm, pseudoaneurysm, dissection, penetrating ulcer, or traumatic disruption in the infrarenal abdominal aorta with or without extension into the iliac artery(ies). The terms, endovascular graft, endoprosthesis, endograft, and stentgraft, refer to a covered stent. The infrarenal aortic endograft may be an aortic tube device, a bifurcated unibody device, a modular bifurcated docking system with docking limb(s), or an aorto-uni-iliac device. Codes 34707 and 34708 describe introduction, positioning, and deployment of an ilio-iliac endograft for treatment of isolated arterial pathology (with or without rupture), such as aneurysm, pseudoaneurysm, arteriovenous malformation, or trauma involving the iliac artery. For treatment of atherosclerotic occlusive disease in the iliac artery(ies) with a covered stent(s), see 37221, 37223. For covered stent placement for atherosclerotic occlusive disease in the aorta, see 37236, 37237.

▶Add-on code 34717 is reported at the time of aorto-iliac artery endograft placement (34703, 34704, 34705, 34706) for deployment of a bifurcated endograft in the common iliac artery with extension(s) into both the internal iliac and external iliac arteries, when performed, to maintain perfusion in both vessels for treatment of iliac artery pathology (with or without rupture), such as aneurysm, pseudoaneurysm, dissection, penetrating ulcer, arteriovenous malformation, or traumatic disruption. The iliac branched endograft is a multi-piece system consisting of a bifurcated device that is placed in the common iliac artery and then additional extension(s) are placed into both the internal iliac artery and external iliac/common femoral arteries as needed, as well as a proximal extension that overlaps with an aorto-iliac endograft, when performed. All additional extensions proximally into the common iliac artery or distally into the external iliac and/or common femoral arteries are inherent to these codes.

Report 34705 or 34706 for simultaneous bilateral iliac artery aneurysm repairs with aorto-bi-iliac endograft. For isolated bilateral iliac artery repair using iliac artery tube endografts, report 34707 or 34708 with modifier 50 appended.◀

Decompressive laparotomy for abdominal compartment syndrome after ruptured abdominal aortic and/or iliac artery aneurysm repair may be separately reported with 49000 in addition to 34702, 34704, 34706, or 34708.

▶The treatment zone for endograft procedures is defined by those vessels that contain an endograft(s) (main body, docking limb[s], and/or extension[s]) deployed during that operative session. Adjunctive procedures outside the treatment zone may be separately reported (eg, angioplasty, endovascular stent placement, embolization). For example, when an endograft terminates in the common iliac artery, any additional treatment performed in the external and/or internal iliac artery may be separately reportable. Placement of a docking limb is inherent to a modular endograft(s), and, therefore, 34709 may not be reported separately if the docking limb extends into the external iliac artery. In addition, any interventions (eg, angioplasty, stenting, additional stent graft extension[s]) in the external iliac artery where the docking limb terminates may not be reported separately. Any catheterization or treatment of the internal iliac artery, such as embolization, may be separately reported. For 34701 and 34702, the abdominal aortic treatment zone is defined as the infrarenal aorta. For 34703 and 34704, the abdominal aortic treatment zone is typically defined as the infrarenal aorta and ipsilateral common iliac artery. For 34705 and 34706, the abdominal aortic treatment zone is typically defined as the infrarenal aorta and both common iliac arteries. For 34707, 34708, 34717, 34718, the treatment zone is defined as the portion of the iliac artery(ies) (eg, common, internal, external iliac arteries) that contains the endograft.◀

Codes 34702, 34704, 34706, 34708 are reported when endovascular repair is performed on ruptured aneurysm in the aorta or iliac artery(ies). Rupture is defined as clinical and/or radiographic evidence of acute hemorrhage for purposes of reporting these codes. A chronic, contained rupture is considered a pseudoaneurysm, and endovascular treatment of a chronic, contained rupture is reported with 34701, 34703, 34705, or 34707.

Code 34709 is reported for placement of extension prosthesis(es) that terminate(s) either in the internal iliac, external iliac, or common femoral artery(ies) or in the abdominal aorta proximal to the renal artery(ies) in conjunction with 34701, 34702, 34703, 34704, 34705, 34706, 34707, 34708. Code 34709 may only be reported once per vessel treated (ie, multiple endograft extensions placed in a single vessel may only be reported once). Endograft extension(s) that terminate(s) in the common iliac arteries are included in 34703, 34704, 34705,

34706, 34707, 34708 and are not separately reported. Treatment zone angioplasty/stenting, when performed, is included in 34709. In addition, proximal infrarenal abdominal aortic extension prosthesis(es) that terminate(s) in the aorta below the renal artery(ies) are also included in 34701, 34702, 34703, 34704, 34705, 34706 and are not separately reportable.

Codes 34710, 34711 are reported for delayed placement of distal or proximal extension prosthesis(es) for endovascular repair of infrarenal abdominal aortic or iliac aneurysm, false aneurysm, dissection, endoleak, or endograft migration. Pre-procedure sizing and device selection, all nonselective catheterization(s), all associated radiological supervision and interpretation, and treatment zone angioplasty/stenting, when performed, are included in 34710 and 34711. Codes 34710 and 34711 may only be reported once per vessel treated (ie, multiple endograft extensions placed in a single vessel may only be reported once).

▶If an aorto-iliac artery endograft (34703, 34704, 34705, 34706) is not being placed during the same operative session, 34718 may be reported for placement of a bifurcated endograft in the common iliac artery with extension(s) into both the internal iliac and external iliac arteries, to maintain perfusion in both vessels for treatment of iliac artery pathology (without rupture), such as aneurysm, pseudoaneurysm, dissection, arteriovenous malformation. The iliac branched endograft is a multi-piece system consisting of a bifurcated device that is placed in the common iliac artery and then additional extension(s) are placed into both the internal iliac artery and external iliac/common femoral arteries as needed as well as a proximal extension that overlaps with an aorto-iliac endograft, when performed. All additional extensions placed proximally into the common iliac artery or distally into the external iliac and/or common femoral arteries are inherent to these codes. For isolated bilateral iliac artery repair using iliac artery branched endografts, use 34718 with modifier 50 appended.

Codes 34709, 34710, 34711 may not be separately reported with 34717, 34718 for ipsilateral extension prosthesis(es). However, 34709, 34710, 34711 may be reported separately for extension prosthesis(es) in the iliac/femoral arteries contralateral to the iliac branched endograft.◀

Nonselective catheterization is included in 34701, 34702, 34703, 34704, 34705, 34706, 34707, 34708 and is not separately reported. However, selective catheterization of the hypogastric artery(ies), renal artery(ies), and/or arterial families outside the treatment zone of the endograft may be separately reported. Intravascular ultrasound (37252, 37253) performed during endovascular aneurysm repair may be separately reported. Balloon angioplasty and/or stenting within the treatment zone of the endograft, either before or after endograft deployment, is not separately reported. Fluoroscopic guidance and radiological supervision and interpretation in conjunction with endograft repair is not separately reported, and includes all intraprocedural imaging (eg, angiography, rotational CT) of the aorta and its branches prior to deployment of the endovascular device, fluoroscopic guidance and roadmapping used in the delivery of the endovascular components, and intraprocedural and completion angiography (eg, confirm position, detect endoleak, evaluate runoff) performed at the time of the endovascular infrarenal aorta and/or iliac repair.

▶Selective arterial catheterization of the internal and external iliac arteries (eg, 36245, 36246, 36247, 36248) ipsilateral to an iliac branched endograft is included in 34717, 34718 and not separately reported. However, selective catheterization of the renal artery(ies), the contralateral hypogastric artery, and/or arterial families outside the treatment zone of the graft may be separately reported. Intravascular ultrasound (37252, 37253) performed during endovascular aneurysm repair may be separately reported. Balloon angioplasty within the target treatment zone of the endograft, either before or after endograft deployment, is not separately reported. Fluoroscopic guidance and radiological supervision and interpretation performed in conjunction with endovascular iliac branched repair is not separately reported. Endovascular iliac branched repair includes all intraprocedural imaging (eg, angiography, rotational CT) of the aorta and its branches prior to deployment of the endovascular device, fluoroscopic guidance in the delivery of the endovascular components, and intraprocedural arterial angiography (eg, confirm position, detect endoleak, evaluate runoff) performed at the time of the endovascular aorto-iliac repair).◀

Codes 34709, 34710, 34711 include nonselective introduction of guidewires and catheters into the treatment zone from peripheral artery access(es). However, selective catheterization of the hypogastric artery(ies), renal artery(ies), and/or arterial families outside the treatment zone may be separately reported. Codes 34709, 34710, 34711 also include balloon angioplasty and/or stenting within the treatment zone of the endograft extension, either before or after deployment of the endograft, fluoroscopic guidance, and all associated radiological supervision and interpretation performed in conjunction with endovascular endograft extension (eg, angiographic diagnostic imaging of the aorta and its branches prior to deployment of the endovascular device, fluoroscopic guidance in the delivery of the endovascular components, and intraprocedural and completion angiography to confirm endograft position, detect endoleak, and evaluate runoff).

Code 34712 describes transcatheter delivery of accessory-enhanced fixation devices to the endograft (eg, anchor, screw, tack), including all associated radiological supervision and interpretation. Code 34712 may only be reported once per operative session.

Vascular access requiring use of closure devices for large sheaths (ie, 12 French or larger) or access requiring open surgical arterial exposure may be separately reported (eg, 34713, 34714, 34715, 34716, 34812, 34820, 34833, 34834). Code 34713 describes percutaneous access and closure of a femoral arteriotomy for delivery of endovascular prosthesis through a large arterial sheath (ie, 12 French or larger). Ultrasound guidance (ie, 76937), when performed, is included in 34713. (Percutaneous access using a sheath smaller than 12 French is included in 34701-34712 and is not separately reported.)

Code 34812 describes open repair and closure of the femoral artery. Extensive repair of an artery (eg, 35226, 35286, 35371) may also be reported separately. Iliac exposure for device delivery through a retroperitoneal incision, open brachial exposure, or axillary or subclavian exposure through an infraclavicular, or supraclavicular or sternotomy incision during endovascular aneurysm repair may be separately reported (eg, 34715, 34812, 34820, 34834). Endovascular device delivery or establishment of cardiopulmonary bypass that requires creation of a prosthetic conduit utilizing a femoral artery, iliac artery with a retroperitoneal incision, or axillary or subclavian artery exposure through an infraclavicular, supraclavicular, or sternotomy incision (34714, 34716, 34833) and oversewing of the conduit at the time of procedure completion may be separately reported during endovascular aneurysm repair or cardiac procedures requiring cardiopulmonary bypass. If a conduit is converted to a bypass, report the bypass (eg, 35665) and not the arterial exposure with conduit (34714, 34716, 34833). Arterial embolization(s) of renal, lumbar, inferior mesenteric, hypogastric or external iliac arteries to facilitate complete endovascular aneurysm exclusion may be separately reported (eg, 37242).

Balloon angioplasty and/or stenting at the sealing zone(s) of an endograft is an integral part of the procedure and is not separately reported. However, balloon angioplasty and/or stent deployment in vessels that do not contain endograft (outside the treatment zone for the endograft), either before or after endograft deployment, may be separately reported (eg, 37220, 37221, 37222, 37223).

Other interventional procedures performed at the time of endovascular abdominal aortic aneurysm repair may be additionally reported (eg, renal transluminal angioplasty, arterial embolization, intravascular ultrasound, balloon angioplasty or stenting of native artery[s] outside the endograft treatment zone, when done before or after deployment of endograft).

(For fenestrated endovascular repair of the visceral aorta, see 34841-34844. For fenestrated endovascular repair of the visceral aorta and concomitant infrarenal abdominal aorta, see 34845-34848)

34707 Endovascular repair of iliac artery by deployment of an ilio-iliac tube endograft including pre-procedure sizing and device selection, all nonselective catheterization(s), all associated radiological supervision and interpretation, and all endograft extension(s) proximally to the aortic bifurcation and distally to the iliac bifurcation, and treatment zone angioplasty/stenting, when performed, unilateral; for other than rupture (eg, for aneurysm, pseudoaneurysm, dissection, arteriovenous malformation)

(For covered stent placement[s] for atherosclerotic occlusive disease of the abdominal aorta, see 37236, 37237)

(For covered stent placement[s] for atherosclerotic occlusive disease of the iliac artery, see 37221, 37223)

34708   for rupture including temporary aortic and/or iliac balloon occlusion, when performed (eg, for aneurysm, pseudoaneurysm, dissection, arteriovenous malformation, traumatic disruption)

▶(For endovascular repair of iliac artery by deployment of an iliac branched endograft, see 34717, 34718)◄

#+● 34717 Endovascular repair of iliac artery at the time of aorto-iliac artery endograft placement by deployment of an iliac branched endograft including pre-procedure sizing and device selection, all ipsilateral selective iliac artery catheterization(s), all associated radiological supervision and interpretation, and all endograft extension(s) proximally to the aortic bifurcation and distally in the internal iliac, external iliac, and common femoral artery(ies), and treatment zone angioplasty/stenting, when performed, for rupture or other than rupture (eg, for aneurysm, pseudoaneurysm, dissection, arteriovenous malformation, penetrating ulcer, traumatic disruption), unilateral (List separately in addition to code for primary procedure)

▶(Use 34717 in conjunction with 34703, 34704, 34705, 34706)◄

▶(34717 may only be reported once per side. For bilateral procedure, report 34717 twice. Do not report modifier 50 in conjunction with 34717)◄

▶(Do not report 34717 in conjunction with 34709 on the same side)◄

▶(Do not report 34717 in conjunction with 34710, 34711)◄

▶(For placement of an iliac branched endograft at a separate setting than aorto-iliac endograft placement, use 34718)◄

Endovascular Repair
34717, 34718

A. Placement of iliac branch endoprosthesis (IBE) associated with placement of aorto-bi-iliac artery endoprosthesis (same session)

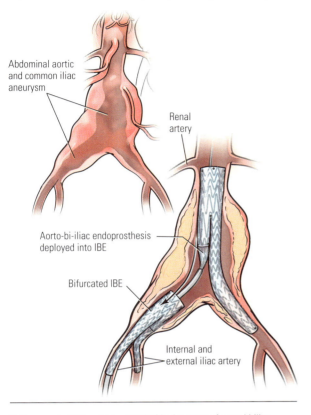

B. Placement of IBE, not associated with placement of aorto-bi-iliac endoprosthesis (different session)

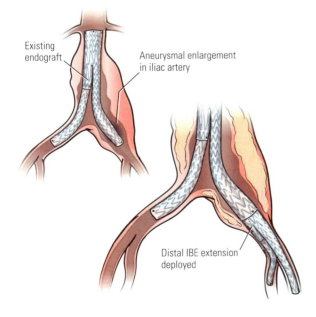

+ 34709 Placement of extension prosthesis(es) distal to the common iliac artery(ies) or proximal to the renal artery(ies) for endovascular repair of infrarenal abdominal aortic or iliac aneurysm, false aneurysm, dissection, penetrating ulcer, including pre-procedure sizing and device selection, all nonselective catheterization(s), all associated radiological supervision and interpretation, and treatment zone angioplasty/stenting, when performed, per vessel treated (List separately in addition to code for primary procedure)

(Use 34709 in conjunction with 34701, 34702, 34703, 34704, 34705, 34706, 34707, 34708)

(34709 may only be reported once per vessel treated [ie, multiple endograft extensions placed in a single vessel may only be reported once])

(Do not report 34709 for placement of a docking limb that extends into the external iliac artery)

▶(For placement of an iliac branched endograft, see 34717, 34718)◀

(For endograft placement into a renal artery that is being covered by a proximal extension, see 37236, 37237)

\# ● 34718 Endovascular repair of iliac artery, not associated with placement of an aorto-iliac artery endograft at the same session, by deployment of an iliac branched endograft, including pre-procedure sizing and device selection, all ipsilateral selective iliac artery catheterization(s), all associated radiological supervision and interpretation, and all endograft extension(s) proximally to the aortic bifurcation and distally in the internal iliac, external iliac, and common femoral artery(ies), and treatment zone angioplasty/stenting, when performed, for other than rupture (eg, for aneurysm, pseudoaneurysm, dissection, arteriovenous malformation, penetrating ulcer), unilateral

▶(For bilateral placement of an iliac branched endograft, report modifier 50)◀

▶(Do not report 34718 in conjunction with 34701, 34702, 34703, 34704, 34705, 34706, 34707, 34708, 34709, 34717)◀

▶(Do not report 34718 in conjunction with 34710, 34711 on the same side)◀

▶(For placement of an iliac branched endograft in the same setting as aorto-iliac endograft placement, use 34717)◀

▶(For placement of an isolated iliac branched endograft for rupture, use 37799)◀

34710 Delayed placement of distal or proximal extension prosthesis for endovascular repair of infrarenal abdominal aortic or iliac aneurysm, false aneurysm, dissection, endoleak, or endograft migration, including pre-procedure sizing and device selection, all nonselective catheterization(s), all associated radiological supervision and interpretation, and treatment zone angioplasty/stenting, when performed; initial vessel treated

+ **34711** each additional vessel treated (List separately in addition to code for primary procedure)

(Use 34711 in conjunction with 34710)

(34710, 34711 may each be reported only once per operative session [ie, multiple endograft extensions placed in a single vessel may only be reported with a single code])

(For decompressive laparotomy, use 49000 in conjunction with 34702, 34704, 34706, 34708, 34710)

(If the delayed revision is a transcatheter enhanced fixation device [eg, anchors, screws], report 34712)

(Do not report 34710, 34711 in conjunction with 34701, 34702, 34703, 34704, 34705, 34706, 34707, 34708, 34709)

▶(Do not report 34710, 34711 in conjunction with 34718 on the same side)◀

(Do not report 34701-34711 in conjunction with 34841, 34842, 34843, 34844, 34845, 34846, 34847, 34848)

▶(For endovascular repair of iliac artery bifurcation [eg, aneurysm, pseudoaneurysm, arteriovenous malformation, trauma] using bifurcated endograft, see 34717, 34718)◀

(Report 37252, 37253 for intravascular ultrasound when performed during endovascular aneurysm repair)

▶(For isolated bilateral iliac artery repair using iliac artery tube endografts, report 34707 or 34708 with modifier 50)◀

▶(For open arterial exposure, report 34714, 34715, 34716, 34812, 34820, 34833, 34834 as appropriate, in conjunction with 34701, 34702, 34703, 34704, 34705, 34706, 34707, 34708, 34710, 34712, 34718)◀

▶(For percutaneous arterial closure, report 34713 as appropriate, in conjunction with 34701, 34702, 34703, 34704, 34705, 34706, 34707, 34708, 34710, 34712, 34718)◀

(For simultaneous bilateral iliac artery aneurysm repairs with aorto-biiliac endograft, see 34705, 34706, as appropriate)

34712 Transcatheter delivery of enhanced fixation device(s) to the endograft (eg, anchor, screw, tack) and all associated radiological supervision and interpretation

(Report 34712 only once per operative session)

+ **34713** Percutaneous access and closure of femoral artery for delivery of endograft through a large sheath (12 French or larger), including ultrasound guidance, when performed, unilateral (List separately in addition to code for primary procedure)

▶(Use 34713 in conjunction with 33880, 33881, 33883, 33884, 33886, 34701, 34702, 34703, 34704, 34705, 34706, 34707, 34708, 34710, 34712, 34718, 34841, 34842, 34843, 34844, 34845, 34846, 34847, 34848, as appropriate. Do not report 34713 in conjunction with 33880, 33881, 33883, 33884, 33886, 34701, 34702, 34703, 34704, 34705, 34706, 34707, 34708, 34710, 34712, 34718, 34841, 34842, 34843, 34844, 34845, 34846, 34847, 34848, for percutaneous closure of femoral artery after delivery of endovascular prosthesis if a sheath smaller than 12 French was used)◀

▶(34713 may only be reported once per side. For bilateral procedure, report 34713 twice. Do not report modifier 50 in conjunction with 34713)◀

(Do not report ultrasound guidance [ie, 76937] for percutaneous vascular access in conjunction with 34713 for the same access)

(Do not report 34713 for percutaneous access and closure of the femoral artery in conjunction with 37221, 37223, 37236, 37237)

(Do not report 34713 in conjunction with 37221, 37223 for covered stent placement[s] for atherosclerotic occlusive disease of the iliac artery[ies])

#+ **34812** Open femoral artery exposure for delivery of endovascular prosthesis, by groin incision, unilateral (List separately in addition to code for primary procedure)

▶(Use 34812 in conjunction with 33880, 33881, 33883, 33884, 33886, 33990, 33991, 34701, 34702, 34703, 34704, 34705, 34706, 34707, 34708, 34710, 34712, 34718, 34841, 34842, 34843, 34844, 34845, 34846, 34847, 34848)◀

▶(34812 may only be reported once per side. For bilateral procedure, report 34812 twice. Do not report modifier 50 in conjunction with 34812)◀

(Do not report 34812 in conjunction with 33953, 33954, 33959, 33962, 33969, 33984, 33987)

+ 34714 Open femoral artery exposure with creation of conduit for delivery of endovascular prosthesis or for establishment of cardiopulmonary bypass, by groin incision, unilateral (List separately in addition to code for primary procedure)

▶(Use 34714 in conjunction with 32852, 32854, 33031, 33120, 33251, 33256, 33259, 33261, 33305, 33315, 33322, 33335, 33390, 33391, 33404, 33405, 33406, 33410, 33411, 33412, 33413, 33414, 33415, 33416, 33417, 33422, 33425, 33426, 33427, 33430, 33440, 33460, 33463, 33464, 33465, 33468, 33474, 33475, 33476, 33478, 33496, 33500, 33502, 33504, 33505, 33506, 33507, 33510, 33511, 33512, 33513, 33514, 33516, 33533, 33534, 33535, 33536, 33542, 33545, 33548, 33600-33688, 33692, 33694, 33697, 33702, 33710, 33720, 33722, 33724, 33726, 33730, 33732, 33736, 33750, 33755, 33762, 33764, 33766, 33767, 33770-33783, 33786, 33788, 33802, 33803, 33814, 33820, 33822, 33824, 33840, 33845, 33851, 33853, 33858, 33859, 33863, 33864, 33871, 33875, 33877, 33880, 33881, 33883, 33884, 33886, 33910, 33916, 33917, 33920, 33922, 33926, 33935, 33945, 33975, 33976, 33977, 33978, 33979, 33980, 33983, 33990, 33991, 34701, 34702, 34703, 34704, 34705, 34706, 34707, 34708, 34710, 34712, 34718, 34841, 34842, 34843, 34844, 34845, 34846, 34847, 34848)◀

▶(34714 may only be reported once per side. For bilateral procedure, report 34714 twice. Do not report modifier 50 in conjunction with 34714)◀

(Do not report 34714 in conjunction with 33362, 33953, 33954, 33959, 33962, 33969, 33984, 34812 when performed on the same side)

#+ 34820 Open iliac artery exposure for delivery of endovascular prosthesis or iliac occlusion during endovascular therapy, by abdominal or retroperitoneal incision, unilateral (List separately in addition to code for primary procedure)

▶(Use 34820 in conjunction with 33880, 33881, 33883, 33884, 33886, 33990, 33991, 34701, 34702, 34703, 34704, 34705, 34706, 34707, 34708, 34710, 34712, 34718, 34841, 34842, 34843, 34844, 34845, 34846, 34847, 34848)◀

▶(34820 may only be reported once per side. For bilateral procedure, report 34820 twice. Do not report modifier 50 in conjunction with 34820)◀

(Do not report 34820 in conjunction with 33953, 33954, 33959, 33962, 33969, 33984)

#+ 34833 Open iliac artery exposure with creation of conduit for delivery of endovascular prosthesis or for establishment of cardiopulmonary bypass, by abdominal or retroperitoneal incision, unilateral (List separately in addition to code for primary procedure)

▶(Use 34833 in conjunction with 32852, 32854, 33031, 33120, 33251, 33256, 33259, 33261, 33305, 33315, 33322, 33335, 33390, 33391, 33404, 33405, 33406, 33410, 33411, 33412, 33413, 33414, 33415, 33416, 33417, 33422, 33425, 33426, 33427, 33430, 33440, 33460, 33463, 33464, 33465, 33468, 33474, 33475, 33476, 33478, 33496, 33500, 33502, 33504, 33505, 33506, 33507, 33510, 33511, 33512, 33513, 33514, 33516, 33533, 33534, 33535, 33536, 33542, 33545, 33548, 33600-33688, 33692, 33694, 33697, 33702, 33710, 33720, 33722, 33724, 33726, 33730, 33732, 33736, 33750, 33755, 33762, 33764, 33766, 33767, 33770-33783, 33786, 33788, 33802, 33803, 33814, 33820, 33822, 33824, 33840, 33845, 33851, 33853, 33858, 33859, 33863, 33864, 33871, 33875, 33877, 33880, 33881, 33883, 33884, 33886, 33910, 33916, 33917, 33920, 33922, 33926, 33935, 33945, 33975, 33976, 33977, 33978, 33979, 33980, 33983, 33990, 33991, 34701, 34702, 34703, 34704, 34705, 34706, 34707, 34708, 34710, 34712, 34718, 34841, 34842, 34843, 34844, 34845, 34846, 34847, 34848)◀

▶(34833 may only be reported once per side. For bilateral procedure, report 34833 twice. Do not report modifier 50 in conjunction with 34833)◀

(Do not report 34833 in conjunction with 33364, 33953, 33954, 33959, 33962, 33969, 33984, 34820 when performed on the same side)

#+ 34834 Open brachial artery exposure for delivery of endovascular prosthesis, unilateral (List separately in addition to code for primary procedure)

▶(Use 34834 in conjunction with 33880, 33881, 33883, 33884, 33886, 33990, 33991, 34701, 34702, 34703, 34704, 34705, 34706, 34707, 34708, 34710, 34712, 34718, 34841, 34842, 34843, 34844, 34845, 34846, 34847, 34848)◀

▶(34834 may only be reported once per side. For bilateral procedure, report 34834 twice. Do not report modifier 50 in conjunction with 34834)◀

(Do not report 34834 in conjunction with 33953, 33954, 33959, 33962, 33969, 33984)

+ 34715 Open axillary/subclavian artery exposure for delivery of endovascular prosthesis by infraclavicular or supraclavicular incision, unilateral (List separately in addition to code for primary procedure)

▶(Use 34715 in conjunction with 33880, 33881, 33883, 33884, 33886, 33990, 33991, 34701, 34702, 34703, 34704, 34705, 34706, 34707, 34708, 34710, 34712, 34718, 34841, 34842, 34843, 34844, 34845, 34846, 34847, 34848)◀

▶(34715 may only be reported once per side. For bilateral procedure, report 34715 twice. Do not report modifier 50 in conjunction with 34715)◀

(Do not report 34715 in conjunction with 33363, 33953, 33954, 33959, 33962, 33969, 33984, 0451T, 0452T, 0455T, 0456T)

+ **34716** Open axillary/subclavian artery exposure with creation of conduit for delivery of endovascular prosthesis or for establishment of cardiopulmonary bypass, by infraclavicular or supraclavicular incision, unilateral (List separately in addition to code for primary procedure)

▶(Use 34716 in conjunction with 32852, 32854, 33031, 33120, 33251, 33256, 33259-33261, 33305, 33315, 33322, 33335, 33390, 33391, 33404, 33405, 33406, 33410, 33411, 33412, 33413, 33414, 33415, 33416, 33417, 33422, 33425, 33426, 33427, 33430, 33440, 33460, 33463, 33464, 33465, 33468, 33474, 33475, 33476, 33478, 33496, 33500, 33502, 33504, 33505, 33506, 33507, 33510, 33511, 33512, 33513, 33514, 33516, 33533, 33534, 33535, 33536, 33542, 33545, 33548, 33600-33688, 33692, 33694, 33697, 33702-33722, 33724, 33726, 33730, 33732, 33736, 33750, 33755, 33762, 33764, 33766, 33767, 33770-33783, 33786, 33788, 33802, 33803, 33814, 33820, 33822, 33824, 33840, 33845, 33851, 33853, 33858, 33859, 33863, 33864, 33871, 33875, 33877, 33880, 33881, 33883, 33884, 33886, 33910, 33916, 33917, 33920, 33922, 33926, 33935, 33945, 33975, 33976, 33977, 33978, 33979, 33980, 33983, 33990, 33991, 34701, 34702, 34703, 34704, 34705, 34706, 34707, 34708, 34710, 34712, 34718, 34841, 34842, 34843, 34844, 34845, 34846, 34847, 34848)◀

▶(34716 may only be reported once per side. For bilateral procedure, report 34716 twice. Do not report modifier 50 in conjunction with 34716)◀

(Do not report 34716 in conjunction with 33953, 33954, 33959, 33962, 33969, 33984, 0451T, 0452T, 0455T, 0456T)

(34800, 34802, 34803, 34804, 34805, 34806 have been deleted. To report, see 34701, 34702, 34703, 34704, 34705, 34706, 34707, 34708)

34717 Code is out of numerical sequence. See 34707-34711

34718 Code is out of numerical sequence. See 34707-34711

+ **34808** Endovascular placement of iliac artery occlusion device (List separately in addition to code for primary procedure)

▶(Use 34808 in conjunction with 34701, 34702, 34703, 34704, 34707, 34708, 34709, 34710, 34813, 34841, 34842, 34843, 34844)◀

Rationale

Several changes have occurred under the Cardiovascular System/Arteries and Veins/Endovascular Repair of Abdominal Aorta and/or Iliac Arteries subsection. In accordance with the deletion of codes 33860 and 33870 and addition of codes 33858, 33859, and 33871, the inclusionary parenthetical notes following codes 34714, 34716, and 34833 have been revised to reflect these changes.

Refer to the codebook and the Rationale for codes 33858, 33859, 33860, 33870, and 33871 for a full discussion of these changes.

Category III code 0254T has been converted to Category I codes 34717 and 34718. New guidelines and parenthetical notes have been added and existing guidelines and parenthetical notes have been revised throughout the code set to provide instruction on the proper reporting of codes 34717 and 34718.

Since the addition of code 0254T in 2011, the performance of iliac artery repair by deployment of an iliac branched endograft has increased to a level that warranted converting it to a Category I code. Code 34717 is an add-on code that describes endovascular repair of the iliac artery using an iliac branched endograft performed at the time of aorto-iliac artery endograft placement (ie, 34703, 34704, 34705, 34706). Code 34718 is a stand-alone code that describes the same procedure, but it is not performed at the time of aorto-iliac artery endograft placement.

Both codes 34717 and 34718 include pre-procedure sizing and device selection; selective iliac artery catheterization(s) performed on the same side (ie, ipsilateral); all associated radiological supervision and interpretation; all endograft extension(s) proximal to (near) the aortic bifurcation and distally (away from aortic bifurcation) in the internal iliac, external iliac, and common femoral artery(ies); and any angioplasty/stenting performed in the treatment zone. Treatment zone is defined by the vessels that contain the endograft(s) (main body, docking limb[s], and/or extension[s]) deployed during the operative session.

In support of the revision to instructions for reporting add-on procedures when performed bilaterally, the instructional parenthetical notes for add-on codes 34713, 34714, 34715, 34716, 34812, 34820, 34833, and 34834 have been revised with new language to not report modifier 50. The new bilateral language was also used for the parenthetical notes following codes 34717 and 34718, which are unilateral procedures. Code 34717 should be reported twice when the procedure is performed bilaterally. However, when code 34718 is performed bilaterally, modifier 50, *Bilateral Procedure,* should be appended as it is not an add-on code. Refer to the codebook and the Rationale for modifier 50, *Bilateral Procedure,* guideline revisions for a full discussion of these changes.

Clinical Example (34717)

A 75-year-old male, who has coronary artery disease (CAD), chronic obstructive pulmonary disease (COPD), asymptomatic infrarenal abdominal aortic, and right common iliac artery aneurysms, undergoes endovascular repair of the iliac artery with an iliac branched endograft during endovascular repair with an aorto-iliac artery endograft. [**Note:** This is an add-on service. Only consider the additional work related to endovascular repair of the iliac artery with an iliac branched endograft.]

Description of Procedure (34717)

Bring the iliac branch endograft, catheters, and introducer sheaths to the operating table after verification of appropriate diameters and lengths once endovascular aneurysm repair (EVR) has been performed. The patient remains systemically anticoagulated. Use the entry wire(s) to enter the pre-existing sheath under fluoroscopic guidance. Place a multisided hole catheter and perform flush aorto-iliac angiography with interpretation. Insert a bifurcated iliac branch device into the common iliac limb after orientation to the internal iliac position. Selective wire access with catheter insertion into the internal iliac artery from a contralateral approach and through the iliac branch device, which has been partially deployed. Place an internal iliac endoprosthesis through the iliac branch bifurcated graft and mate to it above and into the main internal iliac artery below. Deploy the iliac branch device into the external iliac artery. Deploy the external iliac artery endoprosthesis to mate with the bifurcated device and into the distal external iliac or femoral artery. Place a large compliant balloon over the wire and into the iliac endograft(s) to perform balloon dilation at the proximal and distal seal zones of the endograft. Perform an aortogram (do not report separately) and immediately interpret for adequacy of the graft position, patency of appropriate branches (internal iliac, external iliac), presence or absence of endoleaks, and type of endoleak, if present. Assess the patency of collateral vessels (lumbar, internal iliac) that may contribute to persistent endoleaks. Perform adjunctive balloon angioplasty for endoleak treatment, as necessary. When the graft is in appropriate position and free of endoleak on angiogram, remove the catheters and guidewires.

Clinical Example (34718)

A 75-year-old male with CAD and COPD, who had previously undergone endovascular repair with placement of an aorto-iliac artery endograft, now presents with a new right common iliac aneurysm. Endovascular repair with an iliac branched endograft is performed to preserve flow into his pelvis and right leg.

Description of Procedure (34718)

Bring the endograft, catheters, and introducer sheaths to the operating table after verification of appropriate diameters and lengths. Systemically anticoagulate the patient. Use the entry wire(s) to enter the introducer needle under fluoroscopic guidance. Place the sheaths in the access vessels. Place a multisided hole catheter and perform flush aorto-iliac angiography with interpretation. Insert a bifurcated iliac branch device into the common iliac limb after orientation to the internal iliac position. Selective wire access with catheter insertion into the internal iliac artery from a contralateral approach and through the iliac branch device, which has been partially deployed. Place an internal iliac endoprosthesis through the iliac branch bifurcated graft and mate to it above and into the main internal iliac artery below. Deploy the iliac branch device into the external iliac artery. Deploy the external iliac artery endoprosthesis to mate with the bifurcated device and into the distal external iliac or femoral artery. Place a large compliant balloon over the wire into the iliac endograft(s) to perform balloon dilation at the proximal and distal seal zones of the endograft. Perform an aortogram (do not report separately) and immediately interpret for adequacy of the graft position, patency of appropriate branches (internal iliac, external iliac), presence or absence of endoleaks, and type of endoleak if present. Assess the patency of collateral vessels (lumbar, internal iliac) that may contribute to persistent endoleaks. Perform adjunctive balloon angioplasty for endoleak treatment, as necessary. When the graft is in appropriate position and free of endoleak on angiogram, remove the catheters and guidewires.

Fenestrated Endovascular Repair of the Visceral and Infrarenal Aorta

34845 Endovascular repair of visceral aorta and infrarenal abdominal aorta (eg, aneurysm, pseudoaneurysm, dissection, penetrating ulcer, intramural hematoma, or traumatic disruption) with a fenestrated visceral aortic endograft and concomitant unibody or modular infrarenal aortic endograft and all associated radiological supervision and interpretation, including target zone angioplasty, when performed; including one visceral artery endoprosthesis (superior mesenteric, celiac or renal artery)

34846 including two visceral artery endoprostheses (superior mesenteric, celiac and/or renal artery[s])

34847 including three visceral artery endoprostheses (superior mesenteric, celiac and/or renal artery[s])

34848 including four or more visceral artery endoprostheses (superior mesenteric, celiac and/or renal artery[s])

(Do not report 34845, 34846, 34847, 34848 in conjunction with 34701, 34702, 34703, 34704, 34705, 34706, 34841, 34842, 34843, 34844, 35081, 35102)

(Do not report 34845, 34846, 34847, 34848 in conjunction with 34839, when planning services are performed on the day before or the day of the fenestrated endovascular repair procedure)

(Do not report 34841-34848 in conjunction with 37236, 37237 for bare metal or covered stents placed into the visceral branches within the endoprosthesis target zone)

▶(For placement of distal extension prosthesis[es] terminating in the internal iliac, external iliac, or common femoral artery[ies], see 34709, 34710, 34711, 34718)◀

(Use 34845, 34846, 34847, 34848 in conjunction with 37220, 37221, 37222, 37223, only when 37220, 37221, 37222, 37223 are performed outside the target treatment zone of the endoprosthesis)

Rationale

In support of the conversion of Category III code 0254T to Category I codes 34717 and 34718, the cross-reference parenthetical note following code 34848 has been revised by replacing code 0254T with code 34718 when a distal extension prosthesis[es] terminating in the internal iliac, external iliac, or common femoral artery[ies] is placed.

Refer to the codebook and the Rationale for codes 34717 and 34718 for a full discussion of these changes.

Direct Repair of Aneurysm or Excision (Partial or Total) and Graft Insertion for Aneurysm, Pseudoaneurysm, Ruptured Aneurysm, and Associated Occlusive Disease

Procedures 35001-35152 include preparation of artery for anastomosis including endarterectomy.

(For direct repairs associated with occlusive disease only, see 35201-35286)

(For intracranial aneurysm, see 61700 et seq)

(For endovascular repair of abdominal aortic and/or iliac artery aneurysm, see 34701-34716)

▶(For thoracic aortic aneurysm, see 33858-33875)◀

(For endovascular repair of descending thoracic aorta, involving coverage of left subclavian artery origin, use 33880)

35001 Direct repair of aneurysm, pseudoaneurysm, or excision (partial or total) and graft insertion, with or without patch graft; for aneurysm and associated occlusive disease, carotid, subclavian artery, by neck incision

Rationale

In support of the deletion of codes 33860 and 33870 and addition of codes 33858, 33859, and 33871, the cross-reference parenthetical note for thoracic aortic aneurysm procedures at the beginning of the Direct Repair of Aneurysm or Excision (Partial or Total) and Graft Insertion for Aneurysm, Pseudoaneurysm, Ruptured Aneurysm, and Associated Occlusive Disease subsection has been revised to reflect these changes.

Refer to the codebook and the Rationale for codes 33858, 33859, 33860, 33870, and 33871 for a full discussion of these changes.

Bypass Graft

Vein

+ **35572** Harvest of femoropopliteal vein, 1 segment, for vascular reconstruction procedure (eg, aortic, vena caval, coronary, peripheral artery) (List separately in addition to code for primary procedure)

(Use 35572 in conjunction with 33510-33516, 33517-33523, 33533-33536, 34502, 34520, 35001, 35002, 35011-35022, 35102, 35103, 35121-35152, 35231-35256, 35501-35571, 35583, 35585, 35587, 35879-35907)

▶(For bilateral procedure, report 35572 twice. Do not report modifier 50 in conjunction with 35572)◀

Rationale

In support of the revised instructions for reporting add-on procedures when performed bilaterally, the instructional parenthetical note for add-on code 35572 has been revised to indicate that code 35572 should be reported twice when the procedure is performed bilaterally.

Refer to the codebook and the Rationale for modifier 50, *Bilateral Procedure*, guideline revisions for a full discussion of these changes.

Excision, Exploration, Repair, Revision

▲ **35701** Exploration not followed by surgical repair, artery; neck (eg, carotid, subclavian)

▶(Do not report 35701 in conjunction with 35201, 35231, 35261, 35800, when performed on the same side of the neck)◀

● **35702** upper extremity (eg, axillary, brachial, radial, ulnar)

● **35703** lower extremity (eg, common femoral, deep femoral, superficial femoral, popliteal, tibial, peroneal)

▶(When additional surgical procedures are performed at the same setting by the same surgeon, 35701, 35702, 35703 may only be reported when a nonvascular surgical procedure is performed and only when the artery exploration is performed through a separate incision)◀

▶(Do not report 35702, 35703 in conjunction with 35206, 35207, 35236, 35256, 35266, 35286, 35860 in the same extremity)◀

▶(Do not report 35701, 35702, 35703 to explore and identify a recipient artery [eg, external carotid artery] when performed in conjunction with 15756, 15757, 15758, 20955, 20956, 20957, 20962, 20969, 20970, 20972, 20973, 43496, 49906)◀

▶(35721, 35741 have been deleted)◀

▶(To report exploration of lower extremity artery, use 35703)◀

▶(35761 has been deleted)◀

▶(To report vascular exploration not followed by surgical repair, other than neck artery, upper extremity artery, lower extremity artery, chest, abdomen, or retroperitoneal area, use 37799)◀

▶(For vascular exploration of the chest not followed by surgical repair, use 32100)◀

▶(For vascular exploration of the abdomen not followed by surgical repair, use 49000)◀

▶(For vascular exploration of the retroperitoneal area not followed by surgical repair, use 49010)◀

Rationale

Changes have been made for reporting arterial exploration procedures. Code 35701 has been revised, codes 35721, 35741, 35761 have been deleted, and codes 35702 and 35703 have been added. Parenthetical notes have been added to provide instruction on the appropriate reporting of these new codes.

Prior to 2020, codes 35701, 35721, and 35741 specified the arteries explored (ie, carotid artery [35701], femoral artery [35721], and popliteal artery [35741]). As other arteries in the same and other anatomic locations may be explored, the code structure for arterial exploration has been changed to describe the anatomic location rather than the specific arteries. These codes also previously included the language "with or without lysis of artery." However, lysis of the artery during exploration is performed so infrequently that it was determined the language is no longer necessary and has been removed.

Code 35701 has been revised to describe exploration of an artery in the neck. Codes 35721 and 35741 have been deleted and new codes 35702 (exploration of upper extremity artery) and 35703 (exploration of lower extremity artery) have been added. Codes 35701, 35702, and 35703 include examples of the arteries that apply to each code.

Artery exploration is not reported separately when performed on the same side of the neck or in the same extremity with repair of a vessel, with exploration for postoperative hemorrhage, thrombosis, or infection, or with flap or graft procedures. Exclusionary parenthetical notes listing the specific codes for these procedures have been added following codes 35701, 35702, and 35703. Codes 35701, 35702, and 35703 may only be reported with another procedure if it is a nonvascular surgical procedure and only when the artery exploration is performed through a separate incision.

Code 35761, which described exploration of other vessels, has been deleted. Cross-reference parenthetical notes have been added directing users to the appropriate codes for artery exploration in the chest, abdomen, and retroperitoneal areas. A cross-reference parenthetical note has also been added instructing use of the unlisted code 37799 for vascular exploration not followed by surgical repair for any artery other than those in the codes for the specific anatomic locations.

Clinical Example (35701)

A 59-year-old male is admitted to the ICU in septic shock. At the bedside, a central venous catheter is attempted in the right internal jugular vein. Postprocedure X ray appears to show the tip of the catheter in the aortic arch. The patient is taken to the OR where, upon exploration, the catheter is found to be misplaced in the subcutaneous space of the chest. The carotid artery is explored and found to be free of injury.

Description of Procedure (35701)

Under general anesthesia, carefully inspect the location of the catheter or injury. Assess and mark bony and soft tissue landmarks. Create an incision along the sternocleidomastoid muscle and dissect the neck. Carefully evacuate any hematoma and retract the musculature. Carefully dissect down until the carotid sheath is entered. Identify the internal jugular vein and retract for better visualization of the carotid artery. After carefully inspecting for any cranial nerves, mobilize the carotid artery and inspect for injury. Take care to avoid injury to the jugular vein and cranial nerves. Thoroughly inspect the carotid artery for injury. Finding no injury and after hemostasis is achieved, irrigate the wound bed with warm saline. Place a drain, if required. Close the neck in layers.

Clinical Example (35702)

A 74-year-old male had a left brachial artery catheter placed for arterial pressure monitoring for coronary artery bypass grafting. Two days following a successful bypass procedure, the catheter is removed and pressure is held over the insertion site. The patient complains of pain in the left hand and coolness. The patient is taken to the OR where the left brachial artery is explored and found to be free of injury.

Description of Procedure (35702)

Under general anesthesia, palpate the course of the artery (axillary, brachial, radial and/or ulnar) to determine the change in pulse exam. Create an incision along the left bicep and carry dissection through the soft tissue. Carefully evacuate any hematoma. Dissect down until the brachial artery is identified. Take care to avoid injury to surrounding veins and nerves; carefully dissect and ligate side branches and bridging veins as necessary. Mobilize and inspect the brachial artery. Once the artery has been inspected and no apparent injury is visualized, use a Doppler probe to demonstrate multiphasic flow throughout the artery. Finding no evidence of injury and once hemostasis is achieved, irrigate the wound bed with warm saline and close the arm in layers.

Clinical Example (35703)

A 17-year-old male football player is brought to the ER with concerns of a right posterior knee dislocation. CT angiogram appears to show an abnormality in the right popliteal artery. The right popliteal artery is explored and found to be in spasm, but free of injury.

Description of Procedure (35703)

Under general anesthesia, carefully inspect the location of the injury. Assess and mark bony and soft tissue landmarks. Make a gentle S-shape posterior incision over the popliteal artery. Carefully evacuate any previous hematoma. Carefully dissect and mobilize the tibial nerve and popliteal vein, exposing the popliteal artery. Mobilize the artery and inspect throughout the popliteal fossa, examining for injury. After the artery has been inspected and no apparent injury is visualized, use a Doppler probe to demonstrate multiphasic flow throughout the artery. Finding no injury, irrigate the wound with warm saline and close the incision in multiple layers.

Vascular Injection Procedures

Intra-Arterial—Intra-Aortic

36160 Introduction of needle or intracatheter, aortic, translumbar

Diagnostic Studies of Cervicocerebral Arteries: Codes 36221-36228 describe non-selective and selective arterial catheter placement and diagnostic imaging of the aortic arch, carotid, and vertebral arteries. Codes 36221-36226 include the work of accessing the vessel, placement of catheter(s), contrast injection(s), fluoroscopy, radiological supervision and interpretation, and closure of the arteriotomy by pressure, or application of an arterial closure device. Codes 36221-36228 describe arterial contrast injections with arterial, capillary, and venous phase imaging, when performed.

Code 36227 is an add-on code to report unilateral selective arterial catheter placement and diagnostic imaging of the ipsilateral external carotid circulation and includes all the work of accessing the additional vessel, placement of catheter(s), contrast injection(s), fluoroscopy, radiological supervision and interpretation. Code 36227 is reported in conjunction with 36222, 36223, or 36224.

Code 36228 is an add-on code to report unilateral selective arterial catheter placement and diagnostic imaging of the initial and each additional intracranial branch of the internal carotid or vertebral arteries. Code 36228 is reported in conjunction with 36223, 36224, 36225 or 36226. This includes any additional second or third order catheter selective placement in the same primary branch of the internal carotid, vertebral, or basilar artery and includes all the work of accessing the additional vessel, placement of catheter(s), contrast injection(s), fluoroscopy, radiological supervision and interpretation. It is not reported more than twice per side, regardless of the number of additional branches selectively catheterized.

Codes 36221-36226 are built on progressive hierarchies with more intensive services inclusive of less intensive services. The code inclusive of all of the services provided for that vessel should be reported (ie, use the code inclusive of the most intensive services provided). Only one code in the range 36222-36224 may be reported for each ipsilateral carotid territory. Only one code in the range 36225-36226 may be reported for each ipsilateral vertebral territory.

Code 36221 is reported for non-selective arterial catheter placement in the thoracic aorta and diagnostic imaging of the aortic arch and great vessel origins. Codes 36222-36228 are reported for unilateral artery catheterization. Do not report 36221 in conjunction with 36222-36226 as these selective codes include the work of 36221 when performed.

Do not report 36222, 36223, or 36224 together for ipsilateral angiography. Instead, select the code that represents the most comprehensive service using the following hierarchy of complexity (listed in descending order of complexity): 36224>36223>36222.

Do not report 36225 and 36226 together for ipsilateral angiography. Select the code that represents the more comprehensive service using the following hierarchy of complexity (listed in descending order of complexity): 36226>36225.

▶When bilateral carotid and/or vertebral arterial catheterization and imaging is performed, report 36222, 36223, 36224, 36225, 36226 with modifier 50, and report add-on codes 36227, 36228 twice (do not report modifier 50 in conjunction with 36227, 36228) if the same procedure is performed on both sides. For example, bilateral extracranial carotid angiography with selective catheterization of each common carotid artery would be reported with 36222 and modifier 50. However, when different territory(ies) is studied in the same session on both sides of the body, modifiers may be required to report the imaging performed. Use modifier 59 to denote that different carotid and/or vertebral arteries are being studied. For example, when selective right internal carotid artery catheterization accompanied by right extracranial and intracranial carotid angiography is followed by selective left common carotid artery catheterization with left extracranial carotid angiography, use 36224 to report the right side and 36222-59 to report the left side.◀

Diagnostic angiography of the cervicocerebral vessels may be followed by an interventional procedure at the same session. Interventional procedures may be separately reportable using standard coding conventions.

Do not report 36218 or 75774 as part of diagnostic angiography of the extracranial and intracranial cervicocerebral vessels. It may be appropriate to report 36218 and 75774 for diagnostic angiography of upper extremities and other vascular beds of the neck and/or shoulder girdle performed in the same session as vertebral angiography (eg, workup of a neck tumor that requires catheterization and angiography of the vertebral artery as well as other brachiocephalic arteries).

Report 76376 or 76377 for 3D rendering when performed in conjunction with 36221-36228.

Report 76937 for ultrasound guidance for vascular access, when performed in conjunction with 36221-36228.

36200 Introduction of catheter, aorta

(For non-selective angiography of the extracranial carotid and/or cerebral vessels and cervicocerebral arch, when performed, use 36221)

Rationale

In support of the revision to instructions for reporting add-on procedures when performed bilaterally, the guidelines for Vascular Injection Procedures/Intra-Arterial—Intra-Aortic subsection have been revised to clarify that add-on codes 36227 and 36228 should be reported twice when the procedures are performed bilaterally.

Refer to the codebook and the Rationale for modifier 50, *Bilateral Procedure*, guideline revisions for a full discussion of these changes.

Endovascular Revascularization (Open or Percutaneous, Transcatheter)

37220 Revascularization, endovascular, open or percutaneous, iliac artery, unilateral, initial vessel; with transluminal angioplasty

37221 with transluminal stent placement(s), includes angioplasty within the same vessel, when performed

▶(Use 37220, 37221 in conjunction with 34701-34711, 34718, 34845, 34846, 34847, 34848, only when 37220 or 37221 is performed outside the treatment zone of the endograft)◀

+ 37222 Revascularization, endovascular, open or percutaneous, iliac artery, each additional ipsilateral iliac vessel; with transluminal angioplasty (List separately in addition to code for primary procedure)

(Use 37222 in conjunction with 37220, 37221)

+ 37223 with transluminal stent placement(s), includes angioplasty within the same vessel, when performed (List separately in addition to code for primary procedure)

(Use 37223 in conjunction with 37221)

▶(Use 37222, 37223 in conjunction with 34701-34711, 34718, 34845, 34846, 34847, 34848 only when 37222 or 37223 are performed outside the treatment zone of the endograft)◀

Rationale

In support of the conversion of Category III code 0254T to Category I codes 34717 and 34718, the inclusionary parenthetical notes following codes 37221 and 37223 have been revised by replacing code 0254T with code 34718.

Refer to the codebook and the Rationale for codes 34717 and 34718 for a full discussion of these changes.

Intravascular Ultrasound Services

+ 37252 Intravascular ultrasound (noncoronary vessel) during diagnostic evaluation and/or therapeutic intervention, including radiological supervision and interpretation; initial noncoronary vessel (List separately in addition to code for primary procedure)

+ 37253 each additional noncoronary vessel (List separately in addition to code for primary procedure)

(Use 37253 in conjunction with 37252)

▶(Report 37252, 37253 in conjunction with 33361, 33362, 33363, 33364, 33365, 33366, 33367, 33368, 33369, 33477, 33880, 33881, 33883, 33884, 33886, 34701, 34702, 34703, 34704, 34705, 34706, 34707, 34708, 34709, 34710, 34711, 34712, 34718, 34841, 34842, 34843, 34844, 34845, 34846, 34847, 34848, 36010, 36011, 36012, 36013, 36014, 36015, 36100, 36140, 36160, 36200, 36215, 36216, 36217, 36218, 36221, 36222, 36223, 36224, 36225, 36226, 36227, 36228, 36245, 36246, 36247, 36248, 36251, 36252, 36253, 36254, 36481, 36555-36571, 36578, 36580, 36581, 36582, 36583, 36584, 36585, 36595, 36901, 36902, 36903, 36904, 36905, 36906, 36907, 36908, 36909, 37184, 37185, 37186, 37187, 37188, 37200, 37211, 37212, 37213, 37214, 37215, 37216, 37218, 37220, 37221, 37222, 37223, 37224, 37225, 37226, 37227, 37228, 37229, 37230, 37231, 37232, 37233, 37234, 37235, 37236, 37237, 37238, 37239, 37241, 37242, 37243, 37244, 37246, 37247, 37248, 37249, 61623, 75600, 75605, 75625, 75630, 75635, 75705, 75710, 75716, 75726, 75731, 75733, 75736, 75741, 75743, 75746, 75756, 75774, 75805, 75807, 75810, 75820, 75822, 75825, 75827, 75831, 75833, 75860, 75870, 75872, 75885, 75887, 75889, 75891, 75893, 75894, 75898, 75901, 75902, 75956, 75957, 75958, 75959, 75970, 76000, 77001, 0075T, 0076T, 0234T, 0235T, 0236T, 0237T, 0238T, 0338T)◀

(Do not report 37252, 37253 in conjunction with 37191, 37192, 37193, 37197)

Rationale

In support of the conversion of Category III code 0254T to Category I codes 34717 and 34718, the inclusionary parenthetical note following code 37253 has been revised by replacing code 0254T with code 34718.

Refer to the codebook and the Rationale for codes 34717 and 34718 for a full discussion of these changes.

Hemic and Lymphatic Systems

Lymph Nodes and Lymphatic Channels

Radical Lymphadenectomy (Radical Resection of Lymph Nodes)

+ 38746 Thoracic lymphadenectomy by thoracotomy, mediastinal and regional lymphadenectomy (List separately in addition to code for primary procedure)

(On the right, mediastinal lymph nodes include the paratracheal, subcarinal, paraesophageal, and inferior pulmonary ligament)

(On the left, mediastinal lymph nodes include the aortopulmonary window, subcarinal, paraesophageal, and inferior pulmonary ligament)

▶(Report 38746 in conjunction with 21601, 31760, 31766, 31786, 32096-32200, 32220-32320, 32440-32491, 32503-32505, 33025, 33030, 33050-33130, 39200-39220, 39560, 39561, 43101, 43112, 43117, 43118, 43122, 43123, 43351, 60270, 60505)◀

(To report mediastinal and regional lymphadenectomy via thoracoscopy [VATS], see 32674)

Rationale

In support of deletion of code 19260, the parenthetical note following code 38746 has been revised by replacing code 19260 with new code 21601.

Refer to the codebook and the Rationale for breast biopsy procedure codes for a full discussion of these changes.

Digestive System

Esophagus

Repair

43400 Ligation, direct, esophageal varices

▶(43401 has been deleted)◀

Rationale

To ensure that the CPT code set reflects current clinical practice, code 43401, *Transection of esophagus with repair,* for esophageal varices, has been deleted because of low utilization.

Anus

▶For incision of thrombosed external hemorrhoid, use 46083. For ligation of internal hemorrhoid(s), see 46221, 46945, 46946. For excision of internal and/or external hemorrhoid(s), see 46250-46262, 46320. For injection of hemorrhoid(s), use 46500. For destruction of internal hemorrhoid(s) by thermal energy, use 46930. For destruction of hemorrhoid(s) by cryosurgery, use 46999. For transanal hemorrhoidal dearterialization, including ultrasound guidance, with mucopexy, when performed, use 46948. For hemorrhoidopexy, use 46947. Do not report 46600 in conjunction with 46020-46947, 0184T, during the same operative session.◀

Rationale

In support of the conversion of Category III code 0249T into Category I code 46948, instructions have been added to the guidelines within the Digestive System/Anus subsection that direct users to the correct codes to report for transanal hemorrhoidal dearterialization. In addition, in support of the deletion of Category III code 0377T, the Digestive System/Anus subsection introductory guidelines have also been updated by removing the deleted code.

Refer to the codebook and the Rationale for codes 46948 and 0377T for a full discussion of these changes.

Incision

46020 Placement of seton

▶(Do not report 46020 in conjunction with 46060, 46280, 46600)◀

Rationale

In support of the conversion of Category III code 0249T into Category I code 46948, this code has been deleted from the exclusionary parenthetical note following code 46020.

Refer to the codebook and the Rationale for code 46948 for a full discussion of these changes.

Excision

46221 Hemorrhoidectomy, internal, by rubber band ligation(s)

(Do not report 46221 in conjunction with 45350, 45398)

#▲ **46945** Hemorrhoidectomy, internal, by ligation other than rubber band; single hemorrhoid column/group, without imaging guidance

#▲ **46946** 2 or more hemorrhoid columns/groups, without imaging guidance

▶(Do not report 46221, 46945, 46946 in conjunction with 46948)◀

▶(Do not report 46945, 46946 in conjunction with 76872, 76942, 76998)◀

#● **46948** Hemorrhoidectomy, internal, by transanal hemorrhoidal dearterialization, 2 or more hemorrhoid columns/groups, including ultrasound guidance, with mucopexy, when performed

▶(Do not report 46948 in conjunction with 76872, 76942, 76998)◀

▶(For transanal hemorrhoidal dearterialization, single hemorrhoid column/group, use 46999)◀

46220 Excision of single external papilla or tag, anus

46260 Hemorrhoidectomy, internal and external, 2 or more columns/groups;

46261 with fissurectomy

46262 with fistulectomy, including fissurectomy, when performed

▶(Do not report 46250-46262 in conjunction with 46948)◀

Rationale

Category III code 0249T has been deleted and converted to Category I code 46948. In addition, guidelines, two Category I codes, and several parenthetical notes have been revised, along with several deleted and added parenthetical notes in the Digestive System/Anus/Excision subsection.

The descriptor for deleted code 0249T has been revised in the new code 46948 to more accurately describe all services inherent in the procedure, including (1) identification and ligation of the terminal branches of the superior rectal artery through an anoscope equipped with an ultrasound probe (ie, the dearterialization and ultrasound guidance); and, when required, (2) deployment of a ring of sutures to pull-up a prolapse (mucopexy). The ultrasound probe allows localization of all the arteries that are to be individually ligated as needed to interrupt hemorrhoid blood supply. The descriptor indicates that at least two columns/groups must be treated to report this code. This procedure is different from a traditional hemorrhoidectomy, which focuses on excising the hemorrhoidal bundle.

The revision of codes and guidelines and revision, deletion, and addition of parenthetical notes throughout the code set provide directions regarding services that are inherently included as part of this procedure, direct users to correct codes to report for other procedures, and reflect the deletion of code 0249T. This includes (1) revising the guidelines in the Digestive System/Anus subsection directing users to hemorrhoidal procedures, including code 46948 for transanal hemorrhoidal dearterialization and to reflect the appropriate range for the codes in this subsection; (2) replacing all references to code 0249T in guidelines and parenthetical notes with code 46948, when appropriate; (3) revising code descriptors of 46945 and 46946 to exclude imaging; (4) adding exclusionary parenthetical notes restricting reporting of ultrasound procedures in conjunction with code 46948; (5) adding a cross-reference directing users to code 46999 for transanal hemorrhoidal dearterialization of a single hemorrhoid column/group; and (6) deleting Category III code 0249T and any parenthetical notes that directed use of this specific code.

Clinical Example (46945)

A 50-year-old male with a single symptomatic column of internal hemorrhoids undergoes suture ligation of the hemorrhoidal tissue.

Description of Procedure (46945)

After induction of anesthesia, perform a digital rectal examination. Next, place a lubricated operative anoscope in the anal canal. Rotate the anoscope 180° and remove the obturator. Perform visual inspection through the anoscope, which identifies a single hemorrhoid column. Remove fecal matter with suction. Place a Hill Ferguson anal retractor to dilate the anus. Isolate the large friable internal hemorrhoid column. Suture the hemorrhoid column at the apex, middle, and distal portions of the column in order to destroy the blood supply to the hemorrhoid (total of three interrupted sutures). Perform irrigation and suction to remove any remaining blood. At completion of the procedure, remove the retractor.

Clinical Example (46946)

A 50-year-old male with multiple symptomatic columns of internal hemorrhoids undergoes suture ligation of the hemorrhoidal tissue.

Description of Procedure (46946)

After induction of anesthesia, perform a digital rectal examination. Next, place a lubricated operative anoscope in the anal canal. Rotate the anoscope 180° and remove the obturator. Perform visual inspection through the anoscope, which identifies three hemorrhoid columns (right anterior, left lateral, and right posterior). Remove fecal matter with suction. Place a Hill Ferguson anal retractor to dilate the anus. Isolate the first large friable internal hemorrhoid column. Suture at the apex, middle, and distal portions of the column to destroy the blood supply to the hemorrhoid (total of three interrupted sutures). Perform irrigation and suction to remove blood. Move the retractor and repeat this process on the other two columns. At completion of the procedure, remove the retractor.

Clinical Example (46948)

A 50-year-old male with a long history of bright red rectal bleeding due to grade III internal hemorrhoids undergoes ultrasound-guided hemorrhoidal artery ligation with mucopexy as required.

Description of Procedure (46948)

After induction of anesthesia, perform a digital rectal examination. Next, insert a lubricated anoscope with an ultrasound probe attachment and equipped to deliver sutures into the anus. Perform visual inspection. Using the ultrasound probe, perform hemorrhoid artery ligation with figure-of-eight ligation. Use absorbable suture at six positions correlating with the odd numbers of the clock. After the device ties each suture, use ultrasound to confirm artery ligation. If an ultrasound signal is detected after six ligations, perform additional suture ligation, up to a maximum of eight. If significant mucosal/hemorrhoidal prolapse is present, mucopexy may also be performed. Run the previously tied suture in a proximal-to-distal fashion, stopping 1 cm above the dentate line. At this point, tie the suture back to itself at the apex of the hemorrhoidal column (location of initial ultrasound signal), creating a mucopexy of any redundant hemorrhoidal tissue. Repeat this procedure for each of the six terminal branches of the superior rectal artery so that six ligations and pexy sutures are performed. At completion of the procedure, remove the anoscope with ultrasound probe attachment.

Endoscopy

46600 Anoscopy; diagnostic, including collection of specimen(s) by brushing or washing, when performed (separate procedure)

▶(Do not report 46600 in conjunction with 46020-46947, 0184T, during the same operative session)◀

(For diagnostic high-resolution anoscopy [HRA], use 46601)

| 46601 | diagnostic, with high-resolution magnification (HRA) (eg, colposcope, operating microscope) and chemical agent enhancement, including collection of specimen(s) by brushing or washing, when performed |

(Do not report 46601 in conjunction with 69990)

Rationale

In support of the deletion of Category III codes 0249T and 0377T, both codes have been deleted from the exclusionary parenthetical following code 46600.

Refer to the codebook and the Rationale for codes 46948 and 0377T for a full discussion of these changes.

Destruction

| 46948 | Code is out of numerical sequence. See 46200-46230 |

Pancreas

Excision

| 48155 | Pancreatectomy, total |
| 48160 | Pancreatectomy, total or subtotal, with autologous transplantation of pancreas or pancreatic islet cells |

▶(To report pancreatic islet cell transplantation via portal vein catheterization and infusion, see 0584T, 0585T, 0586T)◀

Rationale

In support of the addition of the new Category IIII codes 0584T, 0585T, and 0586T, a parenthetical note has been added following code 48160 directing users to report the new codes for pancreatic islet cell transplantation via portal vein catheterization and infusion.

Refer to the codebook and the Rationale for codes 0584T, 0585T, and 0586T for a full discussion of these changes.

Abdomen, Peritoneum, and Omentum

Incision

| 49000 | Exploratory laparotomy, exploratory celiotomy with or without biopsy(s) (separate procedure) |

(To report wound exploration due to penetrating trauma without laparotomy, use 20102)

| 49002 | Reopening of recent laparotomy |

(To report re-exploration of hepatic wound for removal of packing, use 47362)

▶(To report re-exploration of pelvic wound for removal, including repacking, when performed, use 49014)◀

| 49010 | Exploration, retroperitoneal area with or without biopsy(s) (separate procedure) |

(To report wound exploration due to penetrating trauma without laparotomy, use 20102)

| ● 49013 | Preperitoneal pelvic packing for hemorrhage associated with pelvic trauma, including local exploration |
| ● 49014 | Re-exploration of pelvic wound with removal of preperitoneal pelvic packing, including repacking, when performed |

Rationale

Codes 49013 and 49014 have been established in the Digestive System/Abdomen, Peritoneum, and Omentum/Incision subsection for preperitoneal pelvic packing for hemorrhage associated with pelvic trauma (49013) and re-exploration with removal of packing, and repacking when performed (49014). In addition, an instructional parenthetical note following code 49002 has been added directing users to report code 49014 for re-exploration of pelvic wound for removal of packing including repacking when performed.

These two new codes differ from other exploration procedures in that a laparotomy is not performed. Instead, a Pfannenstiel low-horizontal incision is made just above the pubic rim, with dissection carried out until the urinary bladder is identified, without opening the peritoneum. Code 49014 describes opening the previous incision, removing the pads if bleeding has stopped, including repacking as needed for continued bleeding.

Clinical Example (49013)

A 45-year-old male presents following pelvic trauma with evidence of continued active hemorrhage in the pelvis. Angiographic evaluation is not readily available, and hypotension persists despite active resuscitation. Preperitoneal pelvic packing and local exploration are performed.

Description of Procedure (49013)

Make a Pfannenstiel low horizontal incision just above the pubic rim. Palpate the upper edge of the pubic bone, make a low transverse incision with detachment of the rectus muscles from their insertion on the rami pubic, and carry out dissection until the urinary bladder is identified. Without opening the peritoneum, retract the urinary bladder to one side while manually carrying out blunt dissection to the iliacus muscle. Identification of the extra-peritoneal bladder is critical, as is a retraction of the urinary bladder to the contralateral side in order to directly approach the presacral vessels. Direct packing downward and posteriorly while sliding down the urinary bladder, directing fingers posteriorly and deep into the true pelvis, reaching posteriorly until the sacroiliac joint is palpated. Firmly pack surgical abdominal pads via this route down into the sacroiliac joint. Direct the abdominal pads toward the pelvic venous plexus and branches of the internal iliac artery, which are in close proximity to the sacrum and pelvic bones. Considerable pressure is mandatory in this packing maneuver, so that the abdominal pads are firmly packed on the pelvic ring from the sacrum to the pelvic rim, thus creating pressure directly onto the presacral vessels. Repeat the same maneuver on the contralateral side of the bladder. Take care to avoid compression of the femoral vessels. After the pelvic bleeding is controlled and the patient's vital signs improve, place drains and close the incision with temporary sutures.

Clinical Example (49014)

A 45-year-old male is returned to the OR one or more days following initial preperitoneal packing for active hemorrhage to have the packing removed.

Description of Procedure (49014)

Open the previous incision and debride the wound as needed. Carefully remove the packing, one pad at a time, to confirm bleeding has been controlled. Perform local exploration and irrigation with each pad removal. Close the wound in layers with drains inserted as required.

Repair

Hernioplasty, Herniorrhaphy, Herniotomy

The hernia repair codes in this section are categorized primarily by the type of hernia (inguinal, femoral, incisional, etc).

Some types of hernias are further categorized as "initial" or "recurrent" based on whether or not the hernia has required previous repair(s).

Additional variables accounted for by some of the codes include patient age and clinical presentation (reducible vs. incarcerated or strangulated).

With the exception of the incisional hernia repairs (see 49560-49566) the use of mesh or other prostheses is not separately reported.

The excision/repair of strangulated organs or structures such as testicle(s), intestine, ovaries are reported by using the appropriate code for the excision/repair (eg, 44120, 54520, and 58940) in addition to the appropriate code for the repair of the strangulated hernia.

> (For reduction and repair of intra-abdominal hernia, use 44050)

> (For debridement of abdominal wall, see 11042, 11043)

> ►(Codes 49491-49651 are unilateral procedures. For bilateral procedure, report 49491-49566, 49570-49651 with modifier 50. Report add-on code 49568 twice, when performed biaterally. Do not report modifier 50 in conjunction with 49568)◄

49491 Repair, initial inguinal hernia, preterm infant (younger than 37 weeks gestation at birth), performed from birth up to 50 weeks postconception age, with or without hydrocelectomy; reducible

49492 incarcerated or strangulated

> (Do not report modifier 63 in conjunction with 49491, 49492)

> (Postconception age equals gestational age at birth plus age of infant in weeks at the time of the hernia repair. Initial inguinal hernia repairs that are performed on preterm infants who are older than 50 weeks postconception age and younger than age 6 months at the time of surgery, should be reported using codes 49495, 49496)

Rationale

In support of the revision to instructions for reporting add-on procedures when performed bilaterally, the instructional parenthetical note following Hernioplasty, Herniorrhaphy, and Herniotomy subsection guidelines has been revised to indicate that add-on code 49568 should be reported twice when the procedure is performed bilaterally.

Refer to the codebook and the Rationale for modifier 50, *Bilateral Procedure,* guideline revisions for a full discussion of these changes.

Urinary System

Urethra

Other Procedures

(For 2 or 3 glass urinalysis, use 81020)

53850 Transurethral destruction of prostate tissue; by microwave thermotherapy

53852 by radiofrequency thermotherapy

53854 by radiofrequency generated water vapor thermotherapy

▶(For transurethral ablation of malignant prostate tissue by high-energy water vapor thermotherapy, including intraoperative imaging and needle guidance, use 0582T)◀

53855 Insertion of a temporary prostatic urethral stent, including urethral measurement

(For insertion of permanent urethral stent, use 52282)

Rationale

In support of the establishment of Category III code 0582T (transurethral ablation of malignant prostate tissue), a cross-reference parenthetical note has been added following code 53854 directing users to the new code.

Refer to the codebook and the Rationale for code 0582T for a full discussion of these changes.

Male Genital System

Testis

Repair

54620 Fixation of contralateral testis (separate procedure)

▲ **54640** Orchiopexy, inguinal or scrotal approach

(For bilateral procedure, report 54640 with modifier 50)

(For inguinal hernia repair performed in conjunction with inguinal orchiopexy, see 49495-49525)

54650 Orchiopexy, abdominal approach, for intra-abdominal testis (eg, Fowler-Stephens)

(For laparoscopic approach, use 54692)

Rationale

The descriptor for code 54640 has been revised to delete the text "with or without hernia repair" as this conflicted with the intention of the code to allow separate reporting of inguinal hernia repair when performed—as instructed in the parenthetical note following code 54640. In addition, the term "or scrotal" has been added to the descriptor to better identify all approaches that are typical for the procedure.

Clinical Example (54640)

A six-month-old patient presents with a palpable undescended testis.

Description of Procedure (54640)

Make an incision in the scrotum or the inguinal area from the pubic bone to the upper lateral pelvic area in the skin crease made by the thigh and the lower abdomen. Carry out dissection to find the testis in the inguinal canal. Mobilize the spermatic cord to allow positioning of the testis in the scrotum. In the scrotum, create a small pouch for the testis where the testis is sutured in place to prevent retraction back into the inguinal canal. Close the incision in layers.

Nervous System

Skull, Meninges, and Brain

Craniectomy or Craniotomy

61533 Craniotomy with elevation of bone flap; for subdural implantation of an electrode array, for long-term seizure monitoring

▶(For continuous EEG monitoring, see 95700-95726)◀

61534 for excision of epileptogenic focus without electrocorticography during surgery

61535 for removal of epidural or subdural electrode array, without excision of cerebral tissue (separate procedure)

Rationale

In support of the deletion of codes 95950, 95951, 95953, and 95956 and the establishment of codes 95700-95726, the cross-reference parenthetical note following code 61533 has been revised to reflect these changes.

Refer to the codebook and the Rationale for codes 95950, 95951, 95953, 95956, and 95700-95726 for a full discussion of these changes.

Spine and Spinal Cord

Injection, Drainage, or Aspiration

▶Injection of contrast during fluoroscopic guidance and localization is an inclusive component of 62263, 62264, 62267, 62273, 62280, 62281, 62282, 62302, 62303, 62304, 62305, 62321, 62323, 62325, 62327, 62328, 62329. Fluoroscopic guidance and localization is reported with 77003, unless a formal contrast study (myelography, epidurography, or arthrography) is performed, in which case the use of fluoroscopy is included in the supervision and interpretation codes or the myelography via lumbar injection code. Image guidance and the injection of contrast are inclusive components and are required for the performance of myelography, as described by codes 62302, 62303, 62304, 62305.◀

For radiologic supervision and interpretation of epidurography, use 72275. Code 72275 is only to be used when an epidurogram is performed, images documented, and a formal radiologic report is issued.

Code 62263 describes a catheter-based treatment involving targeted injection of various substances (eg, hypertonic saline, steroid, anesthetic) via an indwelling epidural catheter. Code 62263 includes percutaneous insertion and removal of an epidural catheter (remaining in place over a several-day period), for the administration of multiple injections of a neurolytic agent(s) performed during serial treatment sessions (ie, spanning two or more treatment days). If required, adhesions or scarring may also be lysed by mechanical means. Code 62263 is **not** reported for each adhesiolysis treatment, but should be reported **once** to describe the entire series of injections/infusions spanning two or more treatment days.

▲ 62270 Spinal puncture, lumbar, diagnostic;

#● 62328 with fluoroscopic or CT guidance

▶(Do not report 62270, 62328 in conjunction with 77003, 77012)◀

▶(If ultrasound or MRI guidance is performed, see 76942, 77021)◀

▲ 62272 Spinal puncture, therapeutic, for drainage of cerebrospinal fluid (by needle or catheter);

#● 62329 with fluoroscopic or CT guidance

▶(Do not report 62272, 62329 in conjunction with 77003, 77012)◀

▶(If ultrasound or MRI guidance is performed, see 76942, 77021)◀

62273 Injection, epidural, of blood or clot patch

62328 Code is out of numerical sequence. See 62270-62273

62329 Code is out of numerical sequence. See 62270-62273

Rationale

In support of the changes in reporting spinal puncture procedures with fluoroscopic or CT guidance, codes 62328 and 62329 have been added to the injection, drainage, or aspiration guidelines in the Spine and Spinal Cord subsection.

Codes 62270 and 62272 have been changed to two distinct parent codes by adding a semicolon to ensure language conformity in the descriptors. The new family of codes (62270, 62328) should be used to report diagnostic spinal lumbar puncture with or without fluoroscopic or CT guidance. In addition, the new family of codes (62272, 62329) should be used to report therapeutic spinal puncture for drainage of cerebrospinal fluid with or without fluoroscopic or CT guidance.

Exclusionary parenthetical notes have been added following codes 62328 and 62329 instructing users not to report codes 62270, 62328, 62272, and 62329 in conjunction with fluoroscopic and CT guidance codes 77003 and 77012. To provide further guidance, instructional parenthetical notes following codes 62328 and 62329 have been added to instruct users to see codes 76942 and 77021 for ultrasound or magnetic resonance imaging (MRI) guidance.

Clinical Example (62270)

A 25-year-old female presents with fever and severe headache.

Description of Procedure (62270)

Insert a spinal needle and advance until cerebrospinal fluid (CSF) is obtained, repositioning as necessary. Attach a pressure gauge to the spinal needle. Obtain CSF samples in sterile tubes to be sent for analysis. Then withdraw the needle and apply direct pressure for one minute. Apply a bandage and place the patient on her back.

Clinical Example (62272)

A 25-year-old female presents with severe headache, visual difficulties, and neck stiffness.

Description of Procedure (62272)

Insert the spinal needle at the appropriate position in the lumbar spine and obtain CSF. Connect a manometer and use to measure CSF pressure. Remove a volume of CSF for analysis and/or therapeutic treatment (volume based on indication and clinical judgment). A catheter may be inserted along the needle tract into the subarachnoid space as necessary for greater volume of fluid. Inject therapeutic agents as necessary. Measure a final CSF pressure using the manometer as necessary. Withdraw the spinal needle/catheter and apply direct pressure to the puncture site for one minute.

Clinical Example (62328)

A 60-year-old female with severe degenerative disc disease, scoliosis, and prior failed bedside lumbar puncture presents with fever and severe headache.

Description of Procedure (62328)

Supervise and interpret scout views of the lower back or lumbar spine to select the appropriate field of view. Obtain and interpret preliminary CT or fluoroscopic images of the lower back or lumbar spine to assess the appropriate approach and spinal level(s), evaluate for unexpected findings or interval changes, and adjust patient positioning or protocol as needed. Mark the appropriate skin-entry site, sterilize the skin in the standard fashion, and place sterile drapes as necessary. Anesthetize the skin and subcutaneous tissues using local anesthesia, changing needles as necessary for deeper infiltration. Under intermittent or continuous CT or fluoroscopic guidance, direct the spinal needle to the appropriate position or lumbar level. Reposition as necessary. Confirm satisfactory needle position with CT or fluoroscopic imaging and return of cerebrospinal fluid (CSF). Attach a pressure gauge to the spinal needle if opening pressures is desired. Obtain CSF (volume based on indication and clinical judgment). Store CSF samples in sterile tubes for further analysis as necessary. Withdraw the spinal needle and apply direct pressure to the puncture site for one minute.

Clinical Example (62329)

A 25-year-old female with scoliosis and prior failed bedside lumbar puncture presents with severe headache, visual difficulties, and neck stiffness.

Description of Procedure (62329)

Supervise and interpret scout views of the lower back or lumbar spine to select the appropriate field of view. Obtain and interpret preliminary CT or fluoroscopic images of the lower back or lumbar spine to assess the appropriate approach and spinal level(s), evaluate for unexpected findings or interval changes, and adjust patient positioning or protocol as needed. Mark the appropriate skin-entry site, sterilize the skin in the standard fashion, and place sterile drapes as necessary. Anesthetize the skin and subcutaneous tissues using local anesthesia, changing needles as necessary for deeper infiltration. Under intermittent or continuous CT or fluoroscopic guidance, direct the spinal needle to the appropriate position or lumbar level. Reposition as necessary. Confirm satisfactory needle position with CT or fluoroscopic imaging and return of CSF. Insert catheter along the needle tract into the subarachnoid space as necessary if greater volume of CSF removal is required. Attach a pressure gauge to the spinal needle or catheter if opening pressures are desired. Obtain CSF (volume based on indication and clinical judgment). Store CSF samples in sterile tubes for further analysis as necessary. Inject indicated therapeutic agents when requested. Attach a pressure gauge to the spinal needle or catheter to obtain catheter pressure, if desired. Withdraw the spinal needle/catheter and apply direct pressure to the puncture site for one minute.

Catheter Implantation

▶(For percutaneous placement of intrathecal or epidural catheter, see 62270, 62272, 62273, 62280, 62281, 62282, 62284, 62320, 62321, 62322, 62323, 62324, 62325, 62326, 62327, 62328, 62329)◀

62350　Implantation, revision or repositioning of tunneled intrathecal or epidural catheter, for long-term medication administration via an external pump or implantable reservoir/infusion pump; without laminectomy

62351　　with laminectomy

(For refilling and maintenance of an implantable infusion pump for spinal or brain drug therapy, see 95990, 95991)

Rationale

In support of the revision of codes 62270 and 62272 and the establishment of codes 62328 and 62329, the cross-reference parenthetical note preceding code 62350 has been revised to reflect these changes.

Refer to the codebook and the Rationale for codes 62270, 62272, 62328, and 62329 for a full discussion of these changes.

Surgery | CPT Changes 2020

Posterior Extradural Laminotomy or Laminectomy for Exploration/Decompression of Neural Elements or Excision of Herniated Intervertebral Discs

63020 Laminotomy (hemilaminectomy), with decompression of nerve root(s), including partial facetectomy, foraminotomy and/or excision of herniated intervertebral disc; 1 interspace, cervical

(For bilateral procedure, report 63020 with modifier 50)

63030 1 interspace, lumbar

(For bilateral procedure, report 63030 with modifier 50)

+ 63035 each additional interspace, cervical or lumbar (List separately in addition to code for primary procedure)

(Use 63035 in conjunction with 63020-63030)

▶(For bilateral procedure, report 63035 twice. Do not report modifier 50 in conjunction with 63035)◀

(For percutaneous endoscopic approach, see 0274T, 0275T)

63040 Laminotomy (hemilaminectomy), with decompression of nerve root(s), including partial facetectomy, foraminotomy and/or excision of herniated intervertebral disc, reexploration, single interspace; cervical

(For bilateral procedure, report 63040 with modifier 50)

63042 lumbar

(For bilateral procedure, report 63042 with modifier 50)

+ 63043 each additional cervical interspace (List separately in addition to code for primary procedure)

(Use 63043 in conjunction with 63040)

▶(For bilateral procedure, report 63043 twice. Do not report modifier 50 in conjunction with 63043)◀

+ 63044 each additional lumbar interspace (List separately in addition to code for primary procedure)

(Use 63044 in conjunction with 63042)

▶(For bilateral procedure, report 63044 twice. Do not report modifier 50 in conjunction with 63044)◀

Rationale

In support of the revision to instructions for reporting add-on procedures when performed bilaterally, the instructional parenthetical notes for add-on codes 63035, 63043, and 63044 have been revised to indicate that add-on codes should be reported twice when the procedure is performed bilaterally.

Refer to the codebook and the Rationale for modifier 50, *Bilateral Procedure,* guideline revisions for a full discussion of these changes.

Extracranial Nerves, Peripheral Nerves, and Autonomic Nervous System

Introduction/Injection of Anesthetic Agent (Nerve Block), Diagnostic or Therapeutic

(For destruction by neurolytic agent or chemodenervation, see 62280-62282, 64600-64681)

(For epidural or subarachnoid injection, see 62320, 62321, 62322, 62323, 62324, 62325, 62326, 62327)

▶(64400-64455, 64461, 64462, 64463, 64479, 64480, 64483, 64484, 64490-64495 are unilateral procedures. For bilateral procedures, report 64400, 64405, 64408, 64415, 64416, 64417, 64418, 64420, 64425-64455, 64461, 64463, 64479, 64483, 64490, 64493 with modifier 50. Report add-on codes 64421, 64462, 64480, 64484, 64491, 64492, 64494, 64495 twice, when performed bilaterally. Do not report modifier 50 in conjunction with 64421, 64462, 64480, 64484, 64491, 64492, 64494, 64495)◀

Rationale

In support of the revision to instructions for reporting add-on procedures when performed bilaterally, the instructional parenthetical note in the Introduction/Injection of Anesthetic Agent (Nerve Block), Diagnostic or Therapeutic subsection has been revised to clarify that add-on codes 64421, 64462, 64480, 64484, 64491, 64492, 64494, and 64495 should be reported twice when the procedure is performed bilaterally.

Refer to the codebook and the Rationale for modifier 50, *Bilateral Procedure,* guideline revisions for a full discussion of these changes.

Somatic Nerves

▶Codes 64400-64489 describe the introduction/injection of an anesthetic agent and/or steroid into the somatic nervous system for diagnostic or therapeutic purposes. For injection or destruction of genicular nerve branches, see 64454, 64624, respectively.

Codes 64400-64450, 64454 describe the injection of an anesthetic agent(s) and/or steroid into a nerve plexus, nerve, or branch. These codes are reported once per nerve plexus, nerve, or branch as described in the descriptor regardless of the number of injections performed along the nerve plexus, nerve, or branch described by the code.

Imaging guidance and localization may be reported separately for 64400-64450. Imaging guidance and any injection of contrast are inclusive components of 64451 and 64454.

Codes 64455, 64479, 64480, 64483, 64484 are reported for single or multiple injections on the same site. For 64479, 64480, 64483, 64484, imaging guidance (fluoroscopy or CT) and any injection of contrast are inclusive components and are not reported separately. For 64455, imaging guidance (ultrasound, fluoroscopy, CT) and localization may be reported separately.

Codes 64461, 64462, 64463 describe injection of a paravertebral block (PVB). Codes 64486, 64487, 64488, 64489 describe injection of a transversus abdominis plane (TAP) block. Imaging guidance and any injection of contrast are inclusive components of 64461, 64462, 64463, 64486, 64487, 64488, 64489 and are not reported separately.◄

▲ 64400   Injection(s), anesthetic agent(s) and/or steroid; trigeminal nerve, each branch (ie, ophthalmic, maxillary, mandibular)

►(64402 has been deleted. To report injection of anesthetic agent and/or steroid to the facial nerve, use 64999)◄

▲ 64405   greater occipital nerve

▲ 64408   vagus nerve

►(64410, 64413 have been deleted. To report injection of anesthetic agent and/or steroid to the phrenic nerve, cervical plexus, use 64999)◄

▲ 64415   brachial plexus

▲ 64416   brachial plexus, continuous infusion by catheter (including catheter placement)

(Do not report 64416 in conjunction with 01996)

▲ 64417   axillary nerve

▲ 64418   suprascapular nerve

►Extracranial Nerves, Peripheral Nerves, and Autonomic Nervous System			
Introduction/Injection of Anesthetic Agent (Nerve Block), Diagnostic or Therapeutic			
Code(s)	Unit	Image Guidance Included	Image Guidance Separately Reported, When Performed
Somatic Nerve			
64400-64450	1 unit per plexus, nerve, or branch injected regardless of the number of injections		X
64451	1 unit for any number of nerves innervating the sacroiliac joint injected regardless of the number of injections	X	
64454	1 unit for any number of genicular nerve branches, with a required minimum of three nerve branches	X	
64455	1 or more injections per level		X
64479	1 or more injections per level	X	
+64480	1 or more additional injections per level (add-on)	X	
64483	1 or more injections per level	X	
+64484	1 or more additional injections per level (add-on)	X	
64461	1 injection site	X	
+64462	1 or more additional injections per code (add-on)	X	
64463	1 or more injections per code	X	
64486-64489	By injection site	X	
Destruction by Neurolytic Agent (Eg, Chemical, Thermal, Electrical, or Radiofrequency), Chemodenervation			
Code(s)	Unit	Image Guidance Included	Image Guidance Separately Reported, When Performed
Somatic Nerves			
64624	1 unit for any number of genicular nerve branches, with a required minimum of three nerve branches	X◄	

▲ = Revised code   ● = New code   ►◄ = Contains new or revised text   ✶ = Duplicate PLA test   ↕ = Category I PLA

▲ 64420		intercostal nerve, single level
+▲ 64421		intercostal nerve, each additional level (List separately in addition to code for primary procedure)

▶(Use 64421 in conjunction with 64420)◀

▲ 64425		ilioinguinal, iliohypogastric nerves
▲ 64430		pudendal nerve
▲ 64435		paracervical (uterine) nerve
▲ 64445		sciatic nerve
▲ 64446		sciatic nerve, continuous infusion by catheter (including catheter placement)

(Do not report 64446 in conjunction with 01996)

▲ 64447		femoral nerve

(Do not report 64447 in conjunction with 01996)

▲ 64448		femoral nerve, continuous infusion by catheter (including catheter placement)

(Do not report 64448 in conjunction with 01996)

▲ 64449		lumbar plexus, posterior approach, continuous infusion by catheter (including catheter placement)

(Do not report 64449 in conjunction with 01996)

▲ 64450		other peripheral nerve or branch

▶(For injection, anesthetic agent, nerves innervating the sacroiliac joint, use 64451)◀

● 64451		nerves innervating the sacroiliac joint, with image guidance (ie, fluoroscopy or computed tomography)

▶(Do not report 64451 in conjunction with 64493, 64494, 64495, 77002, 77003, 77012, 95873, 95874)◀

▶(For injection, anesthetic agent, nerves innervating the sacroiliac joint, with ultrasound, use 76999)◀

▶(For bilateral procedure, report 64451 with modifier 50)◀

● 64454		genicular nerve branches, including imaging guidance, when performed

▶(Do not report 64454 in conjunction with 64624)◀

▶(64454 requires injecting all of the following genicular nerve branches: superolateral, superomedial, and inferomedial. If all 3 of these genicular nerve branches are not injected, report 64454 with modifier 52)◀

Rationale

New guidelines have been added to the Introduction/Injection of Anesthetic Agent (Nerve Block), Diagnostic or Therapeutic, Somatic Nerves subsection. In addition, codes 64400-64450 have been revised, codes 64402, 64410, and 64413 have been deleted, and codes 64451 and 64454 have been added along with a new instructional table. These changes provide standardization of the code descriptors and clarify reporting of sacroiliac joint nerve and genicular nerve branch injections.

Codes 64402, 64410, and 64413 have been deleted because these services are not commonly performed. Parenthetical notes have been added directing users to unlisted code 64999 when injections of facial, phrenic, and cervical nerves are performed. Code 64421 has been changed to an add-on code. This code may be reported in conjunction with code 64420, for each additional level of intercostal nerves injected. An instructional table has been added to specify how many units may be reported and if imaging guidance is included and/or if it could be reported separately.

Code 64451 has been added to describe injection(s) into nerves innervating the sacroiliac joint, with image guidance. New code 64451 inherently includes fluoroscopy or CT guidance. For injection of anesthetic agent to nerves innervating the sacroiliac joint using ultrasound guidance, an instructional parenthetical note following code 64451 has been added to see code 76999 (unlisted ultrasound procedure). An exclusionary parenthetical note has also been added following code 64451 to instruct users not to report code 64451 in conjunction with codes 64493, 64494, 64495, 77002, 77003, 77012, 95873, and 95874. Because code 64451 may be performed bilaterally, an instructional parenthetical note has been added to direct the use of modifier 50 when the procedure is performed bilaterally.

Code 64454 has been established to report injecting the superolateral, superomedial, and inferomedial genicular nerve branches. If all three of the listed nerve branches are not injected, then code 64454 should be reported with modifier 52 appended to indicate a reduction in service. An exclusionary parenthetical note has been added to preclude reporting code 64454 with new code 64624 (destruction by neurolytic agent of genicular nerve branches).

In support of the changes, instructional parenthetical notes have been added following codes 64450 and 64493.

Clinical Example (64400)

A patient with a normal neurologic examination reports headaches that include pain in one or more branches of the trigeminal nerve (ophthalmic, maxillary, or mandibular). An injection of local anesthetic with or without a steroid is performed for nerve blockade.

Description of Procedure (64400)

Identify the appropriate skin and bony landmarks bordering the procedure area. Create and place a local anesthetic wheal at the site of the injection. Penetrate the skin with the needle and inject the contents of the syringe along the course of the supraorbital nerve near the medial border of the eyebrow around the supraorbital notch. Remove the needle and observe the site for bleeding, then covered it with a sterile occlusive dressing.

Clinical Example (64408)

A 55-year-old female presents with a neurogenic cough. Injection of an anesthetic agent to the vagus nerve is performed.

Description of Procedure (64408)

Palpate the lateral neck landmarks. Guide spinal needle into paralaryngeal area. After aspiration for blood and air is performed to ensure extraluminal and extravascular position, deliver the injectant solution. Remove injection needle, then apply pressure to the injection site if needed to stop bleeding. Inspect the neck for signs of hematoma or other complications.

Clinical Example (64416)

A 54-year-old female has a six-month history of tumor that is infiltrating her arm, which is causing constant trials, and she has been unable to tolerate physical therapy (PT) or perform normal activities of daily living (ADLs) with her arm. Due to her persistent, debilitating pain, a brachial plexus block with a catheter and a continuous infusion of local anesthetic is scheduled to relieve her pain and allow her to participate in PT to improve her function.

Description of Procedure (64416)

Identify the appropriate skin and bony landmarks bordering the brachial plexus and place at the site of injection. Create a local anesthetic skin wheal. Advance a needle toward the brachial plexus and confirm correct position. Advance a catheter to lie next to the brachial plexus and subsequently infiltrate a local anesthetic and steroid into the fascial plane containing the brachial plexus using intermittent aspiration and injection. Remove the needle and observe the site for bleeding. Cover with a sterile occlusive dressing.

Clinical Example (64417)

A 68-year-old male has a three-year history of a painful mass in his deltoid that is interfering with his ability to complete ADLs. He has had poor control of his pain despite multiple medication trials and PT. Due to his persistent, debilitating pain, an axillary nerve block is scheduled to relieve his pain and improve his function.

Description of Procedure (64417)

Identify the appropriate skin and bony landmarks and place at the site of the injection. Create a local anesthetic skin wheal. Advance a needle toward the axillary nerve and confirm correct position. Infiltrate a local anesthetic and steroid around the nerve using intermittent aspiration and injection. Remove the needle and observe the site for bleeding. Cover with a sterile occlusive dressing.

Clinical Example (64420)

A 48-year-old female has a two-year history of rib pain that is interfering with her ability to complete ADLs. She has had poor control of her pain despite multiple medication trials and PT. Due to her persistent, debilitating pain, a trial of intercostal nerve block is scheduled to relieve her pain and improve her function.

Description of Procedure (64420)

Identify the appropriate skin and bony landmarks and place at the site of the injection. Create a local anesthetic skin wheal. Advance a needle at an angle of approximately 20° cephalad to the skin until the rib is contacted. With the same angle of insertion, walk the needle off the inferior border of the rib and advance 3 mm to place the tip in the space containing the neurovascular bundle between the internal and innermost intercostal muscles. After negative aspiration, inject a local anesthetic. Remove the needle and observe the site for bleeding. Cover with a sterile occlusive dressing.

Clinical Example (64421)

A 48-year-old female has a three-year history of persistent rib pain following a fall that resulted in multiple rib fractures. The pain is interfering with her ability to complete ADLs. She has had poor control of her pain despite multiple medication trials and PT. Due to her persistent, debilitating pain, a trial of intercostal nerve blocks involving multiple intercostal spaces is scheduled to relieve her pain and improve her function.

Description of Procedure (64421)

After the initial intercostal nerve block, perform additional intercostal nerve blocks at other levels. After cleaning the skin with an antiseptic solution, infiltrate 1 to 2 ml of dilute local anesthetic subcutaneously at the planned injection site at the inferior border of the rib. Advance a needle at an angle of approximately 20° cephalad to the skin until the rib is contacted. With the same angle of insertion, walk the needle off the inferior border of the rib and advance 3 mm to place the tip in the space containing the neurovascular bundle between the internal and innermost intercostal muscles. After negative aspiration, deposit local anesthetic at each of the sites. Remove the needle and cover the sites with a sterile occlusive dressing.

Clinical Example (64425)

A 48-year-old male has a three-year history of pain in his groin following an open inguinal hernia repair that is interfering with his ability to complete ADLs. He has had poor control of his pain despite multiple medication trials and PT. Due to persistent, debilitating pain, a trial of ilioinguinal or iliohypogastric nerve block is scheduled to relieve pain and improve function.

Description of Procedure (64425)

Identify the appropriate skin and bony landmarks. Palpate the anterior superior iliac spine and mark the target insertion site 2-cm medial and 2-cm inferior to the anterior superior iliac spine. Create a local anesthetic skin wheal. Advance a needle through the external oblique muscle. A loss of resistance is appreciated as the needle passes through the muscle to lie between it and the internal oblique. After the initial loss of resistance, advance the needle again until a loss of resistance is encountered as the needle passes through the internal oblique muscle and is in the plane between the internal oblique and the transversus abdominus muscle. Following negative aspiration, inject a local anesthetic and steroid. Remove the needle and observe the site for bleeding. Cover with a sterile occlusive dressing.

Clinical Example (64430)

A 48-year-old female has a two-year history of pudendal neuralgia that is interfering with her ability to complete ADLs. She has had poor control of her pain despite multiple medication trials and PT. Due to her persistent, debilitating pain, a trial of pudendal nerve block is scheduled to relieve her pain and improve her function.

Description of Procedure (64430)

Perform a bimanual examination to determine internal pelvic anatomy. Perform concentrated digital evaluation of the levator muscles, pelvic ligaments, and ischial spines. Proceed with povidone cleansing of the entire vaginal canal and cervix. Remove the speculum. Fill a 10-cc control syringe with local anesthetic with or without epinephrine. Attach a spinal needle to the 10-cc syringe. Don sterile gloves and again palpate the ischial spine and sacrospinous ligament. Perform introduction of the needle guide or trumpet, aligning with the digital palpation of the injection site. Direct the spinal needle into the needle guide. Perform an initial injection of the anesthetic into the vaginal tissue. Advance the needle through the vaginal epithelium to the sacrospinous ligament. Perform aspiration to ensure no vascular perforation has occurred and perform further injection. Advance the needle again, slightly monitoring for loss of resistance, signifying complete penetration of the sacrospinous ligament and entrance into the region of the pudendal nerve. Perform aspiration again to ensure no perforation of the major pelvic vessels. Inject the anesthetic slowly to monitor adverse effects of possible intravascular injection. Remove the trumpet and needle. Place a speculum and confirm hemostasis at the injection site. The physician may choose to use more than 10 cc of anesthetic; therefore, the syringe may require refilling and repeat injection, or a second syringe may be used. If bleeding is encountered, hold a large proctoswab in place to exert pressure on any bleeding sites. Use proctoswabs to clean the posterior fourchette of any blood or extruded anesthetic.

Clinical Example (64435)

A 34-year-old female with an intrauterine device (IUD) presented for IUD removal. The IUD string was not identified on examination, and initial probing of the cervical canal was not tolerated by the patient. Cervical dilation under cervical anesthesia is required for retrieval.

Description of Procedure (64435)

Physician places a speculum into the vagina. Position the speculum so that the cervix is centered in the operative field. Clean the cervix and lateral vagina with an appropriate solution. Fill a 10-cc syringe with local anesthetic with or without epinephrine. Place a single-tooth tenaculum at the 12-o'clock position of the cervix to stabilize the organ. Attach a spinal needle to the 10-cc syringe. Initial aspirations and then injections of the anesthetic are placed into the cervix at the 3- and 9-o'clock positions, or the 2-, 4-, 8-, and 10-o'clock positions. Inject the anesthetic slowly to ascertain infiltration of the stroma of the cervix. Confirm hemostasis at each injection site after injection. After the procedure, bleeding is often encountered from the injection site, causing the need to hold pressure with proctoswabs until stable. Once the procedure is complete, wait for complete anesthetic effect.

Clinical Example (64445)

A 25-year-old female has just undergone a right trimalleolar fracture open reduction and fixation, and the surgeon consults the anesthesiologist for pain management in the recovery room. The planned technique is a sciatic nerve block, to which the patient consents.

Description of Procedure (64445)

Identify the appropriate skin and bony landmarks. Create and place a local anesthetic skin wheal at injection site. Anesthetize the skin at the proposed entry site with a small amount of local anesthetic via a small-gauge needle. Insert an insulated stimulating needle through the skin in the gluteal region. Turn a nerve stimulator on and monitor the patient for reports of paresthesia or appropriate muscle twitches in the leg in response to nerve stimulation. Reduce the current on the nerve stimulator to confirm proximity of the needle to the sciatic nerve and to reposition if necessary to maintain a muscle twitch in the appropriate distribution with a low current. Once correct needle position is obtained, aspirate the needle to confirm the absence of blood. Following negative aspiration, administer a small test-dose of local anesthetic, monitor the patient's vital signs (VS), and question the patient about symptoms of intravascular local anesthetic injection. If there are no signs or symptoms of intravascular injection, inject local anesthetic in incremental doses with frequent aspiration to avoid intravascular injection. After completion of the injection, remove the needle. Observe the patient for any signs or symptoms of local anesthetic toxicity. After several minutes have passed, evaluate the initial effects of the sciatic nerve block by physical examination to determine if the patient is developing weakness, numbness, and pain relief in the expected nerve distribution.

Clinical Example (64446)

A 30-year-old male suffers a crushed left foot in an automobile accident. He undergoes major reconstruction of his left foot and ankle under general anesthesia. The surgeon requests a block with continuous infusion to manage postoperative pain and facilitate rehabilitation. In order to provide postoperative pain control, a continuous sciatic nerve block is performed.

Description of Procedure (64446)

Identify the appropriate skin and bony landmarks. Create a local anesthetic skin wheal at the planned needle insertion site. Advance a Tuohy needle toward the sciatic nerve. Attach a nerve stimulator to the needle and advance the needle until it is close to the nerve. A brisk motor response in the ankle, foot, or toes is noted with less than 0.4-mA stimulation. Advance a catheter through the Tuohy needle until it is 3 to 10 cm beyond its tip. Transfer the electrical connection to the catheter and evaluate nerve stimulation to confirm that the catheter is lying next to the nerve. Remove the Tuohy needle, secure the catheter in place, and inject 15 to 20 ml of a local anesthetic through the catheter. Assess block of the sciatic nerve over the next 15 to 30 minutes and start an infusion of a dilute local anesthetic.

Subcutaneous tunneling, affixation, and dressing of the catheter must be done carefully as this area is prone to bacterial contamination, both during and after the procedure.

Clinical Example (64447)

A 30-year-old male undergoes a right anterior cruciate ligament repair under general anesthesia. In order to provide postoperative pain control and increase mobility in his knee, a femoral nerve block is performed. This block will allow earlier discharge from the recovery room, decreased postoperative pain, and earlier ambulation.

Description of Procedure (64447)

Identify the appropriate skin and bony landmarks. Create a local anesthetic skin wheal at the injection site. Anesthetize the skin at the proposed entry site with a small amount of local anesthetic via a small-gauge needle. Advance an insulated stimulating needle through the skin in the groin. Turn the nerve stimulator on and monitor the patient for reports of paresthesia or appropriate muscle twitches in the quadriceps in response to nerve stimulation. Reduce the current on the nerve stimulator to confirm proximity of the needle to the femoral nerve. Reposition the needle if necessary to maintain a muscle twitch in the appropriate distribution with a low current. Once correct needle position is obtained, aspirate the needle to confirm the absence of blood. Following negative aspiration, administer a small test-dose of local anesthetic, monitor the patient's VS, and question the patient about symptoms of intravascular local anesthetic injection. If there are no signs or symptoms of intravascular injection, inject local anesthetic in incremental doses with frequent aspiration to avoid intravascular injection. After completion of the injection, remove the needle. Observe the patient for any signs or symptoms of local anesthetic toxicity. After several minutes have passed, evaluate the initial effects of the femoral nerve block by physical examination to determine if the patient is developing weakness, numbness, and pain relief in the expected nerve distribution.

Clinical Example (64448)

A 65-year-old male undergoes a right total knee replacement (27447) under general anesthesia. The surgeon requests a block with continuous infusion to manage postoperative pain and facilitate rehabilitation. In order to provide postoperative pain control and increased mobility in his knee, a continuous femoral nerve block is performed.

Description of Procedure (64448)

Identify the appropriate skin and bony landmarks. Create a local anesthetic skin wheal. Insert an insulated Tuohy needle through the skin and advance toward the femoral nerve. Confirm proper location of the needle with the use of a nerve stimulator. Advance a catheter through the needle to lie next to the femoral nerve. Next, inject a local anesthetic through the catheter with frequent aspiration and monitoring of the electrocardiogram (ECG) and pulse oximeter to avoid the possibility of intravascular injection. Secure the catheter in place and apply a sterile dressing. Then initiate a dilute local anesthetic infusion. Subcutaneous tunneling, affixation, and dressing of the catheter must be done carefully because this area is prone to bacterial contamination, both during and after the procedure.

Clinical Example (64449)

A 62-year-old female undergoes a left total knee replacement (27447) under general anesthesia. The surgeon requests a block with a continuous infusion to manage postoperative pain and facilitate rehabilitation. In order to provide postoperative pain control and increased mobility in her knee, a continuous lumbar plexus block is performed.

Description of Procedure (64449)

Identify the appropriate skin and bony landmarks. Create and place a local anesthetic skin wheal at the injection site. After infiltrating the skin and deeper tissues with local anesthetic using a small-gauge needle, connect a Tuohy needle designed to allow the introduction of a catheter to a peripheral nerve stimulator. Advance to obtain stimulation of the lumbar plexus. At this point, careful aspiration for blood and CSF is performed. Administer a test-dose of local anesthetic to rule out intravenous (IV) or intrathecal injection. Slowly inject between 15 and 30 ml of dilute local anesthetic through the needle, followed by insertion of an infusion catheter through the needle (about 5 cm past the tip of the needle). Observe the patient for signs of undesired epidural spread and associated hemodynamic changes, and for analgesia of the left leg and hip. Check the catheter for intravascular and intrathecal placement and secure in place. Once correct function of the catheter is confirmed, start a continuous infusion of a dilute local anesthetic.

Clinical Example (64451)

A 68-year-old male has a five-year history of persistent right sacroiliac pain that is interfering with his ability to complete ADLs. He has had poor control of his pain despite multiple medication trials and PT. Due to his persistent, debilitating pain, a trial of diagnostic nerve blocks to the sacroiliac joint is scheduled to relieve his pain and improve his function.

Description of Procedure (64451)

Perform the procedure under fluoroscopic guidance. Target the L5 dorsal ramus nerve at the junction of the sacral ala and S1 superior articular process. Target the S1, S2, and S3 nerves at the posterior lateral foramen of the S1, S2, and S3 foramen, respectively. Under imaging guidance, approach the target areas by introducing a spinal needle to each of the appropriate fluoroscopic landmarks. After negative aspiration, deposit local anesthetic at each of the sites. Remove the needle and stylet.

Clinical Example (64454)

A 78-year-old female has a five-year history of persistent right knee pain that is interfering with her ability to complete ADLs. She has had poor control of her pain despite multiple medication trials and PT. Due to her persistent, debilitating pain, a trial of genicular nerve blocks is scheduled to relieve her pain and improve her function.

Description of Procedure (64454)

Identify the appropriate skin and bony landmarks. Perform the procedure under fluoroscopic guidance. Target the superolateral, superomedial, and inferomedial genicular nerves adjacent to the periosteum on the medial aspect of the tibia, and at both the medial and lateral aspects of the femur at the junctions of the shaft and the epicondyle. Under imaging guidance, approach the target areas by introducing a spinal needle from either an anteroposterior or lateral entry point with the final position residing adjacent to the bone. After negative aspiration, deposit local anesthetic at each of the sites. Remove the needle and stylet.

64455 Injection(s), anesthetic agent and/or steroid, plantar common digital nerve(s) (eg, Morton's neuroma)

(Do not report 64455 in conjunction with 64632)

(Imaging guidance [fluoroscopy or CT] and any injection of contrast are inclusive components of 64479-64484. Imaging guidance and localization are required for the performance of 64479-64484)

(64470-64476 have been deleted. To report, see 64490-64495)

64479 Injection(s), anesthetic agent and/or steroid, transforaminal epidural, with imaging guidance (fluoroscopy or CT); cervical or thoracic, single level

(For transforaminal epidural injection under ultrasound guidance, use 0228T)

+ 64480	cervical or thoracic, each additional level (List separately in addition to code for primary procedure)

(Use 64480 in conjunction with 64479)

(For transforaminal epidural injection under ultrasound guidance, use 0229T)

(For transforaminal epidural injection at the T12-L1 level, use 64479)

64483	lumbar or sacral, single level

(For transforaminal epidural injection under ultrasound guidance, use 0230T)

+ 64484	lumbar or sacral, each additional level (List separately in addition to code for primary procedure)

(Use 64484 in conjunction with 64483)

(For transforaminal epidural injection under ultrasound guidance, use 0231T)

▶(64479-64484 are unilateral procedures. For bilateral procedures, report 64479, 64483 with modifier 50. Report add-on codes 64480, 64484 twice, when performed bilaterally. Do not report modifier 50 in conjunction with 64480, 64484)◀

Rationale

In support of the revision to instructions for reporting add-on procedures when performed bilaterally, the instructional parenthetical note referencing the laterality of codes 64479-64484 has been revised. As stated in the revised note, modifier 50 should be appended to codes 64479 and 64483 when performed bilaterally. However, because codes 64480 and 64484 are add-on codes, they should be reported twice when the procedure is performed bilaterally.

Refer to the codebook and the Rationale for modifier 50, *Bilateral Procedure*, guideline revisions for a full discussion of these changes.

Paravertebral Spinal Nerves and Branches

(Image guidance [fluoroscopy or CT] and any injection of contrast are inclusive components of 64490-64495. Imaging guidance and localization are required for the performance of paravertebral facet joint injections described by codes 64490-64495. If imaging is not used, report 20552-20553. If ultrasound guidance is used, report 0213T-0218T)

▶(For bilateral paravertebral facet injection procedures, report 64490, 64493 with modifier 50. Report add-on codes 64491, 64492, 64494, 64495 twice, when performed bilaterally. Do not report modifier 50 in conjunction with 64491, 64492, 64494, 64495)◀

(For paravertebral facet injection of the T12-L1 joint, or nerves innervating that joint, use 64490)

Rationale

In support of the revision to instructions for reporting add-on procedures when performed bilaterally, the instructional parenthetical note in the Paravertebral Spinal Nerves and Branches subsection has been revised to indicate that add-on codes 64491, 64492, 64494, and 64495 should be reported twice when the procedure is performed bilaterally.

Refer to the codebook and the Rationale for modifier 50, *Bilateral Procedure*, guideline revisions for a full discussion of these changes.

64490	Injection(s), diagnostic or therapeutic agent, paravertebral facet (zygapophyseal) joint (or nerves innervating that joint) with image guidance (fluoroscopy or CT), cervical or thoracic; single level
+ 64491	second level (List separately in addition to code for primary procedure)

(Use 64491 in conjunction with 64490)

+ 64492	third and any additional level(s) (List separately in addition to code for primary procedure)

(Do not report 64492 more than once per day)

(Use 64492 in conjunction with 64490, 64491)

64493	Injection(s), diagnostic or therapeutic agent, paravertebral facet (zygapophyseal) joint (or nerves innervating that joint) with image guidance (fluoroscopy or CT), lumbar or sacral; single level

▶(For injection, anesthetic agent, nerves innervating the sacroiliac joint, use 64451)◀

Rationale

In support of the establishment of code 64451, a parenthetical note following code 64493 has been added to reflect these changes to direct users to the appropriate code for injection of anesthetic agent of nerves innervating the sacroiliac joint.

Refer to the codebook and the Rationale for code 64451 for a full discussion of these changes.

Surgery | CPT Changes 2020

Neurostimulators (Peripheral Nerve)

For electronic analysis with programming, when performed, of peripheral nerve neurostimulator pulse generator/transmitters, see codes 95970, 95971, 95972. An electrode array is a catheter or other device with more than one contact. The function of each contact may be capable of being adjusted during programming services. Test stimulation to confirm correct target site placement of the electrode array(s) and/or to confirm the functional status of the system is inherent to placement, and is not separately reported as electronic analysis or programming of the neurostimulator system. Electronic analysis (95970) at the time of implantation is not separately reported.

Codes 64553, 64555, and 64561 may be used to report both temporary and permanent placement of percutaneous electrode arrays.

(64550 has been deleted)

(For transcutaneous nerve stimulation [TENS], use 97014 for electrical stimulation requiring supervision only or use 97032 for electrical stimulation requiring constant attendance)

▶(For percutaneous implantation or replacement of integrated neurostimulation system, posterior tibial nerve, use 0587T)◀

Rationale

A parenthetical note directing users to new code 0587T for percutaneous implantation or replacement of an integrated neurostimulation system for the posterior tibial nerve has been added in the Neurostimulators (Peripheral Nerve) subsection.

Refer to the codebook and the Rationale for code 0587T for a full discussion of these changes.

Destruction by Neurolytic Agent (eg, Chemical, Thermal, Electrical or Radiofrequency), Chemodenervation

Codes 64600-64681 include the injection of other therapeutic agents (eg, corticosteroids). Do not report diagnostic/therapeutic injections separately. Do not report a code labeled as destruction when using therapies that are not destructive of the target nerve (eg, pulsed radiofrequency), use 64999. For codes labeled as chemodenervation, the supply of the chemodenervation agent is reported separately.

(For chemodenervation of internal anal sphincter, use 46505)

(For chemodenervation of the bladder, use 52287)

(For chemodenervation for strabismus involving the extraocular muscles, use 67345)

(For chemodenervation guided by needle electromyography or muscle electrical stimulation, see 95873, 95874)

Somatic Nerves

64600   Destruction by neurolytic agent, trigeminal nerve; supraorbital, infraorbital, mental, or inferior alveolar branch

64605   second and third division branches at foramen ovale

64610   second and third division branches at foramen ovale under radiologic monitoring

#● 64624   Destruction by neurolytic agent, genicular nerve branches including imaging guidance, when performed

▶(Do not report 64624 in conjunction with 64454)◀

▶(64624 requires the destruction of each of the following genicular nerve branches: superolateral, superomedial, and inferomedial. If a neurolytic agent for the purposes of destruction is not applied to all of these nerve branches, report 64624 with modifier 52)◀

Rationale

In support of the establishment of new codes to report procedures related to the genicular nerves, code 64624 has been added. Code 64624 requires destruction of the superolateral, superomedial, and inferomedial genicular nerve branches. Code 64624 should be reported with modifier 52 appended to indicate a reduction in service, if a neurolytic agent for the purposes of destruction is not applied to all of these nerve branches. An exclusionary parenthetical note has been added to preclude reporting code 64624 with new code 64454 (injection(s) of anesthetic agent(s) and/or steroid into genicular nerve branches).

Refer to the codebook and the Rationale for codes 64400-64454 for a full discussion of these changes.

Clinical Example (64624)

A 78-year-old female has a five-year history of persistent right knee pain that is interfering with her ability to complete ADLs. She has had poor control of her pain despite multiple medication trials and PT. Due to her persistent, debilitating pain, a trial of genicular nerve blocks was conducted and found to temporarily relieve her pain and improve her function. She is now scheduled for genicular nerve radiofrequency lesioning to provide longer-term, sustained pain relief.

Description of Procedure (64624)

Identify the appropriate skin and bony landmarks. Perform the procedure under fluoroscopic guidance. Target the superolateral, superomedial, and inferomedial genicular nerves adjacent to the periosteum on the medial aspect of the tibia, and at both the medial and lateral aspects of the femur at the junctions of the shaft and the epicondyle. Under imaging guidance, guide a radiofrequency cannula from either an anteroposterior or lateral entry point with the final position residing adjacent to the bone. Perform motor stimulation to ensure the absence of adjacent motor fibers. After positive confirmation of sensory placement and negative motor testing, administer local anesthetic adjacent to the nerve to mitigate pain associated with radiofrequency lesioning. Perform radiofrequency ablation. The target tissue should reach 80°C for 90 seconds. Remove the needle and stylet.

#● **64625** Radiofrequency ablation, nerves innervating the sacroiliac joint, with image guidance (ie, fluoroscopy or computed tomography)

▶(Do not report 64625 in conjunction with 64635, 77002, 77003, 77012, 95873, 95874)◀

▶(For radiofrequency ablation, nerves innervating the sacroiliac joint, with ultrasound, use 76999)◀

▶(For bilateral procedure, report 64625 with modifier 50)◀

Rationale

Code 64625 has been added to report radiofrequency ablation to nerves innervating the sacroiliac joint with image guidance.

New code 64625 inherently includes fluoroscopy or CT guidance. Therefore, fluoroscopic and CT guidance codes 77002, 77003, and 77012 are included in the list of codes in the new exclusionary parenthetical note following code 64625. To provide further guidance, a parenthetical note following code 64625 has been added instructing users to see code 76999, *Unlisted ultrasound procedure*, for radiofrequency ablation to nerves innervating the sacroiliac joint with ultrasound.

Because this procedure may be performed bilaterally, instruction has been added to append modifier 50 when the procedure is performed bilaterally.

Clinical Example (64625)

A 68-year-old male has a five-year history of persistent right sacroiliac joint pain and struggles to complete ADLs. He has had poor pain control despite multiple medication trials and PT. Subsequently, a trial of diagnostic nerve blocks was conducted, which temporarily relieved his pain and improved his function. He is now scheduled for radiofrequency ablation of the nerves innervating the sacroiliac joint to provide longer-term, sustained pain relief.

Description of Procedure (64625)

Perform the procedure under fluoroscopic guidance. Target the L5 dorsal ramus nerve at the junction of the sacral ala and S1 superior articular process. Target the S1, S2, and S3 nerves at multiple points along the posterior lateral foramen of the S1, S2, and S3 foramen, respectively. Under imaging guidance, guide a radiofrequency cannula to the appropriate fluoroscopic landmark. Perform sensory stimulation. After further anesthetic is injected, perform radiofrequency ablation at 60°C for 150 seconds. Remove the needle and stylet.

64624 Code is out of numerical sequence. See 64605-64612

64625 Code is out of numerical sequence. See 64605-64612

64633 Destruction by neurolytic agent, paravertebral facet joint nerve(s), with imaging guidance (fluoroscopy or CT); cervical or thoracic, single facet joint

(For bilateral procedure, report 64633 with modifier 50)

#+ **64634** cervical or thoracic, each additional facet joint (List separately in addition to code for primary procedure)

(Use 64634 in conjunction with 64633)

▶(For bilateral procedure, report 64634 twice. Do not report modifier 50 in conjunction with 64634)◀

64635 lumbar or sacral, single facet joint

(For bilateral procedure, report 64635 with modifier 50)

#+ **64636** lumbar or sacral, each additional facet joint (List separately in addition to code for primary procedure)

(Use 64636 in conjunction with 64635)

▶(For bilateral procedure, report 64636 twice. Do not report modifier 50 in conjunction with 64636)◀

(Do not report 64633-64636 in conjunction with 77003, 77012)

(For destruction by neurolytic agent, individual nerves, sacroiliac joint, use 64640)

Rationale

In support of the revision to instructions for reporting add-on procedures when performed bilaterally, the instructional parenthetical notes for add-on codes 64634 and 64636 have been revised to indicate that these codes should be reported twice when the procedure is performed bilaterally.

Refer to the codebook and the Rationale for modifier 50, *Bilateral Procedure*, guideline revisions for a full discussion of these changes.

Eye and Ocular Adnexa

Anterior Segment

Iris, Ciliary Body

Destruction

66700	Ciliary body destruction; diathermy
66710	cyclophotocoagulation, transscleral
▲ 66711	cyclophotocoagulation, endoscopic, without concomitant removal of crystalline lens

▶(For endoscopic cyclophotocoagulation performed at same encounter as extracapsular cataract removal with intraocular lens insertion, see 66987, 66988)◀

(Do not report 66711 in conjunction with 66990)

66720	cryotherapy
66740	cyclodialysis

Rationale

In support of the revision of codes 66711, 66982, and 66984 and addition of codes 66987 and 66988, a new instructional note has been added following code 66711 directing users to report new codes 66987 and 66988 when endoscopic cyclophotocoagulation is performed at the same encounter as an extracapsular cataract removal with intraocular lens insertion.

Refer to the codebook and the Rationale for codes 66987 and 66988 for a full discussion of these changes.

Clinical Example (66711)

A 66-year-old patient with a history of chronic glaucoma has progressive optic nerve damage and elevated intraocular pressure (IOP) that has not been controlled by medical therapy and a previous filtering operation. The patient is pseudophakic with a miotic pupil.

Description of Procedure (66711)

Insert a lid speculum to allow adequate visualization. Make a multiplanar temporal clear corneal incision into the anterior chamber. Inject a small amount of viscoelastic into the anterior chamber, over the pupil and lens to protect the cornea. Then inject viscoelastic under the iris root for 180°. Use viscodissection to carefully separate the iris adhesions to the lens capsule and intraocular lens (IOL), to facilitate visualization of the ciliary body processes with the endoscope. Insert the endoscope or laser probe through the temporal incision to view the nasal ciliary processes on the heads-up display across the bed from the operating microscope. Re-inject viscoelastic to those areas that need additional release of adhesions under direct visualization with the endoscope. While periodically viewing the position of the handpieces through the operating microscope, and continually having the OR staff manually adjusting and orienting the focus of the image on the endocyclophotocoagulation display from the light-pipe or endoscope laser probe, coagulate the ciliary processes through the endoscope. Move the endoscope slowly in an arc of 180° allowing treatment of each individual ciliary process for several seconds with an endpoint of shrinkage and whitening. Reposition the probe to slowly apply a second row of cyclophotocoagulation to the portion of the pars plicata immediately inferior to the ciliary processes and remove the probe. Make a second multiplanar corneal incision 90° away from the first. Insert the endoscope or laser probe through this second incision and treat the contralateral ciliary processes and pars plicata to complete treatment of 270° of the processes. After completion of laser therapy, remove the viscoelastic material from the anterior segment of the eye with an irrigation and aspiration handpiece, with careful attention to remove viscoelastic trapped behind the iris. Confirm that the IOL remains in proper position. Remove the iris hooks one by one. Perform a peripheral iridectomy, as necessary. Inject a miotic drug into the anterior chamber to produce pupillary miosis, as needed. Inject a corticosteroid drug into the anterior chamber and subconjunctival space. Reform the eye with balanced-salt solution. Test the incisions for leaks. Suture any incisions that leak. Remove the lid speculum. Place an antibiotic ointment on the eye, as necessary. Place a soft patch and a rigid shield on the operative eye.

Intraocular Lens Procedures

▲ **66982** Extracapsular cataract removal with insertion of intraocular lens prosthesis (1-stage procedure), manual or mechanical technique (eg, irrigation and aspiration or phacoemulsification), complex, requiring devices or techniques not generally used in routine cataract surgery (eg, iris expansion device, suture support for intraocular lens, or primary posterior capsulorrhexis) or performed on patients in the amblyogenic developmental stage; without endoscopic cyclophotocoagulation

▶(For complex extracapsular cataract removal with concomitant endoscopic cyclophotocoagulation, use 66987)◀

(For insertion of ocular telescope prosthesis including removal of crystalline lens, use 0308T)

#● **66987** with endoscopic cyclophotocoagulation

▶(For complex extracapsular cataract removal without endoscopic cyclophotocoagulation, use 66982)◀

▶(For insertion of ocular telescope prosthesis including removal of crystalline lens, use 0308T)◀

66983 Intracapsular cataract extraction with insertion of intraocular lens prosthesis (1 stage procedure)

(Do not report 66983 in conjunction with 0308T)

▲ **66984** Extracapsular cataract removal with insertion of intraocular lens prosthesis (1 stage procedure), manual or mechanical technique (eg, irrigation and aspiration or phacoemulsification); without endoscopic cyclophotocoagulation

(For complex extracapsular cataract removal, use 66982)

▶(For extracapsular cataract removal with concomitant endoscopic cyclophotocoagulation, use 66988)◀

(For insertion of ocular telescope prosthesis including removal of crystalline lens, use 0308T)

#● **66988** with endoscopic cyclophotocoagulation

▶(For extracapsular cataract removal without endoscopic cyclophotocoagulation, use 66984)◀

▶(For complex extracapsular cataract removal with endoscopic cyclophotocoagulation, use 66987)◀

▶(For insertion of ocular telescope prosthesis, including removal of crystalline lens, use 0308T)◀

66987 Code is out of numerical sequence. See 66940-66984

66988 Code is out of numerical sequence. See 66983-66986

Rationale

Codes 66711, 66982, and 66984 have been revised to clarify reporting of endoscopic cyclophotocoagulation when performed at the same time as cataract surgery.

Code 66711 has been revised by adding "without concomitant removal of crystalline lens," and codes 66982 and 66984 by adding "without endoscopic cyclophotocoagulation." In addition to revising these codes, instructional parenthetical notes have been added following codes 66711, 66982, and 66984.

Along with revisions to codes 66711, 66982, and 66984, two new codes (66987, 66988) have been created. Code 66987 is a child code to code 66982 with two instructional parenthetical notes added. Code 66988 is a child code to code 66984 with three instructional parenthetical notes added.

With the establishment of child codes 66987 and 66988 from the revision of codes 66982 and 66984, the new child codes have been resequenced. These codes have been revised because code 66711 was typically performed with cataract surgery, and after review by RUC, it was requested that a code for endoscopic cyclophotocoagulation when it is performed with cataract surgery should be created.

Clinical Example (66982)

A 71-year-old female presents with chronic angle closure glaucoma and posterior synechiae with fixed miotic pupil and has now developed a cataract. Cataract removal with IOL placement is recommended with iris hooks to open the small pupil.

Description of Procedure (66982)

Insert a lid speculum. Position the microscope. Make a side-port incision 45° to 90° away from the intended site of the surgical incision. Fill the anterior chamber with viscoelastic. Create a temporal multiplanar limbal or corneal incision into the anterior chamber. Make four additional 1-mm incisions at the limbus in order to place iris hooks in a diamond pattern around the eye. One by one, insert the iris hooks into the incisions and manipulate to retract the iris. Reposition the iris hooks in the areas of loose zonules to better support the iris and capsule during subsequent steps of cataract removal. Enter the eye through the main incision with a sharp, bent needle to open the anterior capsule, followed by forceps to fashion a circular opening in the anterior capsule of the cataract. Insert a cannula into the eye to perform hydrodissection by injecting balanced-salt solution between the lens cortex and capsule, loosening the nuclear and cortical layers of the lens in the process, while maintaining the integrity of the capsule. Hydrodelineate as needed by injecting balanced-salt solution between the lens cortex and nucleus. Inject additional viscoelastic into the anterior chamber of the eye before phacoemulsification. Check the function of the phacoemulsification handpiece and the machine settings. Remove bubbles by tapping the handpiece with irrigation on. Insert the phacoemulsification tip into the eye and a second instrument through the side-port incision. Using both hands, as well as the foot-actuated phaco pedal, carefully perform phacoemulsification with simultaneous aspiration of the lens nuclear material. Rotate and disassemble the lens to avoid inadvertent trauma to the cornea, lens capsule, or iris. Add viscoelastic as needed to maintain a safe working space. Remove the phacoemulsification tip and the second instrument from the eye once all of the nuclear material has been removed. Introduce an irrigation and aspiration tip into the eye to aspirate the remainder of the cortical lens material. Then carefully vacuum and polish the interior surface of the thin-lens capsule in an attempt to avoid future secondary-membrane formation. Assess the integrity of the capsule and zonules and determine how much additional support the capsular bag and intraocular lens (IOL) will require. Enlarge incisions and create scleral flaps as needed for the IOL and support system chosen. Insert and suture a capsular tension ring or segment as needed. While maintaining traction on the eye via the side-port incision, insert the tip of the IOL injection device into the main incision and place the IOL in the eye. Once in the eye, allow the IOL to unfold without damage to the cornea. Properly position and center the IOL using a lens hook. Suture the IOL and/or capsular bag or zonular complex, as needed. Remove the viscoelastic material from the anterior segment of the eye with an irrigation and aspiration handpiece. Remove the iris hooks one by one. Perform a peripheral iridectomy, as necessary. Inject a miotic drug into the anterior chamber to produce pupillary miosis, as needed. Reform the eye with balanced-salt solution and adjust the intraocular pressure to a physiologic range. Test the incisions for leaks. Suture any incisions that leak. Remove the lid speculum. Place an antibiotic ointment on the eye, as necessary. Place a soft patch and a rigid shield on the operative eye.

Clinical Example (66984)

A 70-year-old female complains of vision problems. Examination reveals that a cataract in her right eye has progressed to the point of visual impairment. She has difficulty reading and recently failed a driving test.

Description of Procedure (66984)

Insert a lid speculum. Position the microscope. Make a side-port incision 45° to 90° away from the intended site of the surgical incision. Fill the anterior chamber with viscoelastic. Create a temporal multiplanar limbal or corneal incision into the anterior chamber. Enter the eye through the main incision with a sharp, bent needle to open the anterior capsule, followed by forceps to fashion a circular opening in the anterior capsule of the cataract. Insert a cannula into the eye to perform hydrodissection by injecting balanced-salt solution between the lens cortex and capsule, loosening the nuclear and cortical layers of the lens in the process, while maintaining the integrity of the capsule. Hydrodelineate as needed by injecting fluid between the lens cortex and nucleus. Inject additional viscoelastic into the anterior chamber prior to phacoemulsification. Check the function of the phacoemulsification handpiece and machine settings. Remove bubbles by tapping the handpiece with irrigation on. Insert the phacoemulsification tip into the eye and a second instrument through the side-port incision. Using both hands and the foot-actuated phaco pedal, carefully perform phacoemulsification with simultaneous aspiration of the lens nuclear material. Rotate and disassemble the lens to avoid inadvertent trauma to the cornea, lens capsule, or iris. Add viscoelastic as needed to maintain a safe working space. Remove the phacoemulsification tip and second instrument from the eye. Introduce an irrigation and aspiration tip into the eye to aspirate the remainder of the cortical lens material. Then carefully vacuum and polish the interior surface of the thin-lens capsule in an attempt to avoid future secondary-membrane formation. Adjust the size of the incision as needed to accommodate the intraocular lens (IOL). While maintaining traction on the eye via the side-port incision, insert the tip of the IOL injection device into the main incision and place the IOL in the eye. Once in the eye, allow the IOL to unfold without damage to the cornea. Properly position and center the IOL into the capsular bag using a lens hook. Remove the viscoelastic material from the anterior segment of the eye with an irrigation and aspiration handpiece. Inject a miotic drug into the anterior chamber to produce pupillary miosis, as needed. Reform the eye with balanced-salt solution and adjust the intraocular pressure to a physiologic range. Test the incisions for leaks. Suture any incisions that leak. Remove the lid speculum. Place an antibiotic ointment on the eye, as necessary. Place a soft patch and a rigid shield on the operative eye.

Clinical Example (66987)

A 66-year-old female with a history of visually significant cataract and chronic glaucoma that is not controlled by current therapy. Combined cataract removal, IOL implantation, and treatment of the ciliary processes with endoscopic cyclophotocoagulation to reduce aqueous production are recommended.

Description of Procedure (66987)

Insert a lid speculum. Make a side-port incision remote from the anticipated surgical incision. Fill the anterior chamber with viscoelastic. Create a temporal multiplanar limbal or corneal incision into the anterior chamber. Make four additional 1-mm incisions at the limbus in order to place iris hooks in a diamond pattern around the eye. One by one, insert the iris hooks into the incisions and manipulate to retract the iris. Reposition the iris hooks in the areas of loose zonules to better support the iris and capsule during subsequent steps of cataract removal. Use a sharp, bent needle and forceps to fashion an opening in the anterior capsule of the cataract. Perform hydrodissection by injecting fluid between the lens cortex and capsule, loosening the lens in the process. Hydrodelineate as needed by injecting fluid between the lens cortex and nucleus. Inject additional viscoelastic into the anterior chamber before phacoemulsification. Check the function of the phacoemulsification handpiece and machine settings. Remove bubbles by tapping the handpiece with irrigation on. Insert the phacoemulsification tip into the eye. Perform phacoemulsification with simultaneous aspiration of the lens nuclear material. Rotate and disassemble the lens to avoid inadvertent trauma to the cornea, lens capsule, or iris. Use the side-port incision to allow access for a second instrument to aid in the disassembly process. Remove the phacoemulsification tip from the eye once all of the nuclear material has been removed. Introduce an irrigation-aspiration tip into the eye to aspirate the remainder of the cortical lens material. Then carefully vacuum and polish the thin posterior lens capsule in an attempt to avoid future secondary-membrane formation. Assess the integrity of the capsule and zonules and determine how much additional support the capsular bag and IOL will require. Enlarge incisions and create scleral flaps as needed for the IOL and support system chosen. Insert and suture a capsular tension ring or segment as needed. Place the IOL in the eye using an injection device. Once in the eye, position and center the lens properly using a lens hook. Suture the IOL and/or capsular bag or zonular complex as needed. Re-inject a small amount of viscoelastic into the anterior chamber, over the pupil and lens to protect the cornea. Then inject viscoelastic under the iris root for 180° to facilitate visualization of the ciliary body processes with the endoscope. Insert the endoscope or laser probe through the temporal incision to view the nasal ciliary processes on the heads-up display across the bed from the operating microscope. While periodically viewing the position of the handpieces through the operating microscope, and continually having the OR staff manually adjusting and orienting the focus of the image on the endocyclophotocoagulation display from the light-pipe probe, coagulate the ciliary processes through the endoscope with the endpoint of shrinkage and whitening. Move the endoscope slowly in an arc, allowing treatment of each individual process over an arc of 180°, and remove the probe. Make a second corneal incision 90° away from the first or enlarge the prior side-port incision if it is properly positioned. Insert the endoscope or laser probe through this second incision and treat the contralateral ciliary processes to complete treatment of 270° to 360° of the processes. After completion of laser therapy, remove the viscoelastic material from the anterior segment of the eye with an irrigation and aspiration handpiece, with careful attention to remove viscoelastic trapped behind the iris. Confirm that the IOL remains in the proper position. Remove the iris hooks one by one. Perform a peripheral iridectomy, as necessary. Inject a miotic drug into the anterior chamber to produce pupillary miosis, as needed. Inject a corticosteroid drug into the anterior chamber. Reform the eye with balanced-salt solution. Test the incisions for leaks. Suture any incisions that leak. Remove the lid speculum. Place an antibiotic ointment on the eye, as necessary. Place a soft patch and a rigid shield on the operative eye.

Clinical Example (66988)

A 66-year-old male with a history of visually significant cataract and chronic glaucoma that is not controlled by current therapy. Combined cataract removal, IOL implantation, and treatment of the ciliary processes to reduce aqueous production are recommended.

Description of Procedure (66988)

Insert a lid speculum. Position the microscope. Make a side-port incision away from the intended site of the surgical incision. Fill the anterior chamber with viscoelastic. Create a temporal multiplanar limbal or corneal incision into the anterior chamber. Use a sharp, bent needle and forceps to fashion an opening in the anterior capsule of the cataract. Perform hydrodissection by injecting fluid between the lens cortex and capsule, loosening the lens in the process. Hydrodelineate as needed by injecting fluid between the lens cortex and nucleus. Inject additional viscoelastic into the anterior chamber before phacoemulsification. Check the function of the phacoemulsification handpiece and machine settings. Remove bubbles by tapping the handpiece with irrigation on. Insert the phacoemulsification tip into the eye. Perform phacoemulsification with simultaneous aspiration of the lens nuclear material. Rotate and disassemble the lens to avoid inadvertent trauma to the cornea, lens capsule, or iris. Use the side-port incision to allow access for a second instrument to aid in the disassembly process. Remove the phacoemulsification tip from the eye. Introduce an irrigation-aspiration tip into the eye to aspirate the remainder of the cortical lens material. Then carefully vacuum and polish the thin posterior lens capsule in an attempt to avoid future secondary-membrane formation. Adjust the size of the incision as needed to accommodate the IOL. Place the IOL in the eye using an injection device. Once in the eye, properly position and center the IOL using a lens hook. Re-inject a small amount of viscoelastic into the anterior chamber, over the pupil and lens to protect the cornea. Then inject viscoelastic under the iris root for 180° to facilitate visualization of the ciliary body processes with the endoscope. Insert the endoscope or laser probe through the temporal incision, viewing the nasal ciliary processes on the heads-up display across the bed from the operating microscope. While periodically viewing the position of the handpieces through the operating microscope, and continually having the OR staff manually adjusting and orienting the focus of the image on the endocyclophotocoagulation display from the light-pipe probe, coagulate the ciliary processes through the endoscope with the endpoint of shrinkage and whitening. Move the endoscope slowly in an arc, allowing treatment of each individual process over an arc of 180°, and remove the probe. Make a second corneal incision 90° away from the first or enlarge the prior side-port incision if it is properly positioned. Insert the endoscope or laser probe through this second incision and treat the contralateral ciliary processes to complete treatment of 270° to 360° of the processes. After completion of laser therapy, remove the viscoelastic material from the anterior segment of the eye with an irrigation and aspiration handpiece, with careful attention to remove viscoelastic trapped behind the iris. Confirm that the IOL remains in the proper position. Remove the iris hooks one by one. Perform a peripheral iridectomy, as necessary. Inject a miotic drug into the anterior chamber to produce pupillary miosis, as needed. Inject a corticosteroid drug into the anterior chamber. Reform the eye with balanced-salt solution. Test the incisions for leaks. Suture any incisions that leak. Remove the lid speculum. Place an antibiotic ointment on the eye, as necessary. Place a soft patch and a rigid shield on the operative eye.

Ocular Adnexa

Eyelids

Repair (Brow Ptosis, Blepharoptosis, Lid Retraction, Ectropion, Entropion)

67911 Correction of lid retraction

▶(For obtaining autologous graft materials, see 15769, 20920, 20922)◀

▶(For correction of lid defects using fat harvested via liposuction technique, see 15773, 15774)◀

(For correction of trichiasis by mucous membrane graft, use 67835)

67912 Correction of lagophthalmos, with implantation of upper eyelid lid load (eg, gold weight)

Rationale

In support of the deletion of code 20926 and addition of codes 15769, 15773, and 15774, the parenthetical note following code 67911 has been revised by replacing the deleted code with new autologous soft tissue grafting code 15769. In addition, a new cross-reference parenthetical note has been added directing users to the new autologous fat grafting codes 15773 and 15774.

Refer to the codebook and the Rationale for codes 15769, 15773, 15774, and 20926 for a full discussion of these changes.

Conjunctiva

Incision and Drainage

68040 Expression of conjunctival follicles (eg, for trachoma)

(To report automated evacuation of meibomian glands, use 0207T)

▶(For manual evacuation of meibomian glands, use 0563T)◀

Rationale

In support of the addition of code 0563T, a cross-reference parenthetical note has been added following code 68040 directing users to the appropriate code to report manual evacuation of meibomian glands.

Refer to the codebook and the Rationale for code 0563T for a full discussion of these changes.

Auditory System

Middle Ear

Incision

69433 Tympanostomy (requiring insertion of ventilating tube), local or topical anesthesia

(For bilateral procedure, report 69433 with modifier 50)

▶(For tympanostomy requiring insertion of ventilating tube, with iontophoresis, using an automated tube delivery system, use 0583T)◀

69436 Tympanostomy (requiring insertion of ventilating tube), general anesthesia

(For bilateral procedure, report 69436 with modifier 50)

Rationale

In support of the establishment of new Category III code 0583T to report tympanostomy with iontophoresis, a parenthetical note has been added following code 69433 directing users to the appropriate code to report tympanostomy requiring insertion of ventilating tube with iontophoresis using an automated tube-delivery system.

Refer to the codebook and the Rationale for code 0583T for a full discussion of these changes.

Operating Microscope

▶The surgical microscope is employed when the surgical services are performed using the techniques of microsurgery. Code 69990 should be reported (without modifier 51 appended) in addition to the code for the primary procedure performed. Do not use 69990 for visualization with magnifying loupes or corrected vision. Do not report 69990 in addition to procedures where use of the operating microscope is an inclusive component (15756-15758, 15842, 19364, 19368, 20955-20962, 20969-20973, 22551, 22552, 22856-22861, 26551-26554, 26556, 31526, 31531, 31536, 31541, 31545, 31546, 31561, 31571, 43116, 43180, 43496, 46601, 46607, 49906, 61548, 63075-63078, 64727, 64820-64823, 64912, 64913, 65091-68850, 0184T, 0308T, 0402T, 0583T).◀

+ **69990** Microsurgical techniques, requiring use of operating microscope (List separately in addition to code for primary procedure)

Rationale

In support of the establishment of new Category III code 0583T to report tympanostomy with iontophoresis, the guidelines in the Operating Microscope subsection have been revised to include new code 0583T to restrict reporting with code 69990 (microsurgical techniques).

Refer to the codebook and the Rationale for code 0583T for a full discussion of these changes.

Notes

Radiology

Summary of Additions, Deletions, and Revisions

The summary of changes shows the actual changes that have been made to the code descriptors.

New codes appear with a bullet (●) and are indicated as "Code added." Revised codes are preceded with a triangle (▲). Within revised codes, or if a code symbol has been deleted, the deleted language and code symbol appear with a ~~strikethrough~~ (⊖), while new text appears underlined.

The ∕ symbol is used to identify codes for vaccines that are pending FDA approval. The # symbol is used to identify codes that have been resequenced. CPT add-on codes are annotated by the + symbol. The ⊘ symbol is used to identify codes that are exempt from the use of modifier 51. The ★ symbol is used to identify codes that may be used for reporting telemedicine services. The ⋈ is used to identify proprietary laboratory analyses (PLA) test that has an identical descriptor as another PLA test. A PLA code that satisfies Category I code criteria and has been accepted by the CPT Editorial Panel is annotated with the ↑↓ symbol.

Code	Description
▲74022	Radiologic examination, ~~abdomen;~~ complete acute abdomen series, including <u>2 or more views of the abdomen (eg,</u> supine, erect, ~~and/or~~ decubitus ~~views~~), and a single view chest
▲74210	Radiologic examination<u>, pharynx and/or cervical esophagus, including scout neck radiograph(s) and delayed image(s), when performed, contrast (eg, barium) study</u>; ~~pharynx and/or cervical esophagus~~
▲74220	Radiologic examination<u>, esophagus, including scout chest radiograph(s) and delayed image(s), when performed</u>; ~~esophagus~~<u>single-contrast (eg, barium) study</u>
●74221	Code added
▲74230	~~Swallowing~~<u>Radiologic examination, swallowing</u> function, with cineradiography/videoradiography<u>, including scout neck radiograph(s) and delayed image(s), when performed, contrast (eg, barium) study</u>
▲74240	Radiologic examination, <u>upper</u> gastrointestinal tract<u>, including scout abdominal radiograph(s) and delayed image(s),</u> ~~upper~~<u>when performed</u>; ~~with or without delayed images~~<u>single-contrast (eg,</u> ~~without KUB~~<u>barium) study</u>
~~74241~~	~~with or without delayed images, with KUB~~
~~74245~~	~~with small intestine, includes multiple serial images~~
▲74246	~~with or without delayed images~~<u>double-contrast (eg, high-density barium and effervescent agent) study, including glucagon,</u> ~~without KUB~~<u>when administered</u>
~~74247~~	~~with or without delayed images, with KUB~~
+●74248	Code added
~~74249~~	~~with small intestine follow-through~~
▲74250	Radiologic examination, small intestine, ~~includes~~<u>including</u> multiple serial images <u>and scout abdominal radiograph(s), when performed</u>; single-contrast (eg, barium) study
▲74251	<u>double-contrast (eg, high-density barium and air</u> via enteroclysis tube<u>) study, including glucagon, when administered</u>
~~74260~~	~~Duodenography, hypotonic~~
▲74270	Radiologic examination, colon<u>, including scout abdominal radiograph(s) and delayed image(s), when performed</u>; single-contrast (eg, barium) ~~enema, with or without KUB~~<u>study</u>

Radiology

Code	Description
▲74280	air double-contrast with specific (eg, high density barium and air) study, with or without glucagon including glucagon, when administered
76930	Ultrasonic guidance for pericardiocentesis, imaging supervision and interpretation
78205	Liver imaging (SPECT);
78206	with vascular flow
78320	tomographic (SPECT)
#●78429	Code added
#●78430	Code added
#●78431	Code added
#●78432	Code added
#●78433	Code added
#+●78434	Code added
▲78459	Myocardial imaging, positron emission tomography (PET), metabolic evaluation study (including ventricular wall motion[s] and/or ejection fraction[s], when performed), single study;
▲78491	Myocardial imaging, positron emission tomography (PET), perfusion study (including ventricular wall motion[s] and/or ejection fraction[s], when performed); single study, at rest or stress (exercise or pharmacologic)
▲78492	multiple studies at rest and/or stress (exercise or pharmacologic)
78607	Brain imaging, tomographic (SPECT)
78647	tomographic (SPECT)
78710	tomographic (SPECT)
▲78800	Radiopharmaceutical localization of tumor, inflammatory process or distribution of radiopharmaceutical agent(s) (includes vascular flow and blood pool imaging, when performed); limited planar, single area (eg, head, neck, chest, pelvis), single day imaging
▲78801	multiple planar, 2 or more areas (eg, abdomen and pelvis, head and chest), 1 or more days imaging or single area imaging over 2 or more days
▲78802	planar, whole body, single day imaging
▲78803	tomographic (SPECT), single area (eg, head, neck, chest, pelvis), single day imaging
▲78804	planar, whole body, requiring 2 or more days imaging
78805	Radiopharmaceutical localization of inflammatory process; limited area
78806	whole body
78807	tomographic (SPECT)
#●78830	Code added
#●78831	Code added
#●78832	Code added
#+●78835	Code added

Radiology

Diagnostic Radiology (Diagnostic Imaging)

Chest

71045 Radiologic examination, chest; single view

71046 2 views

71047 3 views

71048 4 or more views

▶(For complete acute abdomen series that includes 2 or more views of the abdomen [eg, supine, erect, decubitus], and a single view chest, use 74022)◀

(For concurrent computer-aided detection [CAD] performed in addition to 71045, 71046, 71047, 71048, use 0174T)

(Do not report 71045, 71046, 71047, 71048 in conjunction with 0175T for computer-aided detection [CAD] performed remotely from the primary interpretation)

Rationale

In support of the editorial revision of code 74022, the cross-reference parenthetical note following code 71048 has been revised to be consistent with the revised language in code 74022.

Refer to the codebook and the Rationale for code 74022 for a full discussion of these changes.

Abdomen

▲ **74022** Radiologic examination, complete acute abdomen series, including 2 or more views of the abdomen (eg, supine, erect, decubitus), and a single view chest

Rationale

Code 74022 has been editorially revised to provide clarification of the views included in a complete acute abdomen series. Prior to 2020, code 74022 did not specify the number of abdominal views included in a complete acute abdomen series. Effective 2020, code 74022 specifies that two or more views of the abdomen and a single view of the chest are included.

Gastrointestinal Tract

(For percutaneous placement of gastrostomy tube, use 43246)

▲ **74210** Radiologic examination, pharynx and/or cervical esophagus, including scout neck radiograph(s) and delayed image(s), when performed, contrast (eg, barium) study

▲ **74220** Radiologic examination, esophagus, including scout chest radiograph(s) and delayed image(s), when performed; single-contrast (eg, barium) study

▶(Do not report 74220 in conjunction with 74221, 74240, 74246, 74248)◀

● **74221** double-contrast (eg, high-density barium and effervescent agent) study

▶(Do not report 74221 in conjunction with 74220, 74240, 74246, 74248)◀

▲ **74230** Radiologic examination, swallowing function, with cineradiography/videoradiography, including scout neck radiograph(s) and delayed image(s), when performed, contrast (eg, barium) study

▶(For otorhinolaryngologic services fluoroscopic evaluation of swallowing function, use 92611)◀

74235 Removal of foreign body(s), esophageal, with use of balloon catheter, radiological supervision and interpretation

(For procedure, use 43499)

▲ **74240** Radiologic examination, upper gastrointestinal tract, including scout abdominal radiograph(s) and delayed image(s), when performed; single-contrast (eg, barium) study

▶(Do not report 74240 in conjunction with 74220, 74221, 74246)◀

▶(74241 has been deleted. To report, use 74240)◀

▶(74245 has been deleted. To report, see 74240, 74248)◀

▲ **74246** double-contrast (eg, high-density barium and effervescent agent) study, including glucagon, when administered

▶(Do not report 74246 in conjunction with 74220, 74221, 74240)◀

▶(74247 has been deleted. To report, use 74246)◀

+● **74248** Radiologic small intestine follow-through study, including multiple serial images (List separately in addition to code for primary procedure for upper GI radiologic examination)

▶(Use 74248 in conjunction with 74240, 74246)◀

▶(Do not report 74248 in conjunction with 74250, 74251)◀

▶(74249 has been deleted. To report, see 74246, 74248)◀

▲ **74250** Radiologic examination, small intestine, including multiple serial images and scout abdominal radiograph(s), when performed; single-contrast (eg, barium) study

▶(Do not report 74250 in conjunction with 74248, 74251)◀

▲ **74251** double-contrast (eg, high-density barium and air via enteroclysis tube) study, including glucagon, when administered

▶(For placement of enteroclysis tube, see 44500, 74340)◀

▶(Do not report 74251 in conjunction with 74248, 74250)◀

▶(74260 has been deleted. To report, use 74251)◀

74261 Computed tomographic (CT) colonography, diagnostic, including image postprocessing; without contrast material

74262 with contrast material(s) including non-contrast images, if performed

(Do not report 74261, 74262 in conjunction with 72192-72194, 74150-74170, 74263, 76376, 76377)

74263 Computed tomographic (CT) colonography, screening, including image postprocessing

(Do not report 74263 in conjunction with 72192-72194, 74150-74170, 74261, 74262, 76376, 76377)

▲ **74270** Radiologic examination, colon, including scout abdominal radiograph(s) and delayed image(s), when performed; single-contrast (eg, barium) study

▶(Do not report 74270 in conjunction with 74280)◀

▲ **74280** double-contrast (eg, high density barium and air) study, including glucagon, when administered

▶(Do not report 74280 in conjunction with 74270)◀

Rationale

Many revisions have been made to the Diagnostic Radiology (Diagnostic Imaging), Gastrointestinal Tract subsection, which includes revisions to codes 74210, 74220, 74230, 74240, 74246, 74250, 74251, 74270, and 74280; deletion of codes 74241, 74245, 74247, 74249, and 74260; and addition of codes 74221 and 74248 to provide further granularity to the code family. Parenthetical notes describing the appropriate reporting of the revised codes and new codes have been added.

The AMA Specialty Society Relative Value Services (RVS) Update Committee (RUC) Relativity Assessment Workgroup (RAW) screen identified codes 74210, 74220, 74230, 74240, 74241, 74245, 74246, 74247, 74249, 74250, 74251, 74260, 74270, and 74280 for high-volume growth, and a recommendation was made to revise these codes to reflect current practice.

Prior to 2020, the existing codes omitted key information regarding study types and provided inconsistent guidance on whether certain components were included in each code. The revisions and additions to this code family now address the limitations and reflect the work inherent in each examination.

Code 74210 has been revised to include specific components of the radiologic examination, such as the use of oral contrast.

Code 74220 has been revised from a child code to a parent code to include the use of oral contrast, and a new child code (74221) has been added. For this type of examination, two different methods (single and double contrast) are performed and for different clinical indications. Code 74220 is intended for single-contrast study and code 74221 for double-contrast study. These services may not be reported in conjunction with each other or with codes 74240, 74246, and 74248.

Code 74230 was inconsistent with the rest of the codes in this family. Therefore, it has been revised to provide specifics on the type of radiologic examination for swallowing function. An instructional parenthetical note has been added to direct users to code 92611 when an otorhinolaryngologic fluoroscopic evaluation of swallowing function is performed.

Codes 74240 and 74241 were inconsistent with barium enema codes (74270, 74280), which include scout radiographs (KUB [kidneys, ureters, urinary bladder]) when performed. Therefore, code 74240 has been revised to remove KUB and include the use of oral contrast. An exclusionary parenthetical note has been added to preclude the use of code 74240 with codes 74220, 74221, and 74246. Code 74241 has been deleted because the services included in this code will be captured in code 74240. Code 74246 has been revised to include double-contrast studies and as a child code to code 74240. An exclusionary parenthetical note has been added after code 74246 to preclude the reporting of code 74246 with codes 74220, 74221, and 74240. Code 74248 has been added as an add-on code and should be reported in addition to codes 74240 and 74246. This will include small intestine follow-through study and multiple serial images.

Codes 74245 and 74249 have been deleted as the codes for small-bowel follow-through with upper gastrointestinal (GI) studies have been simplified into codes 74240, 74246, and 74248, and because the work inherent to this additional component is similar for both single-contrast and double-contrast upper GI examinations.

Code 74247 has been deleted as the work included overlaps with code 74246.

Code 74250 did not specify whether or not a scout abdominal radiograph is included; therefore, it has been revised to specify that scout abdominal radiographs are included.

Code 74251 has been revised to include double-contrast and glucagon. Because of the revisions to code 74251, code 74260 has been deleted as it represents an infrequently performed procedure that included key components found in code 74251.

Codes 74270 and 74280 have been revised to include a new structure and delayed images. Prior to this revision, codes 74270 and 74280 did not specify performance of delayed radiographs contained in other codes.

Clinical Example (74220)

A 65-year-old female presents with dysphagia and odynophagia. A single-contrast esophagus study is requested for evaluation of possible esophageal spasm or achalasia.

Description of Procedure (74220)

Position the patient. Obtain scout fluoroscopic image of the chest and upper abdomen. Direct the administration of oral contrast agents by the patient. Observe patient swallow contrast liquids, using different consistencies as needed, in multiple positions for the thoracic esophagus, and take multiple additional spot views. Direct the patient to various positions to better visualize the thoracic esophagus, and continue to perform intermittent fluoroscopy with spot radiographs and dynamic fluoroscopic recording as needed until contrast passes the gastroesophageal junction. Observe patient under fluoroscopic guidance and perform additional maneuvers as needed, swallow water to assess for gastroesophageal reflux. Observe patient swallow a 13-mm barium tablet under fluoroscopic guidance, if needed. Supervise the acquisition of overhead radiographs obtained by the technologist. Review final images and appropriate comparisons while dictating the final report.

Clinical Example (74221)

A 71-year-old male with history of gastroesophageal reflux presents with worsening odynophagia and chest pain. A double-contrast esophagram is requested for evaluation of possible esophageal ulcer or mass.

Description of Procedure (74221)

Position the patient. Obtain scout fluoroscopic image of the chest. Direct the administration of effervescent sodium bicarbonate crystals and water. Direct the administration of oral contrast agents by the patient.

Observe patient under fluoroscopic guidance swallow thin and thick liquids in multiple positions for the thoracic esophagus, and take multiple additional spot views. Repeat swallowing attempts, and direct the patient to various positions to distribute barium along all mucosal surfaces. Direct the patient to various positions to better visualize the thoracic esophagus, and continue to perform intermittent fluoroscopy with spot radiographs and dynamic fluoroscopic recording as needed until contrast passes the gastroesophageal junction. Observe patient under fluoroscopic guidance perform additional maneuvers as needed, swallow water to assess for gastroesophageal reflux. Observe patient under fluoroscopic guidance swallow a 13-mm barium tablet, if needed. Supervise the acquisition of overhead radiographs obtained by the technologist. Review final images and appropriate comparisons while dictating the final report.

Clinical Example (74240)

A 76-year-old female presents with dysphagia. A single-contrast upper gastrointestinal examination is requested for evaluation of possible esophageal dysmotility or hiatal hernia.

Description of Procedure (74240)

Position the patient. Obtain scout fluoroscopic image of the abdomen. Direct the administration of oral contrast agents by the patient. Observe patient under fluoroscopic guidance swallow liquids, of different consistencies as needed, in multiple positions for the thoracic esophagus, stomach, and duodenum, and take multiple additional spot views. Repeat swallowing attempts, and direct the patient to various positions to distribute barium along all mucosal surfaces. Direct the patient to various positions to better visualize the thoracic esophagus, stomach, and duodenum, and continue to perform intermittent fluoroscopy with spot radiographs and dynamic fluoroscopic recording as needed until contrast has passed the duodenojejunal junction. Observe patient under fluoroscopic guidance and perform additional maneuvers as needed, swallow water to assess for gastroesophageal reflux. Supervise the acquisition of overhead radiographs obtained by the technologist. Review final images and appropriate comparisons while dictating the final report.

Clinical Example (74246)

A 65-year-old male presents with chronic anemia and abdominal pain. A double-contrast upper gastrointestinal examination is requested for evaluation of possible gastric or duodenal ulcer or mass.

Description of Procedure (74246)

Position the patient. Obtain scout fluoroscopic image of the chest and abdomen. Direct the administration of effervescent sodium bicarbonate crystals and water. Direct the administration of glucagon as needed. Direct the administration of oral contrast agents by the patient. Observe patient under fluoroscopic guidance swallow thin and thick liquids in multiple positions for the thoracic esophagus, stomach, and duodenum, and take multiple additional spot views. Repeat swallowing attempts and direct the patient to various positions to distribute barium along all mucosal surfaces. Direct the patient to various positions to better visualize the thoracic esophagus, stomach, and duodenum, and continue to perform intermittent fluoroscopy with spot radiographs and dynamic fluoroscopic recording as needed until contrast has passed the duodenojejunal junction. Use paddle palpation to assist visualization of gastric and proximal small bowel folds, as needed. Observe patient under fluoroscopic guidance and perform additional maneuvers as needed swallow water to assess for gastroesophageal reflux. Supervise the acquisition of overhead radiographs obtained by the technologist. Review final images and appropriate comparisons while dictating the final report.

Clinical Example (74248)

A 67-year-old male with abdominal pain and concern for hiatal hernia, during a single-contrast upper gastrointestinal study under fluoroscopic guidance, requires additional evaluation of dilated small bowel loops discovered during the study and undergoes small intestine follow-through study. [**Note:** This is an add-on service. Only consider the additional work related to small intestine follow-through study.]

Description of Procedure (74248)

Position the patient. Direct the administration of effervescent sodium bicarbonate crystals and water as needed. Direct the administration of glucagon as needed. Direct the administration of oral contrast agents by the patient. Direct the patient to various positions to better visualize the duodenum, and proximal, mid, and distal small bowel in all four quadrants and distribute barium along all mucosal surfaces. Continue to perform intermittent fluoroscopy with spot radiographs and dynamic fluoroscopic recording as needed until contrast has passed the terminal ileum and reached the cecum. Use paddle palpation to assist visualization of small bowel segments. Supervise the acquisition of overhead radiographs obtained by the technologist. Review final images and appropriate comparisons while dictating the final report.

Clinical Example (74250)

A 77-year-old male in the emergency department (ED) with a history of prior abdominal surgery presents with abdominal pain and distension. A single-contrast small intestine study is requested for evaluation of possible small bowel obstruction due to adhesions.

Description of Procedure (74250)

Position the patient. Direct the administration of oral contrast by the patient. After allowing time for contrast to reach the small bowel, take a spot radiograph of the abdomen. Evaluate proximal, mid, and distal small bowel segments under fluoroscopy and take multiple additional spot views. Continue to perform intermittent fluoroscopy and spot radiographs until the contrast has reached the colon. Direct the patient to various positions to better visualize small bowel loops in all four abdominal quadrants. Use paddle palpation to assist visualization of small bowel segments. Supervise the acquisition of overhead radiographs obtained by the technologist. Compare the current imaging to all pertinent available prior studies. Dictate a report.

Clinical Example (74251)

A 66-year-old male presents with abdominal pain and weight loss. Double-contrast small intestine study is requested for evaluation of suspected malabsorption syndrome.

Description of Procedure (74251)

Position the patient. Insert the enteric catheter. Monitor the advancement of the catheter under fluoroscopy until the catheter tip is positioned in the duodenum. Administer barium through the catheter using a syringe until barium reaches the distal small bowel. Administer air through the catheter using a pump. Evaluate proximal, mid, and distal small bowel loops under fluoroscopy and take multiple spot views. Continue to perform intermittent fluoroscopy and spot radiographs until the contrast has reached the colon. Direct the patient to various positions to better visualize small bowel segments through the abdomen and in any particular area of interest. Use paddle palpation to assist visualization and separation of bowel segments. Remove the enteric catheter. Supervise the acquisition of overhead radiographs obtained by the technologist. Compare the current imaging to all pertinent available prior studies. Dictate a report.

Clinical Example (74270)

An 81-year-old male presents to the emergency department (ED) with worsening abdominal pain, distension, and melena. A single-contrast colon study is requested for evaluation of suspected colonic obstruction.

Description of Procedure (74270)

Position the patient. Review the scout abdominal radiograph(s) to ensure the colon is clear of stool. Perform a digital rectal examination to assess for rectal mass or stricture. Insert the rectal tube. With the patient in decubitus position, start the administration of barium under fluoroscopic visualization. Direct the patient to various positions to allow filling to the level of the cecum. Take multiple spot views including a lateral rectosigmoid view, the splenic and hepatic flexures, the cecum, and ileocecal region. Assess for reflux of barium into the terminal ileum. Use paddle palpation to assist visualization of the terminal ileum. Supervise the acquisition of overhead and decubitus films and postevacuation films obtained by the technologist. Compare the current imaging to all pertinent available prior studies. Dictate a report.

Clinical Example (74280)

A 65-year-old male presents with a history of colon polyps and recent episodes of hematochezia. A double-contrast colon study is ordered following an incomplete colonoscopy.

Description of Procedure (74280)

Position the patient. Review the scout abdominal radiograph(s) to ensure the colon is clear of stool. Perform a digital rectal examination to assess for rectal mass or stricture. Insert the rectal tube. With the patient in decubitus position, start the administration of barium and some air under fluoroscopic visualization. Direct the patient to various positions to allow filling to the level of the cecum. Return the patient to the upright position and drain excess barium. Move the patient to the prone and supine positions to distribute air and barium along all mucosal surfaces. Take multiple spot views including a lateral rectosigmoid view, the splenic and hepatic flexures, the cecum, and ileocecal region. Assess for reflux of barium into the terminal ileum. Use paddle palpation to assist visualization of the terminal ileum and any overlapping colonic segments. Supervise the acquisition of overhead and decubitus films and post-evacuation films obtained by the technologist. Compare the current imaging to all pertinent available prior studies. Dictate a report.

Vascular Procedures

Transcatheter Procedures

75902 Mechanical removal of intraluminal (intracatheter) obstructive material from central venous device through device lumen, radiologic supervision and interpretation

(For procedure, use 36596)

(For venous catheterization, see 36010-36012)

▶(75952, 75953, 75954 have been deleted. To report, see 34701-34711, 34718)◀

Rationale

In accordance with the conversion of Category III code 0254T to Category 1 codes 34717 and 34718, the deletion parenthetical note following code 75902 has been revised by replacing code 0254T with code 34718.

Refer to the codebook and the Rationale for codes 34717 and 34718 for a full discussion of these changes.

75989 Radiological guidance (ie, fluoroscopy, ultrasound, or computed tomography), for percutaneous drainage (eg, abscess, specimen collection), with placement of catheter, radiological supervision and interpretation

▶(Do not report 75989 in conjunction with 10030, 32554, 32555, 32556, 32557, 33017, 33018, 33019, 47490, 49405, 49406, 49407)◀

Rationale

In accordance with the establishment of codes 33017, 33018, and 33019, the exclusionary parenthetical note following code 75989 has been revised to preclude the use of codes 33017, 33018, and 33019 with code 75989.

Refer to the codebook and the Rationale for codes 33017, 33018, and 33019 for a full discussion of these changes.

Other Procedures

76376 3D rendering with interpretation and reporting of computed tomography, magnetic resonance imaging, ultrasound, or other tomographic modality with image postprocessing under concurrent supervision; not requiring image postprocessing on an independent workstation

(Use 76376 in conjunction with code[s] for base imaging procedure[s])

Radiology   CPT Changes 2020

▶(Do not report 76376 in conjunction with 31627, 34839, 70496, 70498, 70544, 70545, 70546, 70547, 70548, 70549, 71275, 71555, 72159, 72191, 72198, 73206, 73225, 73706, 73725, 74174, 74175, 74185, 74261, 74262, 74263, 75557, 75559, 75561, 75563, 75565, 75571, 75572, 75573, 75574, 75635, 76377, 77046, 77047, 77048, 77049, 77061, 77062, 77063, 78012-78999, 93355, 0523T, 0559T, 0560T, 0561T, 0562T)◀

76377   requiring image postprocessing on an independent workstation

(Use 76377 in conjunction with code[s] for base imaging procedure[s])

▶(Do not report 76377 in conjunction with 34839, 70496, 70498, 70544, 70545, 70546, 70547, 70548, 70549, 71275, 71555, 72159, 72191, 72198, 73206, 73225, 73706, 73725, 74174, 74175, 74185, 74261, 74262, 74263, 75557, 75559, 75561, 75563, 75565, 75571, 75572, 75573, 75574, 75635, 76376, 77046, 77047, 77048, 77049, 77061, 77062, 77063, 78012-78999, 93355, 0523T, 0559T, 0560T, 0561T, 0562T)◀

(76376, 76377 require concurrent supervision of image postprocessing 3D manipulation of volumetric data set and image rendering)

Rationale

In accordance with the establishment of Category III codes 0559T and 0560T (anatomic model/guide) and 0561T and 0562T (three-dimensional [3D] printing), the exclusionary parenthetical notes following codes 76376 and 76377 have been revised to preclude the use of codes 0559T-0562T with codes 76376 and 76377.

Refer to the codebook and the Rationale for codes 0559T-0562T for a full discussion of these changes.

Diagnostic Ultrasound

Genitalia

76872   Ultrasound, transrectal;

▶(Do not report 76872 in conjunction with 45341, 45342, 45391, 45392, 46948, 0421T)◀

76873   prostate volume study for brachytherapy treatment planning (separate procedure)

Rationale

In addition to the conversion of code 0249T to Category I code 46948, the exclusionary parenthetical note following code 76872 has been revised by replacing code 0249T with code 46948.

Refer to the codebook and the Rationale for code 46948 for a full discussion of these changes.

Ultrasonic Guidance Procedures

▶(76930 has been deleted. To report, see 33016, 33017, 33018)◀

76940   Ultrasound guidance for, and monitoring of, parenchymal tissue ablation

▶(Do not report 76940 in conjunction with 20982, 20983, 32994, 32998, 50250, 50542, 76942, 76998, 0582T)◀

(For ablation, see 47370-47382, 47383, 50592, 50593)

Rationale

In support of the establishment of codes 33017, 33018, and 33019, code 76930 (ultrasound guidance for pericardiocentesis) has been deleted, and a parenthetical note has been added directing users to the new codes. In addition, new code 0582T has been added to the exclusionary parenthetical note following code 76940.

Refer to the codebook and the Rationale for codes 33017, 33018, 33019, and 0582T for a full discussion of these changes.

76941   Ultrasonic guidance for intrauterine fetal transfusion or cordocentesis, imaging supervision and interpretation

(For procedure, see 36460, 59012)

76942   Ultrasonic guidance for needle placement (eg, biopsy, aspiration, injection, localization device), imaging supervision and interpretation

▶(Do not report 76942 in conjunction with 10004, 10005, 10006, 10021, 10030, 19083, 19285, 20604, 20606, 20611, 27096, 32554, 32555, 32556, 32557, 37760, 37761, 43232, 43237, 43242, 45341, 45342, 46948, 55874, 64479, 64480, 64483, 64484, 64490, 64491, 64493, 64494, 64495, 76975, 0213T, 0214T, 0215T, 0216T, 0217T, 0218T, 0228T, 0229T, 0230T, 0231T, 0232T, 0481T, 0582T)◀

(For harvesting, preparation, and injection[s] of platelet rich plasma, use 0232T)

Rationale

In support of the conversion of code 0249T to Category I code 46948 (hemorrhoidectomy) and the addition of Category III code 0582T (transurethral ablation of malignant prostate tissue), the exclusionary parenthetical note following code 76942 has been revised to reflect these changes.

Refer to the codebook and the Rationale for codes 46948 and 0582T for a full discussion of these changes.

Other Procedures

76998 Ultrasonic guidance, intraoperative

▶(Do not report 76998 in conjunction with 36475, 36479, 37760, 37761, 46948, 47370, 47371, 47380, 47381, 47382, 0515T, 0516T, 0517T, 0518T, 0519T, 0520T)◀

(For ultrasound guidance for open and laparoscopic radiofrequency tissue ablation, use 76940)

76999 Unlisted ultrasound procedure (eg, diagnostic, interventional)

Rationale

In conjunction with the conversion of code 0249T into Category I code 46948, the exclusionary parenthetical note following code 76998 has been revised by replacing code 0249T with code 46948.

Refer to the codebook and the Rationale for code 46948 for a full discussion of these changes.

Radiologic Guidance

Fluoroscopic Guidance

+ 77003 Fluoroscopic guidance and localization of needle or catheter tip for spine or paraspinous diagnostic or therapeutic injection procedures (epidural or subarachnoid) (List separately in addition to code for primary procedure)

▶(Use 77003 in conjunction with 61050, 61055, 62267, 62273, 62280, 62281, 62282, 62284, 64510, 64517, 64520, 64610, 96450)◀

▶(Do not report 77003 in conjunction with 62270, 62272, 62320, 62321, 62322, 62323, 62324, 62325, 62326, 62327, 62328, 62329)◀

Rationale

In support of the revision of codes 62270 and 62272 and the establishment of codes 62328 and 62329, the parenthetical notes following code 77003 have been revised to reflect these changes.

Refer to the codebook and the Rationale for codes 62270, 62272, 62328, and 62329 for a full discussion of these changes.

Computed Tomography Guidance

77012 Computed tomography guidance for needle placement (eg, biopsy, aspiration, injection, localization device), radiological supervision and interpretation

(Do not report 77011, 77012 in conjunction with 22586)

▶(Do not report 77012 in conjunction with 10009, 10010, 10030, 27096, 32554, 32555, 32556, 32557, 62270, 62272, 62328, 62329, 64479, 64480, 64483, 64484, 64490, 64491, 64492, 64493, 64494, 64495, 64633, 64634, 64635, 64636, 0232T, 0481T)◀

(For harvesting, preparation, and injection[s] of platelet-rich plasma, use 0232T)

77013 Computed tomography guidance for, and monitoring of, parenchymal tissue ablation

(Do not report 77013 in conjunction with 20982, 20983, 32994, 32998)

(For percutaneous ablation, see 47382, 47383, 50592, 50593)

Rationale

In support of the revision of codes 62270 and 62272 and the establishment of codes 62328 and 62329, the parenthetical note following code 77012 has been revised to reflect these changes.

Refer to the codebook and the Rationale for codes 62270, 62272, 62328, and 62329 for a full discussion of these changes.

Nuclear Medicine

Diagnostic

Endocrine System

78070	Parathyroid planar imaging (including subtraction, when performed);
78071	with tomographic (SPECT)
78072	with tomographic (SPECT), and concurrently acquired computed tomography (CT) for anatomical localization

▶(Do not report 78070, 78071, 78072 in conjunction with 78800, 78801, 78802, 78803, 78804, 78830, 78831, 78832, 78835)◀

78075 Adrenal imaging, cortex and/or medulla

Rationale

In support of the establishment of new codes 78830, 78831, 78832, and 78835, a parenthetical note to restrict reporting other radiopharmaceutical localization of tumor procedures has been added following code 78072.

Refer to the codebook and the Rationale for codes 78800-78804, 78830, 78831, 78832, and 78835 for a full discussion of these changes.

Gastrointestinal System

78201	Liver imaging; static only
78202	with vascular flow

(For spleen imaging only, use 78185)

▶(78205, 78206 have been deleted. To report, use 78803)◀

78215	Liver and spleen imaging; static only
78216	with vascular flow

Rationale

In accordance with the deletion of codes 78205 and 78206, a parenthetical note to direct users to the appropriate code for reporting liver imaging (single-photon emission computerized tomography [SPECT]) has been added following code 78202.

Refer to the codebook and the Rationale for codes 78830, 78831, 78832, and 78835 for a full discussion of these changes.

Musculoskeletal System

Bone and joint imaging can be used in the diagnosis of a variety of inflammatory processes (eg, osteomyelitis), as well as for localization of primary and/or metastatic neoplasms.

78300	Bone and/or joint imaging; limited area
78305	multiple areas
78306	whole body
78315	3 phase study

▶(78320 has been deleted. To report, use 78803)◀

Rationale

In accordance with the deletion of code 78320, a cross-reference parenthetical note directing users to the appropriate code for reporting bone and/or joint imaging, tomographic (SPECT) has been added following code 78315.

Refer to the codebook and the Rationale for codes 78830, 78831, 78832, and 78835 for a full discussion of these changes.

Cardiovascular System

▶Myocardial perfusion (SPECT and PET) and cardiac blood pool imaging studies may be performed at rest and/or during stress. When performed during exercise and/or pharmacologic stress, the appropriate stress testing code from the 93015-93018 series may be reported in addition to 78430, 78431, 78432, 78433, 78451-78454, 78472, 78491, 78492. PET can be performed on either a dedicated PET machine (which uses a PET source for attenuation correction) or a combination PET/CT camera (78429, 78430, 78431, 78433). A cardiac PET study performed on a PET/CT camera includes examination of the CT transmission images for review of anatomy in the field of view.◀

Rationale

The guidelines for diagnostic nuclear medicine for the cardiovascular system have been revised to direct users to the new and revised cardiac positron emission tomography (PET) codes.

Refer to the codebook and the Rationale for codes 78429, 78430, 78431, 78432, 78433, and 78434 for a full discussion of these changes.

78414	Determination of central c-v hemodynamics (non-imaging) (eg, ejection fraction with probe technique) with or without pharmacologic intervention or exercise, single or multiple determinations		78458	bilateral
		▲	78459	Myocardial imaging, positron emission tomography (PET), metabolic evaluation study (including ventricular wall motion[s] and/or ejection fraction[s], when performed), single study;
78428	Cardiac shunt detection			
78429	Code is out of numerical sequence. See 78458-78468	#●	78429	with concurrently acquired computed tomography transmission scan
78430	Code is out of numerical sequence. See 78483-78496			
78431	Code is out of numerical sequence. See 78483-78496			►(For CT coronary calcium scoring, use 75571)◄
78432	Code is out of numerical sequence. See 78483-78496			►(CT performed for other than attenuation correction and anatomical localization is reported using the appropriate site specific CT code with modifier 59)◄
78433	Code is out of numerical sequence. See 78483-78496			
78434	Code is out of numerical sequence. See 78483-78496		78466	Myocardial imaging, infarct avid, planar; qualitative or quantitative
78445	Non-cardiac vascular flow imaging (ie, angiography, venography)		78468	with ejection fraction by first pass technique
78451	Myocardial perfusion imaging, tomographic (SPECT) (including attenuation correction, qualitative or quantitative wall motion, ejection fraction by first pass or gated technique, additional quantification, when performed); single study, at rest or stress (exercise or pharmacologic)		78469	tomographic SPECT with or without quantification
				(For myocardial sympathetic innervation imaging, see 0331T, 0332T)
				►(Do not report 78469 in conjunction with 78800, 78801, 78802, 78803, 78804, 78830, 78831, 78832, 78835)◄
	►(Do not report 78451 in conjunction with 78800, 78801, 78802, 78803, 78804, 78830, 78831, 78832, 78835)◄	▲	78491	Myocardial imaging, positron emission tomography (PET), perfusion study (including ventricular wall motion[s] and/or ejection fraction[s], when performed); single study, at rest or stress (exercise or pharmacologic)
78452	multiple studies, at rest and/or stress (exercise or pharmacologic) and/or redistribution and/or rest reinjection	#●	78430	single study, at rest or stress (exercise or pharmacologic), with concurrently acquired computed tomography transmission scan
	►(Do not report 78452 in conjunction with 78800, 78801, 78802, 78803, 78804, 78830, 78831, 78832, 78835)◄	▲	78492	multiple studies at rest and stress (exercise or pharmacologic)
		#●	78431	multiple studies at rest and stress (exercise or pharmacologic), with concurrently acquired computed tomography transmission scan

Rationale

In support of the establishment of new codes 78830, 78831, 78832, and 78835, parenthetical notes to restrict reporting other radiopharmaceutical localization of tumor procedures have been added following codes 78451 and 78452.

Refer to the codebook and the Rationale for codes 78800-78804, 78830, 78831, 78832, and 78835 for a full discussion of these changes.

		#●	78432	Myocardial imaging, positron emission tomography (PET), combined perfusion with metabolic evaluation study (including ventricular wall motion[s] and/or ejection fraction[s], when performed), dual radiotracer (eg, myocardial viability);
		#●	78433	with concurrently acquired computed tomography transmission scan
78453	Myocardial perfusion imaging, planar (including qualitative or quantitative wall motion, ejection fraction by first pass or gated technique, additional quantification, when performed); single study, at rest or stress (exercise or pharmacologic)			►(CT performed for other than attenuation correction and anatomical localization is reported using the appropriate site specific CT code with modifier 59)◄
		#+●	78434	Absolute quantitation of myocardial blood flow (AQMBF), positron emission tomography (PET), rest and pharmacologic stress (List separately in addition to code for primary procedure)
78454	multiple studies, at rest and/or stress (exercise or pharmacologic) and/or redistribution and/or rest reinjection			
				►(Use 78434 in conjunction with 78431, 78492)◄
78456	Acute venous thrombosis imaging, peptide			►(For CT coronary calcium scoring, use 75571)◄
78457	Venous thrombosis imaging, venogram; unilateral			►(For myocardial imaging by planar or SPECT, see 78451, 78452, 78453, 78454)◄

▲=Revised code ●=New code ►◄=Contains new or revised text ✣=Duplicate PLA test ↕=Category I PLA

Rationale

The AMA/RUC had recommended a review of code 78492 for high-volume growth. In 2017, a Centers for Medicare & Medicaid Services (CMS) analysis identified utilization of 10,000 or more that has increased by at least 100% from 2009 through 2014. Therefore, RUC recommended that code 78492 and its code family be referred to the CPT Editorial Panel to undergo substantive descriptor changes to reflect newer technology aspects, such as wall motion, ejection fraction, flow reserve, and technology updates for hardware and software. Therefore, six new codes (78429, 78430, 78431, 78432, 78433, 78434) have been added to report myocardial imaging PET studies. Prior to 2020, existing codes (78459, 78491, 78492) did not describe the full extent of the work provided during each service as the technology evolved. The revisions and additions to this section reflect how imaging is now performed. In support of the establishment of codes for myocardial imaging PET studies the guidelines have been revised to include these codes and describe PET and PET/CT studies. Code 78459 has been revised to include ejection fraction, ventricular wall motion, and specify single study. Child code 78429 has been added to capture the work of reading computerized tomography (CT) transmission scan. An instructional parenthetical note directing users to code 75571 when a coronary calcium CT is performed has been added following code 78429.

Code 78491 has been revised to include ejection fraction and ventricular wall motion, when performed, and the type of stress has also been specified as exercise or pharmacologic to be consistent with other nuclear medicine codes. Code 78430 has been added as a child code to code 78491 to include the work of reading the CT transmission scan. Code 78492 (multiple studies) remains a child code to 78491, and, therefore, has also been revised to include ejection fraction and ventricular wall motion, when performed. Similar to code 78491, the type of stress has also been specified as exercise or pharmacologic to be consistent with other nuclear medicine codes. Code 78431 has been added as a child code to code 78491 to identify multiple studies with exercise and concurrently acquired CT transmission scan.

Code 78432 has been added to report a combination of the services included in codes 78459 and 78492. In addition, child code 78433 has been added to code 78432. Code 78433 includes reading CT attenuation map. An instructional parenthetical note that directs users to append modifier 59 when a CT is performed for other than attenuation correction and anatomical localization has been added following code 78433.

Add-on code 78434 has been added to report absolute quantification of myocardial blood flow PET at rest and pharmacologic stress. Code 78434 is distinct from myocardial profusion imaging (78491, 78492) in that the new procedure includes a time domain and uses separate computer processing to generate measures of global and regional absolute myocardial blood flow. This procedure requires separate technologist's work, usually on a separate computer system, and separate physician interpretive work. Absolute quantification of myocardial blood flow is performed in conjunction with code 78431 or 78492. Instructional parenthetical notes to direct users to refer to code 75571 (CT coronary calcium scoring) and to see code 78451, 78452, 78453, or 78454 for myocardial imaging by planar or SPECT have been added following code 78434.

Category III code 0482T, which was previously used to report absolute quantification of myocardial blood flow PET at rest and stress, has been deleted along with all cross-references.

In support of the establishment of new codes 78800-78804, 78830, 78831, 78832, and 78835, a parenthetical note to restrict reporting other radiopharmaceutical localization of tumor procedures has been added following code 78469.

Refer to the codebook and the Rationale for codes 78800-78804, 78830, 78831, 78832, and 78835 for a full discussion of these changes.

Clinical Example (78429)

A 67-year-old male with chronic ischemic heart disease and probable myocardial scar on positron emission tomography (PET) myocardial perfusion imaging is referred for PET cardiac metabolic imaging with combined computed tomography (CT) localization review and registration to help determine myocardial viability.

Description of Procedure (78429)

Physician evaluates the adequacy of the patient diet preparation and reviews the current glucose level for the patient with the nuclear medicine technologist or nurse, and directs technologist or nurse to adjust as necessary. Check blood glucose for all patients prior to the administration of fludeoxyglucose F-18 (FDG). Be available to prescribe, oversee, and direct the oral or intravenous (IV) administration of glucose, IV doses of insulin, and heparin, as appropriate. Instruct and oversee the nuclear medicine technologists in the administration of the radiopharmaceutical including verifying the dosage per Nuclear Regulatory Commission (NRC) and/or state regulations. After the radiopharmaceutical is administered, the patient leaves the area for approximately one hour. Direct the nuclear medicine technologist to adjust the acquisition protocol as necessary for the individual patient. If wall motion and/or ejection fraction are performed, assess the patient's cardiac rhythm. Be available to answer questions for the technologist and to review components of the study throughout the procedure. The study consists of an acquisition of tomographic PET, synchronized (gated) to the patient's electrocardiography (ECG) when performed. The PET acquisition data is followed by a separate limited CT study without moving the patient. Verify the completeness and adequacy of the data sets before completion of the study and order additional imaging as necessary. Review the PET images for artifacts and abnormal extracardiac distribution. Use CT data to generate attenuation corrected images in all three planes. Construct additional fused images from the PET and CT to correlate the anatomic position of radiopharmaceutical accumulation with the current patient anatomy (creating an interpretation display of multiple PET images, multiple CT images, and multiple fused PET images on top of CT images). Review the CT transmission scan data for proper registration, relevant cardiovascular findings or cardiovascular diagnoses, and for anatomy. The low-resolution chest CT attenuation map typically includes, but is not limited to: coronary calcifications (including a visual estimate of severity and extent), pericardial effusions, pleural effusions, pleural calcifications, ascending aortic aneurysms, descending aortic aneurysms, left atrial enlargement, dilation of the pulmonary artery, pericardial thickening and calcifications, thoracic aortic calcification, heavy aortic valve calcification (an adjunctive test for aortic valve stenosis when performed on gated noncontrast CT), large hiatal hernias, elevated hemi-diaphragms, large pneumonias, and lung masses. Assess ventricular function, when performed, by obtaining an overall ejection fraction and evaluating regional wall motion, using a standardized segment model for the data set with each segment scored as normal, mildly hypokinetic, moderately hypokinetic, severely hypokinetic, akinetic, or dyskinetic. Analyze wall motion, when performed, qualitatively for motion and thickening. Use the extent and distribution of wall motion abnormalities to judge the amount of underlying myocardial scar. Next, assess the distribution of radiopharmaceutical uptake and the relationship to vascular geographic territories. For viability assessment, record regions with lack of uptake or uptake less than 50% of normal segments as nonviable. For inflammation assessment, record regions with myocardial uptake as consistent with inflammation. Examine potential sources of error including correct region of interest for ventricular wall motion and digitally obtained ejection fraction and such patient factors as incomplete dietary preparation or persistent insulin resistance that would explain unanticipated distribution of radiotracer. Integrate results of wall motion assessment, radiotracer uptake pattern, and prior perfusion data, when available, to determine the presence of viability, hibernating myocardium, scar/fibrosis, and inflammation, as appropriate. Attribute results to vascular territories. Make comparison to relevant prior studies. Produce a formal consultative report for the medical record.

Clinical Example (78430)

A 68-year-old male without known coronary artery disease has normal resting myocardial perfusion by single photon emission computed tomography (SPECT) myocardial perfusion imaging (MPI). A previous stress SPECT MPI study was nondiagnostic because of attenuation artifact. A single study PET MPI study with combined CT localization review and registration was requested to determine the presence and severity of obstructive coronary artery disease including an estimate of coronary atherosclerotic burden.

Description of Procedure (78430)

Physician instructs and oversees the nuclear medicine technologists in the administration of the radiopharmaceutical, including verifying the dosage per NRC and/or state regulations. Direct the nuclear medicine technologist to adjust the acquisition protocol as necessary for the individual patient. If wall motion and/or ejection fraction are performed, assess the patient's cardiac rhythm. Be available to answer questions for the technologist and to review components of the study throughout the procedure. The study consists of an acquisition of a single resting or stress tomographic PET study, synchronized (gated) to the patient's ECG when performed. The PET acquisition data is followed by a separate limited CT study without moving the patient. Verify the completeness and adequacy of the data sets before completion of the study and order additional imaging as necessary. Review all images for artifacts and abnormal extracardiac distribution. Use CT data to generate attenuation corrected images in all three planes. Construct additional fused images from the PET and CT to correlate the anatomic position of radiopharmaceutical accumulation with the current patient anatomy (creating an interpretation display of multiple PET images, multiple CT images, and multiple fused PET images on top of CT images). Review the CT transmission scan data for proper registration, relevant cardiovascular findings or cardiovascular diagnoses, and for anatomy. The low-resolution chest CT attenuation map typically includes, but is not limited to: coronary calcifications (including a visual estimate of severity and extent), pericardial effusions, pleural effusions, pleural calcifications, ascending aortic aneurysms, descending aortic aneurysms, left atrial enlargement, dilation of the pulmonary artery, pericardial thickening and calcifications, thoracic aortic calcification, heavy aortic valve calcification (an adjunctive test for aortic valve stenosis when performed on gated noncontrast CT), large hiatal hernias, elevated hemidiaphragms, large pneumonias, and lung masses. Interpret the single-study stress or rest PET emission data including myocardial tracer uptake, cardiac wall motion, and left ventricular ejection fraction and examine the PET data. Review reconstructed images in three planes. Verify registration of the attenuation maps. Score images semiquantitatively on a standard segmental model as normal uptake, mildly reduced, moderately reduced, severely reduced, or absent. Attribute findings to coronary vascular territories. Score gated images, when performed, qualitatively for motion and thickening. Analyze the data set in a standardized segmental model as normal, mildly hypokinetic, moderately hypokinetic, severely hypokinetic, akinetic, or dyskinetic. Validate overall left ventricular ejection fraction, when performed, visually by checking the regions of interest that were selected for the calculation. Correlate results of left ventricular function (when performed) and radiotracer uptake (perfusion). Compare results to relevant prior studies. Produce a formal consultative report for the medical record.

Clinical Example (78431)

A 69-year-old female without known coronary artery disease has symptoms suggestive of angina pectoris. A rest/stress PET myocardial perfusion imaging study with combined CT localization review and registration is requested to determine the presence and severity of cardiac ischemia as well as an estimate of coronary atherosclerotic burden.

Description of Procedure (78431)

Physician instructs and oversees the nuclear medicine technologists in the administration of the radiopharmaceutical including verifying the dosage per NRC and/or state regulations. Direct the nuclear medicine technologist to adjust the acquisition protocol as necessary for the individual patient. If wall motion and/or ejection fraction are performed, assess the patient's cardiac rhythm. Be available to answer questions for the technologist and to review components of the study throughout the procedure. The study consists of an acquisition of both resting and stress tomographic PET studies synchronized (gated) to the patient's ECG when performed. The PET acquisition data are each followed by separate limited CT study without moving the patient. Verify the completeness and adequacy of the data sets before completion of the study and order additional imaging as necessary. Review all images for artifacts and abnormal extracardiac distribution. Use CT data to generate attenuation corrected images in all three planes. Construct additional fused images from the PET and CT to correlate the anatomic position of radiopharmaceutical accumulation with the current patient anatomy (creating an interpretation display of multiple PET images, multiple CT images, and multiple fused PET images on top of CT images). Review the CT transmission scan data for proper registration, relevant cardiovascular findings or cardiovascular diagnoses, and for anatomy. The low-resolution chest CT attenuation map typically includes, but is not limited to: coronary calcifications (including a visual estimate of severity and extent), pericardial effusions, pleural effusions, pleural calcifications, ascending aortic aneurysms, descending aortic aneurysms, left atrial enlargement, dilation of the pulmonary artery, pericardial thickening and calcifications, thoracic aortic calcification, heavy aortic valve calcification (an adjunctive test for aortic valve stenosis when performed on gated noncontrast CT), large hiatal hernias, elevated hemidiaphragms, large pneumonias, and lung masses. Interpret and correlate both stress and rest PET emission data, including myocardial tracer uptake, cardiac wall motion, and left ventricular ejection fraction, and examine the PET data. Review reconstructed images in three planes. Verify registration of the attenuation maps. Score images semiquantitatively on a standard segmental model as normal uptake, mildly reduced, moderately reduced, severely reduced, or absent. Attribute findings to coronary vascular territories. Score gated images, when performed, qualitatively for motion and thickening. Analyze the data set in a standardized segmental model as normal, mildly hypokinetic, moderately hypokinetic, severely hypokinetic, akinetic, or dyskinetic. Validate overall left ventricular ejection fraction, when performed, visually by checking the regions of interest that were selected for the calculation. Correlate results of LV function (when performed) and radiotracer uptake (perfusion). Compare results to relevant prior studies. Produce a formal consultative report for the medical record.

Clinical Example (78432)

A 65-year-old female has an ischemic cardiomyopathy with severely diminished left ventricular contractile function and three-vessel occlusive coronary artery disease. A combined metabolic and perfusion PET study(ies) is requested to determine myocardial viability to help guide revascularization therapy.

Description of Procedure (78432)

Physician evaluates the adequacy of the patient diet preparation and reviews the current glucose level for the patient with the nuclear medicine technologist or nurse and directs technologist or nurse to adjust as necessary. Check blood glucose for all patients prior to the administration of F-18 FDG. Be available to prescribe, oversee, and direct the oral or IV administration of glucose and IV doses of insulin and heparin, as appropriate. Instruct and oversee the nuclear medicine technologists in the administration of the radiopharmaceutical including verifying the dosage per NRC and/or state regulations. After the radiopharmaceutical is administered, the patient leaves the area for approximately one hour. Direct the nuclear medicine technologist to adjust the acquisition protocol as necessary for the individual patient. If wall motion and/or ejection fraction are performed, assess the patient's cardiac rhythm. Be available to answer questions for the technologist and to review components of the study throughout the procedure. The dual radiopharmaceutical multiple set of studies typically consists of a resting perfusion plus a complete metabolic study with acquisitions of tomographic PET data sets and synchronized (gated) to the patient's ECG when performed. (This service represents all aspects of code 78491 plus code 78459.) Verify the completeness and adequacy of the data sets before completion of the study and order additional imaging as necessary. Review the PET images for artifacts and abnormal extracardiac distribution and verify registration of the attenuation maps for both perfusion and metabolic data sets. Assess ventricular function, when performed, by obtaining an overall ejection fraction and evaluating regional wall motion, using a standardized segment model for the data set with each segment scored as normal, mildly hypokinetic, moderately hypokinetic, severely hypokinetic, akinetic, or dyskinetic. Analyze wall motion, when performed, qualitatively for motion and thickening. Use the extent and distribution of wall motion abnormalities to judge the amount of underlying myocardial scar. Next, assess the distribution of radiopharmaceutical uptake and the relationship to vascular geographic territories for both perfusion and metabolic images. Examine myocardial tracer uptake on the rest perfusion study. For this, review reconstructed images in three planes. Verify registration of the attenuation maps. Score images are semiquantitatively on a standard segmental model as normal uptake, mildly reduced, moderately reduced, severely reduced, or absent. Attribute findings to coronary vascular territories. Then examine radiotracer uptake on the metabolic images. For viability assessment, record regions with lack of uptake or uptake less than 50% of normal segments as nonviable. For inflammation assessment, record regions with myocardial uptake as consistent with inflammation. Examine potential sources of error, including correct region of interest for ventricular wall motion and digitally obtained ejection fraction and such patient factors as incomplete dietary preparation or persistent insulin resistance that would explain unanticipated distribution of radiotracer. Integrate results of wall motion assessment (when performed), radiotracer uptake pattern on the metabolic image set, and myocardial uptake on the perfusion image set to determine the presence of viability, hibernating myocardium, scar or fibrosis, and inflammation, as appropriate. Attribute results to vascular territories. Make comparison to relevant prior studies. Produce a formal consultative report for the medical record.

Clinical Example (78433)

A 66-year-old male has an ischemic cardiomyopathy with severely diminished left ventricular contractile function and three-vessel occlusive coronary artery disease. A combined metabolic and perfusion PET/CT study with combined localization review and registration is requested to determine myocardial viability to help guide revascularization therapy.

Description of Procedure (78433)

Physician evaluates the adequacy of the patient diet preparation and reviews the current glucose level for the patient with the nuclear medicine technologist or nurse and directs technologist or nurse to adjust as necessary. Blood glucose is checked for all patients prior to the administration of F-18 FDG. The physician is available to prescribe, oversee, and direct the oral or IV administration of glucose, IV doses of insulin and heparin, as appropriate. The physician instructs and oversees the nuclear medicine technologists in the administration of the radiopharmaceutical including verifying the dosage per NRC and/or state regulations. After the radiopharmaceutical is administered the patient leaves the area for approximately 1 hour. The physician directs the nuclear medicine technologist to adjust the acquisition protocol as necessary for the individual patient. If wall motion and/or ejection fraction are performed, the patient's cardiac rhythm is assessed. The physician is available to answer questions for the technologist and to review components of the study throughout the procedure. The dual radiopharmaceutical multiple set of studies typically consists of a resting perfusion plus a complete metabolic study with acquisitions of tomographic PET data sets and synchronized (gated) to the patient's ECG when performed. The PET acquisition data are each followed by separate limited CT study without moving the patient. (This service represents all aspects of code 78430 plus code 78429.) Verify the completeness and adequacy of the data sets before completion of the study and order additional imaging as necessary. Review the PET images for artifacts and abnormal extracardiac distribution and verify registration of the attenuation maps for both perfusion and metabolic data sets. Use CT data to generate attenuation corrected images in all three planes. Construct additional fused images from the PET and CT to correlate the anatomic position of radiopharmaceutical accumulation with the current patient anatomy (creating an interpretation display of multiple PET images, multiple CT images, and multiple fused PET images on top of CT images). Review the CT transmission scan data for proper registration, relevant cardiovascular findings or cardiovascular diagnoses, and for anatomy. The low-resolution chest CT attenuation map typically includes, but is not limited to: coronary calcifications (including a visual estimate of severity and extent), pericardial effusions, pleural effusions, pleural calcifications, ascending aortic aneurysms, descending aortic aneurysms, left atrial enlargement, dilation of the pulmonary artery, pericardial thickening and calcifications, thoracic aortic calcification, heavy aortic valve calcification (an adjunctive test for aortic valve stenosis when performed on gated noncontrast CT), large hiatal hernias, elevated hemidiaphragms, large pneumonias, and lung masses. Assess ventricular function, when performed, by obtaining an overall ejection fraction and evaluating regional wall motion, using a standardized segment model for the data set with each segment scored as normal, mildly hypokinetic, moderately hypokinetic, severely hypokinetic, akinetic, or dyskinetic. Analyze wall motion, when performed, qualitatively for motion and thickening. Use the extent and distribution of wall motion abnormalities to judge the amount of underlying myocardial scar. Next, assess the distribution of radiopharmaceutical uptake and the relationship to vascular geographic territories for both perfusion and metabolic images. Examine myocardial tracer uptake on the rest perfusion study. For this, review reconstructed images in three planes. Verify registration of the attenuation maps. Score images semiquantitatively on a standard segmental model as normal uptake, mildly reduced, moderately reduced, severely reduced, or absent. Attribute findings to coronary vascular territories. Then examine radiotracer uptake on the metabolic images. For viability assessment, record regions with lack of uptake or uptake less than 50% of normal segments as nonviable. For inflammation assessment, record regions with myocardial uptake as consistent with inflammation. Examine potential sources of error, including correct region of interest for ventricular wall motion and digitally obtained ejection fraction and such patient factors as incomplete dietary preparation or persistent insulin resistance that would explain unanticipated distribution of radiotracer. Integrate results of wall motion assessment (when performed), radiotracer uptake pattern on the metabolic image set, and myocardial uptake on the perfusion image set to determine the presence of viability, hibernating myocardium, scar or fibrosis, and inflammation, as appropriate. Attribute results to vascular territories. Make comparison to relevant prior studies. Produce a formal consultative report for the medical record.

Clinical Example (78434)

A 67-year-old male requires additional physiological assessment during a pharmacologic stress/rest PET or PET/CT myocardial perfusion imaging, and undergoes absolute quantitation of myocardial blood flow (AQMBF) imaging. [**Note:** This is an add-on service. Only consider the additional work related to AQMBF.]

Description of Procedure (78434)

Under the direction of the physician, following stress/rest PET or PET/CT myocardial perfusion imaging the nuclear medicine technologist acquires images for PET myocardial perfusion imaging in a manner that will also allow for AQMBF imaging (eg, images are acquired in 3D and list mode). Then re-bin the data to allow AQMBF and export the data set to a dedicated computer with software program for AQMBF. Transfer the processed data set and quality control information to the interpreting physician. Then review the quality control for AQMBF (eg, the bolus duration, peak, and plateau waveforms) and, if quality is acceptable, review the numeric output for AQMBF in ml/g/min for rest, stress, and indexed/reserve flow for each coronary bed and for the global left ventricular. Also review the interactive polar map display. Integrate the AQMBF data with the static perfusion image data, attenuation maps, clinical data, and generate an overall report.

Clinical Example (78459)

A 66-year-old male with ischemic cardiomyopathy and reduced LV function is being considered for coronary revascularization. PET myocardial metabolic evaluation is requested to determine viability of some left ventricular segments to guide therapy.

Description of Procedure (78459)

The study consists of an acquisition of tomographic PET data set and synchronized (gated) to the patient's ECG when performed. Verify the completeness and adequacy of the data sets before completion of the study and order additional imaging as necessary. Physician reviews the PET images for artifacts and abnormal extracardiac distribution and verifies registration of the attenuation maps. Assess ventricular function, when performed, by obtaining an overall ejection fraction and evaluating regional wall motion, using a standardized segment model for the data set with each segment scored as normal, mildly hypokinetic, moderately hypokinetic, severely hypokinetic, akinetic, or dyskinetic. Analyze wall motion, when performed, qualitatively for motion and thickening. Use the extent and distribution of wall motion abnormalities to judge the amount of underlying myocardial scar. Next, assess the distribution of radiopharmaceutical uptake and the relationship to vascular geographic territories. For viability assessment, record regions with lack of uptake or uptake less than 50% of normal segments as nonviable. For inflammation assessment, record regions with myocardial uptake as consistent with inflammation. Potential sources of error are examined including correct region of interest for ventricular wall motion and digitally obtained ejection fraction and patient factors such as incomplete dietary preparation or persistent insulin resistance that would explain unanticipated distribution of radiotracer. Results of wall motion assessment, radiotracer uptake pattern and prior perfusion data, when available, are integrated to determine the presence of viability, hibernating myocardium, scar/fibrosis, and inflammation, as appropriate. Results are attributed to vascular territories. Comparison is made to relevant prior studies. A formal consultative report is produced for the medical record.

Clinical Example (78491)

A 68-year-old male has normal resting myocardial perfusion by SPECT MPI, but a previous stress SPECT MPI study was nondiagnostic because of attenuation artifact. A single-study PET MPI study was requested to determine the presence and severity of obstructive coronary artery disease.

Description of Procedure (78491)

Physician instructs and oversees the nuclear medicine technologists in the administration of the radiopharmaceutical including verifying the dosage per NRC and/or state regulations. Direct the nuclear medicine technologist to adjust the acquisition protocol as necessary for the individual patient. If wall motion and/or ejection fraction are performed, assess the patient's cardiac rhythm. Be available to answer questions for the technologist and to review components of the study throughout the procedure. The study consists of an acquisition of a single resting or stress tomographic PET study synchronized (gated) to the patient's ECG when performed. Verify the completeness and adequacy of the data sets before completion of the study and order additional imaging as necessary. Review all images for artifacts and abnormal extracardiac distribution. Interpret the single-study stress or rest PET emission data, including myocardial tracer uptake, cardiac wall motion, and left ventricular ejection fraction, and examine the PET data. Review reconstructed images in three planes. Verify registration of the attenuation maps. Score images semiquantitatively on a standard segmental model as normal uptake, mildly reduced, moderately reduced, severely reduced, or absent. Attribute findings to coronary vascular territories. Score gated images, when performed, qualitatively for motion and thickening. Analyze the data set in a standardized segmental model as normal, mildly hypokinetic, moderately hypokinetic, severely hypokinetic, akinetic, or dyskinetic. Validate overall left ventricular ejection fraction, when performed, visually by checking the regions of interest that were selected for the calculation. Correlate results of LV function (when performed) and radiotracer uptake (perfusion). Compare results to relevant prior studies. Produce a formal consultative report for the medical record.

Clinical Example (78492)

A 69-year-old female has known coronary artery disease and left bundle branch block on ECG and symptoms suggestive of angina pectoris. A rest/stress PET myocardial perfusion imaging study is requested to determine the presence and severity of cardiac ischemia.

Description of Procedure (78492)

Physician instructs and oversees the nuclear medicine technologists in the administration of the radiopharmaceutical including verifying the dosage per NRC and/or state regulations. Direct the nuclear medicine technologist to adjust the acquisition protocol as necessary for the individual patient. If wall motion and/or ejection fraction are performed, assess the patient's cardiac rhythm. Be available to answer questions for the technologist and to review components of the study throughout the procedure. The study consists of acquisitions of both resting and stress tomographic PET studies synchronized (gated) to the patient's ECG when performed. Verify the completeness and adequacy of the data sets before completion of the study and order additional imaging as necessary. Review all images for artifacts and abnormal extracardiac distribution. Interpret and correlate both stress and rest PET emission data, including myocardial tracer uptake, cardiac wall motion, and left ventricular ejection fraction, and examine the PET data. Review reconstructed images in three planes. Verify registration of the attenuation maps. Score images semiquantitatively on a standard segmental model as normal uptake, mildly reduced, moderately reduced, severely reduced, or absent. Perform this for rest and stress images. Integrate the information derived from rest and stress images to determine the presence of normal perfusion, reversible defects indicating ischemia, fixed defects indicating infarction, or a combination thereof. Attribute findings to coronary vascular territories. Note abnormal changes in left ventricular size between rest and stress images if present. Score gated images, when performed, qualitatively for motion and thickening for both rest and stress images. Analyze the data set in a standardized segmental model as normal, mildly hypokinetic, moderately hypokinetic, severely hypokinetic, akinetic, or dyskinetic. Note normal increase or, if present, abnormal decline in global left ventricular function or changes in regional wall motion between rest and stress. Validate overall left ventricular ejection fraction, when performed, visually by checking the regions of interest that were selected for the calculation. Correlate results of LV function (when performed), LV size, and radiotracer uptake (perfusion) at rest and stress to make a final assessment of myocardial perfusion, inducible ischemia, and ventricular function and determine the presence or absence of high risk findings. Compare results to relevant prior studies. Produce a formal consultative report for the medical record.

78494 Cardiac blood pool imaging, gated equilibrium, SPECT, at rest, wall motion study plus ejection fraction, with or without quantitative processing

▶(Do not report 78494 in conjunction with 78800, 78801, 78802, 78803, 78804, 78830, 78831, 78832, 78835)◀

Rationale

In support of the establishment of new codes 78830, 78831, 78832, and 78835, a parenthetical note to restrict reporting other radiopharmaceutical localization of tumor procedures has been added following code 78494.

Refer to the codebook and the Rationale for codes 78800-78804, 78830, 78831, 78832, and 78835 for a full discussion of these changes.

Nervous System

78600	Brain imaging, less than 4 static views;
78601	with vascular flow
78605	Brain imaging, minimum 4 static views;
78606	with vascular flow

▶(78607 has been deleted. To report, use 78803)◀

Rationale

In support of the deletion of code 78607, a parenthetical note to direct users to the appropriate code for reporting brain imaging, tomographic (SPECT) has been added following code 78606.

Refer to the codebook and the Rationale for codes 78800-78804, 78830, 78831, 78832, and 78835 for a full discussion of these changes.

78608	Brain imaging, positron emission tomography (PET); metabolic evaluation
78609	perfusion evaluation
78610	Brain imaging, vascular flow only
78630	Cerebrospinal fluid flow, imaging (not including introduction of material); cisternography

(For injection procedure, see 61000-61070, 62270-62327)

78635	ventriculography

(For injection procedure, see 61000-61070, 62270-62294)

78645	shunt evaluation

(For injection procedure, see 61000-61070, 62270-62294)

▶(78647 has been deleted. To report, use 78803)◀

Rationale

In accordance with the deletion of code 78647, a cross-reference parenthetical note directing users to the appropriate code for reporting cerebrospinal fluid flow imaging, tomographic (SPECT) has been added following code 78645.

Refer to the codebook and the Rationale for codes 78800-78804, 78830, 78831, 78832, and 78835 for a full discussion of these changes.

Genitourinary System

78700	Kidney imaging morphology;
78701	with vascular flow
78707	with vascular flow and function, single study without pharmacological intervention
78708	with vascular flow and function, single study, with pharmacological intervention (eg, angiotensin converting enzyme inhibitor and/or diuretic)
78709	with vascular flow and function, multiple studies, with and without pharmacological intervention (eg, angiotensin converting enzyme inhibitor and/or diuretic)

(For introduction of radioactive substance in association with renal endoscopy, use 77778)

▶(78710 has been deleted. To report, use 78803)◀

78725	Kidney function study, non-imaging radioisotopic study

Rationale

In accordance with the deletion of code 78710, a cross-reference parenthetical note to direct users to the appropriate code for reporting kidney imaging morphology, tomographic (SPECT) has been added following code 78709.

Refer to the codebook and the Rationale for codes 78800-78804, 78830, 78831, 78832, and 78835 for a full discussion of these changes.

Other Procedures

(For specific organ, see appropriate heading)

▲ **78800** Radiopharmaceutical localization of tumor, inflammatory process or distribution of radiopharmaceutical agent(s) (includes vascular flow and blood pool imaging, when performed); planar, single area (eg, head, neck, chest, pelvis), single day imaging

(For specific organ, see appropriate heading)

▲ 78801 planar, 2 or more areas (eg, abdomen and pelvis, head and chest), 1 or more days imaging or single area imaging over 2 or more days

▲ 78802 planar, whole body, single day imaging

#▲ 78804 planar, whole body, requiring 2 or more days imaging

▲ 78803 tomographic (SPECT), single area (eg, head, neck, chest, pelvis), single day imaging

78804 Code is out of numerical sequence. See 78801-78811

▶(78805, 78806, 78807 have been deleted. To report, see 78300, 78305, 78306, 78315, 78800, 78801, 78802, 78803, 78830, 78831, 78832)◀

▶(For imaging bone infectious or inflammatory disease with a bone imaging radiopharmaceutical, see 78300, 78305, 78306, 78315)◀

#● 78830 tomographic (SPECT) with concurrently acquired computed tomography (CT) transmission scan for anatomical review, localization and determination/detection of pathology, single area (eg, head, neck, chest, pelvis), single day imaging

#● 78831 tomographic (SPECT), minimum 2 areas (eg, pelvis and knees, abdomen and pelvis), single day imaging, or single area imaging over 2 or more days

#● 78832 tomographic (SPECT) with concurrently acquired computed tomography (CT) transmission scan for anatomical review, localization and determination/detection of pathology, minimum 2 areas (eg, pelvis and knees, abdomen and pelvis), single day imaging, or single area imaging over 2 or more days

▶(For cerebrospinal fluid studies that require injection procedure, see 61055, 61070, 62320, 62321, 62322, 62323)◀

#+● 78835 Radiopharmaceutical quantification measurement(s) single area (List separately in addition to code for primary procedure)

▶(Use 78835 in conjunction with 78830, 78832)◀

▶(Report multiple units of 78835 if quantitation is more than 1 area or more than 1 day imaging)◀

▶(Report myocardial SPECT imaging with 78451, 78452, 78469, 78494)◀

▶(For all nuclear medicine codes, select the organ/system-specific code[s] first; if there is no organ/system-specific code[s], see 78800, 78801, 78802, 78803, 78830, 78831, 78832)◀

▶(For parathyroid imaging, see 78070, 78071, 78072)◀

78830 Code is out of numerical sequence. See 78801-78811

78831 Code is out of numerical sequence. See 78801-78811

78832 Code is out of numerical sequence. See 78801-78811

78835 Code is out of numerical sequence. See 78801-78811

Rationale

In response to an analysis of resources of the major set of imaging procedures, significant changes have been made in the Radiology, Nuclear Medicine subsection of the CPT code set. Three new codes (78830, 78831, 78832) have been added to report tomographic (SPECT) studies, and one new code (78835) has been added to report radiopharmaceutical quantification measurement(s). In support of the establishment of codes 78830, 78831, 78832, and 78835, radiopharmaceutical localization of inflammatory process codes 78805 (limited area), 78806 (whole body), and 78807 (tomographic [SPECT]) have been deleted. In addition, radiopharmaceutical localization tumor codes (78800, 78801, 78802, 78803, 78804) have been revised. These significant changes have been made to (1) address current gaps in coding for several types of SPECT-CT studies; and (2) differentiate between planar radiopharmaceutical localization procedures and SPECT-CT radiopharmaceutical localization procedures.

The newly structured generic family of codes (78800, 78801, 78802, 78803, 78804, 78830, 78831, 78832, 78835) provides two methods for radiopharmaceutical localization of tumors, either by planar or by tomographic (SPECT) technique. In particular, the radiopharmaceutical localization tumor codes (78800, 78801, 78802, 78803, 78804) have been revised to specify the body areas and the time it takes to perform the study. Similarly, the new tomographic (SPECT) codes (78803, 78830, 78831, 78832) specify the body areas and the time it takes to perform the study.

In addition, new add-on code (78835) describes radiopharmaceutical quantification measurement(s) for a single area. Code 78835 should be used in conjunction with tomographic (SPECT) codes 78830 and 78832. If quantitation involves more than one area or more than one day of imaging, multiple units of code 78835 should be reported. Two parenthetical notes have been added to support these instructions. To further support, instruct, and clarify the numerous changes made in the Nuclear Medicine subsection, instructional, exclusionary, inclusionary, deletion, and cross-reference parenthetical notes have been added and revised throughout the code set to support accurate reporting of the new and deleted codes.

Clinical Example (78800)

A 60-year-old male with swollen digit on the right foot and positive bone scan uptake recently presents for indium-labeled white blood cell (WBC) scan imaging performed at 24 hours after radiotracer re-injection. A single area of imaging is performed to evaluate for active infection and/or osteomyelitis.

Description of Procedure (78800)

Physician instructs and oversees the nuclear medicine technologists in the administration of the radiopharmaceutical including verifying the dosage per NRC and/or state regulations. Direct the nuclear medicine technologist to adjust the acquisition protocol as necessary for the individual patient. Be available to answer questions for the technologist and to review components of the study throughout the procedure. Determine the adequacy of the planar limited study and the patient positioning. Interpret the planar images obtained. Correlate the findings to previous imaging, medical information, and clinical story, and generate a report for the medical record.

Clinical Example (78801)

A 55-year-old female with history of prior sternotomy and pain with elevated sedimentation rate and suspected infection presents for Tc99m-labeled WBC planar imaging of the sternum, at 2 hours and 24 hours post radiotracer re-injection (administration) to evaluate for active infection and/or osteomyelitis.

Description of Procedure (78801)

Physician instructs and oversees the nuclear medicine technologists in the administration of the radiopharmaceutical including verifying the dosage per NRC and/or state regulations. Direct the nuclear medicine technologist to adjust the acquisition protocol as necessary for the individual patient. After review of day 1 images, determine the sequence and timing of imaging for the second day (day 2). Be available to answer questions for the technologist and to review components of the study throughout the procedure. Determine the adequacy of the day 2 planar images and the patient positioning. Interpret the 2 days/areas of planar images obtained. Correlate the findings to previous imaging, medical information, and clinical story, and generate a report for the medical record.

Clinical Example (78802)

A 61-year-old female with suspected sepsis of undetermined site based on fever, leukocytosis, and positive culture presents for indium-111 WBC evaluation of the body, performed on one day (24 hours post radiopharmaceutical administration) to determine the locus of infection.

Description of Procedure (78802)

Physician instructs and oversees the nuclear medicine technologists in the administration of the radiopharmaceutical including verifying the dosage per NRC and/or state regulations. Direct the nuclear medicine technologist to adjust the acquisition protocol as necessary for the individual patient's clinical situation and diagnosis. Be available to answer questions for the technologist and patient and to review components of the study throughout the procedure. Determine the adequacy of the initial planar images, the need for additional focused planar views, and the patient positioning. Review any additional planar views or images and then interpret whole-body planar and any additional focused images. Correlate the findings to previous imaging studies, medical information, and clinical story, and generate a report for the medical record.

Clinical Example (78803)

A 70-year-old confused male with shortness of breath and lower extremity deep vein thrombosis is evaluated for segmental pulmonary thromboembolism and determination of extent of lung involvement. A lung perfusion SPECT study is performed.

Description of Procedure (78803)

Physician instructs and oversees the nuclear medicine technologists in the administration of the radiopharmaceutical including verifying the dosage per NRC and/or state regulations. Directs the nuclear medicine technologist to adjust the acquisition protocol as necessary for the individual patient clinical situation and diagnosis. The physician is available to answer questions for the technologist and patient and to review components of the study throughout the procedure. Verify the completeness and adequacy of the SPECT data sets before completion of the study and order additional imaging as necessary. Review all images for artifacts and abnormal distribution. Review reconstructed images in three planes. Review the cinegraphic images and apply filters necessary for the patient protocol. Verify registration of the attenuation maps, if utilized. Compare results to relevant prior studies, laboratory, or other electronic record information. Produce a formal consultative report for the medical record.

Clinical Example (78804)

A 62-year-old male with history of metastatic, well-differentiated neuroendocrine cancer presents for indium-111 pentetreotide whole-body imaging performed over two days (two body scans performed), to determine response to ongoing therapy.

Description of Procedure (78804)

Physician instructs and oversees the nuclear medicine technologists in the administration of the radiopharmaceutical including verifying the dosage per NRC and/or state regulations. Direct the nuclear medicine technologist to adjust the acquisition protocol as necessary for the individual patient clinical situation and diagnosis. Be available to answer questions for the technologist and patient and to review components of the study throughout the procedure. Determine the adequacy of the day 1 planar images and the patient positioning and need for any additional planar images to be obtained. Initially correlate the findings to previous imaging, medical information, and clinical story and determine the appropriateness and timing of the day 2 whole-body planar imaging. Determine the adequacy of the multiple day planar studies (on both days) and the patient positioning and need for additional planar or other images. Interpret multiple-day, whole-body planar images obtained. Correlate the findings to early and late imaging, previous imaging, medical information, and clinical story, and generate a report for the medical record.

Clinical Example (78830)

A 66-year-old female with chronic low-back pain, status post lumbar laminectomy 18 months prior with posterolateral bone graft fusion and hardware level L2-S1, presents for bone SPECT-CT imaging of the lumbar spine (single study) performed to determine the presence of stress fractures and pseudoarthosis of the bone fusion graft, and/or determination of fixation hardware motion-loosening or other pathology.

Description of Procedure (78830)

Physician instructs and oversees the nuclear medicine technologists in the administration of the radiopharmaceutical including verifying the dosage per NRC and/or state regulations. Direct the nuclear medicine technologist to adjust the acquisition protocol as necessary for the individual patient clinical situation and diagnosis. Be available to answer questions for the technologist and patient and to review components of the study throughout the procedure. Oversee the administration of the diagnostic radiopharmaceutical and instruct technologist with initial protocol choice based on patient history. Determine the adequacy of the SPECT-CT study and the patient positioning, looking for motion artifact. Review the cinegraphic images and CT transmission for proper registration and apply filters as necessary for the individual study. Interpret the single area SPECT-CT images obtained, including evaluation and review of three planes of SPECT images for determination of radiopharmaceutical-based physiology uptake and pathology. Review three planes of (cross-sectional) CT for anatomy, incidental findings, and CT pathology (including hardware or surgical grafts, if present). Correlate the fused SPECT-CT images. Compare the SPECT-CT findings to previous imaging, medical information, and clinical story, and generate a report for the medical record, including recording any relevant CT incidental or relevant findings.

Clinical Example (78831)

A 58-year-old male with metastatic papillary thyroid cancer with a prior radioiodine body scan indicating suspected nodal or bone involvement in the thorax and nonspecific activity in the pelvis presents for two SPECT studies performed (same day) following body scan to anatomically localize thorax pathology and to help localize pathology in the pelvis.

Description of Procedure (78831)

Physician instructs and oversees the nuclear medicine technologists in the administration of the radiopharmaceutical including verifying the dosage per NRC and/or state regulations. Direct the nuclear medicine technologist to adjust the acquisition protocol as necessary for the individual patient. Be available to answer questions for the technologist and to review components of the study throughout the procedure. Review the history, physical examination, and prior medical records and evaluate the adequacy of patient for procedure ordered. Oversee the administration of the diagnostic radiopharmaceutical and instruct technologist with protocol choice based on patient history. Determine the adequacy of the SPECT studies and the patient positioning, looking for motion artifact. Review the two sets of cinegraphic images, apply filters necessary for each SPECT for the patient protocol, and perform visual and/or software merging of correlative prior imaging studies (eg, MR, diagnostic CT). Interpret two sets of SPECT images obtained, and correlate the findings to previous imaging, medical information, and clinical story, and generate a report for the medical record.

Clinical Example (78832)

An 82-year-old female with vascular grafts and sepsis, and with possible discitis in the cervical and lumbar spine suggested by prior imaging, presents for multiple (two or more) gallium-67 SPECT-CT studies required over one to two days to detect and anatomically localize multiple sites of infection suspected in the spine.

Description of Procedure (78832)

Physician instructs and oversees the nuclear medicine technologists in the administration of the radiopharmaceutical including verifying the dosage per NRC and/or state regulations. Direct the nuclear medicine technologist to adjust the acquisition protocol as necessary for the individual patient. Be available to answer questions for the technologist and to review components of the study throughout the procedure. Oversee the administration of the diagnostic radiopharmaceutical and instruct technologist with initial protocol choice based on patient history. After completion of the initial SPECT-CT study, review the image sets and determine the region and timing of the second (or more) SPECT-CT study. After completion, determine the adequacy of the second SPECT-CT study and the patient positioning, looking for motion artifact. Review the cinegraphic images and CT transmission for proper registration and apply filters as necessary for the individual study. Interpret the two (or more) areas of SPECT-CT images obtained, including evaluation and review of three planes of SPECT images for determination of radiopharmaceutical-based physiology uptake and pathology. Review three planes of (cross-sectional) CT for anatomy, incidental findings, and CT pathology (including hardware or surgical grafts, if present). Correlate the fused SPECT-CT images. Compare the two (or more) SPECT-CT studies' results and findings to previous imaging, medical information, and clinical story, and generate a comprehensive report for the medical record, including recording any incidental or relevant CT findings.

Clinical Example (78835)

A 70-year-old male with metastatic prostate cancer to the bones on staging/restaging bone scanning is considered for undergoing immunotherapy and other high-cost therapies. Bone SPECT-CT quantification is requested to determine the extent of therapeutic response rate in the metastatic lesions, and to determine whether to stop, continue, or change therapeutic intervention. [**Note:** This is an add-on service. Only consider the additional work related to quantitation.]

Description of Procedure (78835)

Acquire SPECT-CT imaging in a manner that will also allow quantitation (eg, images are acquired in 3D and list mode). Then re-bin the data to allow quantitation and export the data set to a dedicated computer with software program. In addition to the usual SPECT-CT imaging processing, then also process the re-binned data for quantitation using a separate software program. The technologist imports the data into a computerized quality control software program for analysis of data quality. Transfer the processed data set and quality control information to the interpreting physician. The physician then reviews the quality control for quantitation (eg, bolus duration, peak, and plateau waveforms) and, if quality is acceptable, reviews the numeric data. Then integrate the quantitation data with the SPECT-CT image data, attenuation maps, clinical data, and generate an overall report for the medical record.

Pathology and Laboratory

Summary of Additions, Deletions, and Revisions

The summary of changes shows the actual changes that have been made to the code descriptors.

New codes appear with a bullet (●) and are indicated as "Code added." Revised codes are preceded with a triangle (▲). Within revised codes, or if a code symbol has been deleted, the deleted language and code symbol appear with a ~~strikethrough~~ (⊖), while new text appears underlined.

The ⟋ symbol is used to identify codes for vaccines that are pending FDA approval. The # symbol is used to identify codes that have been resequenced. CPT add-on codes are annotated by the + symbol. The ⊘ symbol is used to identify codes that are exempt from the use of modifier 51. The ★ symbol is used to identify codes that may be used for reporting telemedicine services. The ⋈ is used to identify proprietary laboratory analyses (PLA) test that has an identical descriptor as another PLA test. A PLA code that satisfies Category I code criteria and has been accepted by the CPT Editorial Panel is annotated with the ↑↓ symbol.

Code	Description
●80145	Code added
●80187	Code added
#●80230	Code added
#●80235	Code added
#●81277	Code added
#●80280	Code added
#●80285	Code added
#●81307	Code added
#●81308	Code added
#●81309	Code added
▲81350	UGT1A1 (UDP glucuronosyltransferase 1 family, polypeptide A1) (eg, ~~irinotecan~~ drug metabolism, hereditary unconjugated hyperbilirubinemia [Gilbert syndrome])~~,~~ gene analysis, common variants (eg, *28, *36, *37)
▲81404	Molecular pathology procedure, Level 5 (eg, analysis of 2-5 exons by DNA sequence analysis, mutation scanning or duplication/deletion variants of 6-10 exons, or characterization of a dynamic mutation disorder/triplet repeat by Southern blot analysis)
	~~PIK3CA (phosphatidylinositol-4,5-bisphosphate 3-kinase, catalytic subunit alpha) (eg, colorectal cancer), targeted sequence analysis (eg, exons 9 and 20)~~
	UGT1A1 (UDP glucuronosyltransferase 1 family, polypeptide A1) (eg, hereditary unconjugated hyperbilirubinemia [Crigler-Najjar syndrome]) full gene sequence
▲81406	Molecular pathology procedure, Level 7 (eg, analysis of 11-25 exons by DNA sequence analysis, mutation scanning or duplication/deletion variants of 26-50 exons~~, cytogenomic array analysis for neoplasia~~)
	~~Cytogenomic microarray analysis, neoplasia (eg, interrogation of copy number, and loss-of-heterozygosity via single nucleotide polymorphism [SNP]-based comparative genomic hybridization [CGH] microarray analysis)~~
	~~PALB2 (partner and localizer of BRCA2) (eg, breast and pancreatic cancer), full gene sequence~~

Pathology and Laboratory

Code	Description
▲81407	Molecular pathology procedure, Level 8 (eg, analysis of 26-50 exons by DNA sequence analysis, mutation scanning or duplication/deletion variants of >50 exons, sequence analysis of multiple genes on one platform) *APOB (apolipoprotein B)* (eg, familial hypercholesterolemia type B) full gene sequence
#●81522	Code added
●81542	Code added
●81552	Code added
●87563	Code added
▲0008U	Helicobacter pylori detection and antibiotic resistance, DNA, 16S and 23S rRNA, gyrA, pbp1, rdxA and rpoB, next generation sequencing, formalin-fixed paraffin-embedded or fresh tissue or fecal sample, predictive, reported as positive or negative for resistance to clarithromycin, fluoroquinolones, metronidazole, amoxicillin, tetracycline, and rifabutin
0020U	~~Drug test(s), presumptive, with definitive confirmation of positive results, any number of drug classes, urine, with specimen verification including DNA authentication in comparison to buccal DNA, per date of service~~
0028U	~~CYP2D6 (cytochrome P450, family 2, subfamily D, polypeptide 6) (eg, drug metabolism) gene analysis, copy number variants, common variants with reflex to targeted sequence analysis~~
0057U	~~Oncology (solid organ neoplasia), mRNA, gene expression profiling by massively parallel sequencing for analysis of 51 genes, utilizing formalin-fixed paraffin-embedded tissue, algorithm reported as a normalized percentile rank~~
●0062U	Code added
●0063U	Code added
●0064U	Code added
●0065U	Code added
●0066U	Code added
●0067U	Code added
●0068U	Code added
●0069U	Code added
●0070U	Code added
+●0071U	Code added
+●0072U	Code added
+●0073U	Code added
+●0074U	Code added
+●0075U	Code added
+●0076U	Code added
●0077U	Code added
●0078U	Code added
●0079U	Code added
●0080U	Code added

CPT Changes 2020 — Pathology and Laboratory

Code	Description
0081U	Oncology (uveal melanoma), mRNA, gene expression profiling by real-time RT-PCR of 15 genes (12 content and 3 housekeeping genes), utilizing fine needle aspirate or formalin-fixed paraffin-embedded tissue, algorithm reported as risk of metastasis
●0082U	Code added
●0083U	Code added
●0084U	Code added
●0085U	Code added
●0086U	Code added
●0087U	Code added
●0088U	Code added
●0089U	Code added
●0090U	Code added
●0091U	Code added
●0092U	Code added
●0093U	Code added
●0094U	Code added
●0095U	Code added
●0096U	Code added
●0097U	Code added
●0098U	Code added
●0099U	Code added
●0100U	Code added
●0101U	Code added
●0102U	Code added
●0103U	Code added
0104U	Hereditary pan cancer (eg, hereditary breast and ovarian cancer, hereditary endometrial cancer, hereditary colorectal cancer), genomic sequence analysis panel utilizing a combination of NGS, Sanger, MLPA, and array CGH, with mRNA analytics to resolve variants of unknown significance when indicated (32 genes [sequencing and deletion/duplication], *EPCAM* and *GREM1* [deletion/duplication only])
●0105U	Code added
●0106U	Code added
●0107U	Code added
●0108U	Code added
●0109U	Code added
●0110U	Code added

▲ = Revised code ● = New code ▶◀ = Contains new or revised text ✕ = Duplicate PLA test ↕ = Category I PLA

Code	Description
●0111U	Code added
●0112U	Code added
●0113U	Code added
●0114U	Code added
●0115U	Code added
●0116U	Code added
●0117U	Code added
●0118U	Code added
●0119U	Code added
●0120U	Code added
●0121U	Code added
●0122U	Code added
●0123U	Code added
●0124U	Code added
●0125U	Code added
●0126U	Code added
●0127U	Code added
●0128U	Code added
●0129U	Code added
+●0130U	Code added
+●0131U	Code added
+●0132U	Code added
+●0133U	Code added
+●0134U	Code added
+●0135U	Code added
+●0136U	Code added
+●0137U	Code added
+●0138U	Code added

Pathology and Laboratory

Therapeutic Drug Assays

Therapeutic Drug Assays are performed to monitor clinical response to a known, prescribed medication.

The material for examination is whole blood, serum, plasma, or cerebrospinal fluid. Examination is quantitative. Coding is by parent drug; measured metabolites of the drug are included in the code, if performed.

●	80145	Adalimumab
	80150	Amikacin
	80173	Haloperidol
#●	80230	Infliximab
#●	80235	Lacosamide
	80175	Lamotrigine
	80185	Phenytoin; total
	80186	free
●	80187	Posaconazole
	80188	Primidone
	80202	Vancomycin
#●	80280	Vedolizumab
#●	80285	Voriconazole
	80203	Zonisamide
	80230	Code is out of numerical sequence. See 80170-80176
	80235	Code is out of numerical sequence. See 80170-80176
	80280	Code is out of numerical sequence. See 80201-80299
	80285	Code is out of numerical sequence. See 80201-80299
	80299	Quantitation of therapeutic drug, not elsewhere specified

Rationale

Six new codes have been added to the Therapeutic Drug Assays subsection. Each of these codes has been added to identify a specific drug that previously lacked specific codes for identification. As is noted within the existing guidelines, the materials tested may be from various sources and are quantitative in nature. Performance of the testing procedure is not limited to a particular method; therefore, the specific method of testing for the noted substance may vary.

Clinical Example (80145)

A 22-year-old female with Crohns disease presents with increased bowel movements a few weeks prior to the next adalimumab self-injection. Her physician is wondering about loss of response to therapy. Blood draw is obtained at trough. Adalimumab quantitation is low at 4 mcg/mL, and antibodies-to-adalimumab are borderline positive. Results are reported back to the ordering physician, who added an immunomodulator to the therapeutic regimen.

Description of Procedure (80145)

The adalimumab quantitation test is an enzyme-linked immunosorbent assay (ELISA) to determine free adalimumab in serum. Free adalimumab from the sample is bound to the specific monoclonal anti-adalimumab antibody followed by a washing step and peroxidase-labeled antibody. If the result is 5.0 mcg/mL or less, then perform an adalimumab antibody test. Report quantitative adalimumab results.

Clinical Example (80187)

A 51-year-old female cadaveric-kidney transplant recipient developed an infection with Aspergillus fumigatus, which was resistant to voriconazole but sensitive to posaconazole. After one week of therapy, target trough serum posaconazole concentrations were achieved, with no therapeutic response. Dosage was changed and a repeat posaconazole trough level was ordered.

Description of Procedure (80187)

Process a serum sample with acetonitrile to precipitate proteins. Remove the supernatant, and analyze posaconazole by liquid chromatography or mass spectrometry. Report quantitative posaconazole results.

Clinical Example (80230)

A 38-year-old male with Crohns disease presents with blood in stool shortly before the next infliximab infusion. His physician obtains a trough level to evaluate for loss of response to therapy.

Description of Procedure (80230)

Perform pre-analytical sample preparation to remove nonimmunoglobulin proteins from the serum matrix and cleave all immunoglobulin proteins using trypsin digestion. Subject the sample to liquid chromatography–tandem mass spectrometry (LC-MS/MS). If the result is below 5.1 mcg/mL, perform testing for antibodies to infliximab. Report quantitative infliximab results.

Clinical Example (80235)

A 36-year-old male with refractory epilepsy was being treated with carbamazepine, and lacosamide therapy was added. His physician orders a lacosamide trough level to evaluate for loss of response to therapy.

Description of Procedure (80235)

Process the patient's serum sample and subject it to high-performance LC-MS/MS. Report quantitative lacosamide results.

Clinical Example (80280)

A 75-year-old male with Crohns disease presents with multiple episodes daily of bloody diarrhea. After four months on vedolizumab, his physician orders a trough level to evaluate for loss of response to therapy. A blood draw is obtained at trough.

Description of Procedure (80280)

Perform pre-analytical immunopurification of the serum sample. Then subject the immune-enriched and reduced sample to LC-MS/MS. Report quantitative vedolizumab results.

Clinical Example (80285)

A 21-year-old male with subacute liver failure was diagnosed with pulmonary aspergillosis and treated with voriconazole. He developed tremors, lip twitching, and hair loss, potentially due to the drug. Plasma voriconazole trough concentration testing is ordered to inform future dosing.

Description of Procedure (80285)

Dilute serum samples in acetonitrile containing an internal standard. Centrifuge the protein precipitate. Dilute a portion of the supernatant with mobile phase for detection using tandem mass spectrometry. Report quantitative voriconazole results.

Molecular Pathology

Tier 1 Molecular Pathology Procedures

81228 Cytogenomic constitutional (genome-wide) microarray analysis; interrogation of genomic regions for copy number variants (eg, bacterial artificial chromosome [BAC] or oligo-based comparative genomic hybridization [CGH] microarray analysis)

81229 interrogation of genomic regions for copy number and single nucleotide polymorphism (SNP) variants for chromosomal abnormalities

(Do not report 81228 in conjunction with 81229)

(When performing cytogenomic constitutional microarray analysis that is not genome-wide [ie, regionally targeted], report the specific code for the targeted analysis if available [eg, 81405] or the unlisted molecular pathology code [81479])

(Do not report analyte-specific molecular pathology procedures separately in conjunction with 81228, 81229 when the specific analytes are included as part of the microarray analysis)

(Do not report 88271 when performing cytogenomic microarray analysis)

(For genomic sequencing procedures or other molecular multianalyte assays for copy number analysis using circulating cell-free fetal DNA in maternal blood, see 81420, 81422, 81479)

#● **81277** Cytogenomic neoplasia (genome-wide) microarray analysis, interrogation of genomic regions for copy number and loss-of-heterozygosity variants for chromosomal abnormalities

▶(Do not report analyte-specific molecular pathology procedures separately when the specific analytes are included as part of the cytogenomic microarray analysis for neoplasia)◀

▶(Do not report 88271 when performing cytogenomic microarray analysis)◀

81230 Code is out of numerical sequence. See 81225-81229

81277 Code is out of numerical sequence. See 81228-81235

81307 Code is out of numerical sequence. See 81310-81316

81308 Code is out of numerical sequence. See 81310-81316

81309 Code is out of numerical sequence. See 81310-81316

Rationale

Tier 1 code 81277, which describes cytogenomic array analysis for neoplasia, has been added to report microarray analysis for copy number and loss-of-heterozygosity variants for chromosomal abnormalities. In addition, two exclusionary parenthetical notes have been added to restrict separate reporting of analyte-specific molecular pathology procedures and to preclude the use of code 88271 for cytogenomic microarray analysis.

Refer to the codebook and the Rationale for code 81406 for a full discussion of these changes.

Clinical Example (81277)

A 45-year-old female presented with symptoms concerning for acute leukemia. Morphologic and flow cytometry assessment identified B-cell acute lymphoblastic leukemia. Chromosome studies did not yield suitable metaphases, and fluorescence in situ hybridization (FISH) studies revealed some chromosomes in a copy state of 3 and 4 raising concern for a doubled pseudo-hyperdiploid B-ALL clone indicative of a poor prognosis. Cytogenomic array analysis was ordered to distinguish between a doubled pseudo-hyperdiploid and hyperdiploid clone.

Description of Procedure (81277)

Label deoxyribonucleic acid (DNA) extracted from the patient's bone marrow or peripheral blood and hybridize to the microarray. Following hybridization, scan the microarray. Measure the intensity of signals and compare to a reference data set. Use these data to determine copy number changes and regions with loss of heterozygosity. Analyze the data and compose a report specifying the patient's copy number changes and any loss of heterozygosity that may be associated with the neoplastic process. Edit and sign the report. Communicate the results to the ordering physician.

81310	*NPM1 (nucleophosmin)* (eg, acute myeloid leukemia) gene analysis, exon 12 variants
81311	*NRAS (neuroblastoma RAS viral [v-ras] oncogene homolog)* (eg, colorectal carcinoma), gene analysis, variants in exon 2 (eg, codons 12 and 13) and exon 3 (eg, codon 61)
81312	Code is out of numerical sequence. See 81310-81316
# 81306	*NUDT15 (nudix hydrolase 15)* (eg, drug metabolism) gene analysis, common variant(s) (eg, *2, *3, *4, *5, *6)
# 81312	*PABPN1 (poly[A] binding protein nuclear 1)* (eg, oculopharyngeal muscular dystrophy) gene analysis, evaluation to detect abnormal (eg, expanded) alleles
#● 81307	*PALB2 (partner and localizer of BRCA2)* (eg, breast and pancreatic cancer) gene analysis; full gene sequence
#● 81308	known familial variant
81313	*PCA3/KLK3 (prostate cancer antigen 3 [non-protein coding]/kallikrein-related peptidase 3 [prostate specific antigen])* ratio (eg, prostate cancer)

Rationale

Tier 1 codes 81307 and 81308 have been established to report partner and localizer gene analysis for BRCA2. This includes the removal of the PALB2 language from the descriptor of code 81406 for molecular pathology. Prior to establishment of the new Tier 1 codes (81307, 81308), Tier 2 code 81406 was used to identify full-gene sequencing for PALB2. Since the addition of testing for the PALB2 gene to code 81406 within the Tier 2 code set, the frequency of PALB2 tests has increased to the level that is consistent with their clinical uses. Therefore, this test has been removed from code 81406 and it is now reported with Tier 1 codes. Multiple codes have been developed within the Tier 1 code subset for the PALB2 gene to allow testing for full-gene sequence gene analysis (81307) and known familial variant gene analysis (81308).

Clinical Example (81307)

A 40-year-old female with significant family history of breast cancer has been diagnosed with a stage 2, triple negative, left invasive ductal breast cancer and is referred for genetic testing for inherited breast cancer syndromes. Tests for BRCA1 and BRCA2 were negative. Based on her tumor characteristics and family history, her physician orders PALB2 full sequence analysis.

Description of Procedure (81307)

Isolate high-quality genomic DNA from whole blood, and subject it to Sanger sequencing of the PALB2 gene. Analyze the data and compose a report.

Clinical Example (81308)

A 30-year-old pregnant female with family history of breast cancer is referred for PALB2 analysis of a known familial variant. Her physician orders PALB2 testing to determine if she is at increased risk for breast cancer and needs early and more frequent screening.

Description of Procedure (81308)

Isolate high-quality DNA from peripheral whole blood, and subject it to Sanger sequencing of the PALB2 gene for the known familial variant. Analyze the data and compose a report.

81314	*PDGFRA (platelet-derived growth factor receptor, alpha polypeptide)* (eg, gastrointestinal stromal tumor [GIST]), gene analysis, targeted sequence analysis (eg, exons 12, 18)
#● 81309	*PIK3CA (phosphatidylinositol-4, 5-biphosphate 3-kinase, catalytic subunit alpha)* (eg, colorectal and breast cancer) gene analysis, targeted sequence analysis (eg, exons 7, 9, 20)
# 81320	*PLCG2 (phospholipase C gamma 2)* (eg, chronic lymphocytic leukemia) gene analysis, common variants (eg, R665W, S707F, L845F)

Rationale

Code 81309 has been established to report targeted sequence analysis of the PIK3CA gene. This test was previously reported with Tier 2 code 81404. Since the addition of this gene analysis to the Tier 2 code set, the frequency of the test has increased to the level that is consistent with its intended clinical use. Therefore, this test has been removed from code 81404 and is now reported with the Tier 1 code.

Clinical Example (81309)

A 55-year-old female presents with a 2-cm mass in her right breast. Pathological examination of the excised mass supports a diagnosis of HR positive/HER2 negative breast cancer. Adjuvant endocrine therapy is initiated. Subsequently, enlarged peripheral lymph nodes are found and metastatic disease is identified. A tissue sample is sent to the laboratory for PIK3CA mutation detection.

Description of Procedure (81309)

Extract high-quality DNA from tumor tissue. Perform real-time polymerase chain reaction (PCR) to detect PIK3CA mutations in a background of wild-type DNA utilizing fluorescent probe-linked primers specific for each of 11 common mutations in exons 7, 9, and 20 of the PIK3CA gene. Analyze the fluorescent curves that are produced and compose a report that specifies the mutation status of the patient's tumor.

81346	*TYMS (thymidylate synthetase)* (eg, 5-fluorouracil/5-FU drug metabolism), gene analysis, common variant(s) (eg, tandem repeat variant)
▲ 81350	*UGT1A1 (UDP glucuronosyltransferase 1 family, polypeptide A1)* (eg, drug metabolism, hereditary unconjugated hyperbilirubinemia [Gilbert syndrome]) gene analysis, common variants (eg, *28, *36, *37)
81355	*VKORC1 (vitamin K epoxide reductase complex, subunit 1)* (eg, warfarin metabolism), gene analysis, common variant(s) (eg, -1639G>A, c.173+1000C>T)

Rationale

Tier 1 code 81350 has been revised to include examples of common gene analysis for drug metabolism and hereditary unconjugated hyperbilirubinemia. This enabled the inclusion of a new gene to report full-gene sequencing of UGT1A1 within code 81404.

Clinical Example (81350)

A 60-year-old male presents with fatigue and weight loss. The patient is found to have poorly differentiated adenocarcinoma of the colon with unresectable metastases to the liver. Despite 5-FU, leucovorin, and oxaliplatin (FOLFOX) therapy, the patient's disease progresses, and irinotecan therapy is recommended. Prior to beginning irinotecan treatment, an anticoagulated peripheral blood sample is submitted to test the patient's UGT1A1 promoter TA repeat numbers.

Description of Procedure (81350)

Isolate high-quality genomic DNA from whole blood. Subject it to PCR amplification for the region containing the UGT1A1 promoter TA repeat segment. Subject the fluorescent products to analysis using capillary electrophoresis. Evaluate the electropherogram and compare it to a sizing ladder to determine the patient's genotype. Based on this analysis, compose a report that specifies the patient's genotype. Edit and sign the report. Communicate the results to appropriate caregivers.

Tier 2 Molecular Pathology Procedures

▲ 81404 Molecular pathology procedure, Level 5 (eg, analysis of 2-5 exons by DNA sequence analysis, mutation scanning or duplication/deletion variants of 6-10 exons, or characterization of a dynamic mutation disorder/triplet repeat by Southern blot analysis)

ACADS (acyl-CoA dehydrogenase, C-2 to C-3 short chain) (eg, short chain acyl-CoA dehydrogenase deficiency), targeted sequence analysis (eg, exons 5 and 6)

AQP2 (aquaporin 2 [collecting duct]) (eg, nephrogenic diabetes insipidus), full gene sequence

ARX (aristaless related homeobox) (eg, X-linked lissencephaly with ambiguous genitalia, X-linked mental retardation), full gene sequence

AVPR2 (arginine vasopressin receptor 2) (eg, nephrogenic diabetes insipidus), full gene sequence

BBS10 (Bardet-Biedl syndrome 10) (eg, Bardet-Biedl syndrome), full gene sequence

BTD (biotinidase) (eg, biotinidase deficiency), full gene sequence

C10orf2 (chromosome 10 open reading frame 2) (eg, mitochondrial DNA depletion syndrome), full gene sequence

CAV3 (caveolin 3) (eg, CAV3-related distal myopathy, limb-girdle muscular dystrophy type 1C), full gene sequence

CD40LG (CD40 ligand) (eg, X-linked hyper IgM syndrome), full gene sequence

CDKN2A (cyclin-dependent kinase inhibitor 2A) (eg, CDKN2A-related cutaneous malignant melanoma, familial atypical mole-malignant melanoma syndrome), full gene sequence

CLRN1 (clarin 1) (eg, Usher syndrome, type 3), full gene sequence

COX6B1 (cytochrome c oxidase subunit VIb polypeptide 1) (eg, mitochondrial respiratory chain complex IV deficiency), full gene sequence

CPT2 (carnitine palmitoyltransferase 2) (eg, carnitine palmitoyltransferase II deficiency), full gene sequence

CRX (cone-rod homeobox) (eg, cone-rod dystrophy 2, Leber congenital amaurosis), full gene sequence

CYP1B1 (cytochrome P450, family 1, subfamily B, polypeptide 1) (eg, primary congenital glaucoma), full gene sequence

EGR2 (early growth response 2) (eg, Charcot-Marie-Tooth), full gene sequence

EMD (emerin) (eg, Emery-Dreifuss muscular dystrophy), duplication/deletion analysis

EPM2A (epilepsy, progressive myoclonus type 2A, Lafora disease [laforin]) (eg, progressive myoclonus epilepsy), full gene sequence

FGF23 (fibroblast growth factor 23) (eg, hypophosphatemic rickets), full gene sequence

FGFR2 (fibroblast growth factor receptor 2) (eg, craniosynostosis, Apert syndrome, Crouzon syndrome), targeted sequence analysis (eg, exons 8, 10)

FGFR3 (fibroblast growth factor receptor 3) (eg, achondroplasia, hypochondroplasia), targeted sequence analysis (eg, exons 8, 11, 12, 13)

FHL1 (four and a half LIM domains 1) (eg, Emery-Dreifuss muscular dystrophy), full gene sequence

FKRP (fukutin related protein) (eg, congenital muscular dystrophy type 1C [MDC1C], limb-girdle muscular dystrophy [LGMD] type 2I), full gene sequence

FOXG1 (forkhead box G1) (eg, Rett syndrome), full gene sequence

FSHMD1A (facioscapulohumeral muscular dystrophy 1A) (eg, facioscapulohumeral muscular dystrophy), evaluation to detect abnormal (eg, deleted) alleles

FSHMD1A (facioscapulohumeral muscular dystrophy 1A) (eg, facioscapulohumeral muscular dystrophy), characterization of haplotype(s) (ie, chromosome 4A and 4B haplotypes)

GH1 (growth hormone 1) (eg, growth hormone deficiency), full gene sequence

GP1BB (glycoprotein Ib [platelet], beta polypeptide) (eg, Bernard-Soulier syndrome type B), full gene sequence

(For common deletion variants of alpha globin 1 and alpha globin 2 genes, use 81257)

HNF1B (HNF1 homeobox B) (eg, maturity-onset diabetes of the young [MODY]), duplication/deletion analysis

HRAS (v-Ha-ras Harvey rat sarcoma viral oncogene homolog) (eg, Costello syndrome), full gene sequence

HSD3B2 (hydroxy-delta-5-steroid dehydrogenase, 3 beta- and steroid delta-isomerase 2) (eg, 3-beta-hydroxysteroid dehydrogenase type II deficiency), full gene sequence

HSD11B2 (hydroxysteroid [11-beta] dehydrogenase 2) (eg, mineralocorticoid excess syndrome), full gene sequence

HSPB1 (heat shock 27kDa protein 1) (eg, Charcot-Marie-Tooth disease), full gene sequence

INS (insulin) (eg, diabetes mellitus), full gene sequence

KCNJ1 (potassium inwardly-rectifying channel, subfamily J, member 1) (eg, Bartter syndrome), full gene sequence

KCNJ10 (potassium inwardly-rectifying channel, subfamily J, member 10) (eg, SeSAME syndrome, EAST syndrome, sensorineural hearing loss), full gene sequence

LITAF (lipopolysaccharide-induced TNF factor) (eg, Charcot-Marie-Tooth), full gene sequence

MEFV (Mediterranean fever) (eg, familial Mediterranean fever), full gene sequence

MEN1 (multiple endocrine neoplasia I) (eg, multiple endocrine neoplasia type 1, Wermer syndrome), duplication/deletion analysis

MMACHC (methylmalonic aciduria [cobalamin deficiency] cblC type, with homocystinuria) (eg, methylmalonic acidemia and homocystinuria), full gene sequence

MPV17 (MpV17 mitochondrial inner membrane protein) (eg, mitochondrial DNA depletion syndrome), duplication/deletion analysis

NDP (Norrie disease [pseudoglioma]) (eg, Norrie disease), full gene sequence

NDUFA1 (NADH dehydrogenase [ubiquinone] 1 alpha subcomplex, 1, 7.5kDa) (eg, Leigh syndrome, mitochondrial complex I deficiency), full gene sequence

NDUFAF2 (NADH dehydrogenase [ubiquinone] 1 alpha subcomplex, assembly factor 2) (eg, Leigh syndrome, mitochondrial complex I deficiency), full gene sequence

NDUFS4 (NADH dehydrogenase [ubiquinone] Fe-S protein 4, 18kDa [NADH-coenzyme Q reductase]) (eg, Leigh syndrome, mitochondrial complex I deficiency), full gene sequence

NIPA1 (non-imprinted in Prader-Willi/Angelman syndrome 1) (eg, spastic paraplegia), full gene sequence

NLGN4X (neuroligin 4, X-linked) (eg, autism spectrum disorders), duplication/deletion analysis

NPC2 (Niemann-Pick disease, type C2 [epididymal secretory protein E1]) (eg, Niemann-Pick disease type C2), full gene sequence

NR0B1 (nuclear receptor subfamily 0, group B, member 1) (eg, congenital adrenal hypoplasia), full gene sequence

PDX1 (pancreatic and duodenal homeobox 1) (eg, maturity-onset diabetes of the young [MODY]), full gene sequence

PHOX2B (paired-like homeobox 2b) (eg, congenital central hypoventilation syndrome), full gene sequence

PLP1 (proteolipid protein 1) (eg, Pelizaeus-Merzbacher disease, spastic paraplegia), duplication/deletion analysis

PQBP1 (polyglutamine binding protein 1) (eg, Renpenning syndrome), duplication/deletion analysis

PRNP (prion protein) (eg, genetic prion disease), full gene sequence

PROP1 (PROP paired-like homeobox 1) (eg, combined pituitary hormone deficiency), full gene sequence

PRPH2 (peripherin 2 [retinal degeneration, slow]) (eg, retinitis pigmentosa), full gene sequence

PRSS1 (protease, serine, 1 [trypsin 1]) (eg, hereditary pancreatitis), full gene sequence

RAF1 (v-raf-1 murine leukemia viral oncogene homolog 1) (eg, LEOPARD syndrome), targeted sequence analysis (eg, exons 7, 12, 14, 17)

RET (ret proto-oncogene) (eg, multiple endocrine neoplasia, type 2B and familial medullary thyroid carcinoma), common variants (eg, M918T, 2647_2648delinsTT, A883F)

RHO (rhodopsin) (eg, retinitis pigmentosa), full gene sequence

RP1 (retinitis pigmentosa 1) (eg, retinitis pigmentosa), full gene sequence

SCN1B (sodium channel, voltage-gated, type I, beta) (eg, Brugada syndrome), full gene sequence

SCO2 (SCO cytochrome oxidase deficient homolog 2 [SCO1L]) (eg, mitochondrial respiratory chain complex IV deficiency), full gene sequence

SDHC (succinate dehydrogenase complex, subunit C, integral membrane protein, 15kDa) (eg, hereditary paraganglioma-pheochromocytoma syndrome), duplication/deletion analysis

SDHD (succinate dehydrogenase complex, subunit D, integral membrane protein) (eg, hereditary paraganglioma), full gene sequence

SGCG (sarcoglycan, gamma [35kDa dystrophin-associated glycoprotein]) (eg, limb-girdle muscular dystrophy), duplication/deletion analysis

SH2D1A (SH2 domain containing 1A) (eg, X-linked lymphoproliferative syndrome), full gene sequence

SLC16A2 (solute carrier family 16, member 2 [thyroid hormone transporter]) (eg, specific thyroid hormone cell transporter deficiency, Allan-Herndon-Dudley syndrome), duplication/deletion analysis

SLC25A20 (solute carrier family 25 [carnitine/acylcarnitine translocase], member 20) (eg, carnitine-acylcarnitine translocase deficiency), duplication/deletion analysis

SLC25A4 (solute carrier family 25 [mitochondrial carrier; adenine nucleotide translocator], member 4) (eg, progressive external ophthalmoplegia), full gene sequence

SOD1 (superoxide dismutase 1, soluble) (eg, amyotrophic lateral sclerosis), full gene sequence

SPINK1 (serine peptidase inhibitor, Kazal type 1) (eg, hereditary pancreatitis), full gene sequence

STK11 (serine/threonine kinase 11) (eg, Peutz-Jeghers syndrome), duplication/deletion analysis

TACO1 (translational activator of mitochondrial encoded cytochrome c oxidase I) (eg, mitochondrial respiratory chain complex IV deficiency), full gene sequence

THAP1 (THAP domain containing, apoptosis associated protein 1) (eg, torsion dystonia), full gene sequence

TOR1A (torsin family 1, member A [torsin A]) (eg, torsion dystonia), full gene sequence

TP53 (tumor protein 53) (eg, tumor samples), targeted sequence analysis of 2-5 exons

TTPA (tocopherol [alpha] transfer protein) (eg, ataxia), full gene sequence

TTR (transthyretin) (eg, familial transthyretin amyloidosis), full gene sequence

TWIST1 (twist homolog 1 [Drosophila]) (eg, Saethre-Chotzen syndrome), full gene sequence

TYR (tyrosinase [oculocutaneous albinism IA]) (eg, oculocutaneous albinism IA), full gene sequence

▶*UGT1A1 (UDP glucuronosyltransferase 1 family, polypeptide A1)* (eg, hereditary unconjugated hyperbilirubinemia [Crigler-Najjar syndrome]) full gene sequence◀

USH1G (Usher syndrome 1G [autosomal recessive]) (eg, Usher syndrome, type 1), full gene sequence

VHL (von Hippel-Lindau tumor suppressor) (eg, von Hippel-Lindau familial cancer syndrome), full gene sequence

VWF (von Willebrand factor) (eg, von Willebrand disease type 1C), targeted sequence analysis (eg, exons 26, 27, 37)

ZEB2 (zinc finger E-box binding homeobox 2) (eg, Mowat-Wilson syndrome), duplication/deletion analysis

ZNF41 (zinc finger protein 41) (eg, X-linked mental retardation 89), full gene sequence

Rationale

In accordance with the establishment of Tier 1 code 81309, targeted sequence analysis of the PIK3CA gene has been removed from Tier 2 code 81404. In addition, code 81404 has been revised with the addition of UGT1A1 full-gene sequencing for unconjugated hyperbilirubinemia.

Refer to the codebook and the Rationale for code 81309 for a full discussion of these changes.

▲ **81406** Molecular pathology procedure, Level 7 (eg, analysis of 11-25 exons by DNA sequence analysis, mutation scanning or duplication/deletion variants of 26-50 exons)

ACADVL (acyl-CoA dehydrogenase, very long chain) (eg, very long chain acyl-coenzyme A dehydrogenase deficiency), full gene sequence

ACTN4 (actinin, alpha 4) (eg, focal segmental glomerulosclerosis), full gene sequence

AFG3L2 (AFG3 ATPase family gene 3-like 2 [S. cerevisiae]) (eg, spinocerebellar ataxia), full gene sequence

AIRE (autoimmune regulator) (eg, autoimmune polyendocrinopathy syndrome type 1), full gene sequence

ALDH7A1 (aldehyde dehydrogenase 7 family, member A1) (eg, pyridoxine-dependent epilepsy), full gene sequence

ANO5 (anoctamin 5) (eg, limb-girdle muscular dystrophy), full gene sequence

ANOS1 (anosmin-1) (eg, Kallmann syndrome 1), full gene sequence

APP (amyloid beta [A4] precursor protein) (eg, Alzheimer disease), full gene sequence

ASS1 (argininosuccinate synthase 1) (eg, citrullinemia type I), full gene sequence

ATL1 (atlastin GTPase 1) (eg, spastic paraplegia), full gene sequence

ATP1A2 (ATPase, Na+/K+ transporting, alpha 2 polypeptide) (eg, familial hemiplegic migraine), full gene sequence

ATP7B (ATPase, Cu++ transporting, beta polypeptide) (eg, Wilson disease), full gene sequence

BBS1 (Bardet-Biedl syndrome 1) (eg, Bardet-Biedl syndrome), full gene sequence

BBS2 (Bardet-Biedl syndrome 2) (eg, Bardet-Biedl syndrome), full gene sequence

BCKDHB (branched-chain keto acid dehydrogenase E1, beta polypeptide) (eg, maple syrup urine disease, type 1B), full gene sequence

BEST1 (bestrophin 1) (eg, vitelliform macular dystrophy), full gene sequence

BMPR2 (bone morphogenetic protein receptor, type II [serine/threonine kinase]) (eg, heritable pulmonary arterial hypertension), full gene sequence

BRAF (B-Raf proto-oncogene, serine/threonine kinase) (eg, Noonan syndrome), full gene sequence

BSCL2 (Berardinelli-Seip congenital lipodystrophy 2 [seipin]) (eg, Berardinelli-Seip congenital lipodystrophy), full gene sequence

BTK (Bruton agammaglobulinemia tyrosine kinase) (eg, X-linked agammaglobulinemia), full gene sequence

CACNB2 (calcium channel, voltage-dependent, beta 2 subunit) (eg, Brugada syndrome), full gene sequence

CAPN3 (calpain 3) (eg, limb-girdle muscular dystrophy [LGMD] type 2A, calpainopathy), full gene sequence

CBS (cystathionine-beta-synthase) (eg, homocystinuria, cystathionine beta-synthase deficiency), full gene sequence

CDH1 (cadherin 1, type 1, E-cadherin [epithelial]) (eg, hereditary diffuse gastric cancer), full gene sequence

CDKL5 (cyclin-dependent kinase-like 5) (eg, early infantile epileptic encephalopathy), full gene sequence

CLCN1 (chloride channel 1, skeletal muscle) (eg, myotonia congenita), full gene sequence

CLCNKB (chloride channel, voltage-sensitive Kb) (eg, Bartter syndrome 3 and 4b), full gene sequence

CNTNAP2 (contactin-associated protein-like 2) (eg, Pitt-Hopkins-like syndrome 1), full gene sequence

COL6A2 (collagen, type VI, alpha 2) (eg, collagen type VI-related disorders), duplication/deletion analysis

CPT1A (carnitine palmitoyltransferase 1A [liver]) (eg, carnitine palmitoyltransferase 1A [CPT1A] deficiency), full gene sequence

CRB1 (crumbs homolog 1 [Drosophila]) (eg, Leber congenital amaurosis), full gene sequence

CREBBP (CREB binding protein) (eg, Rubinstein-Taybi syndrome), duplication/deletion analysis

DBT (dihydrolipoamide branched chain transacylase E2) (eg, maple syrup urine disease, type 2), full gene sequence

DLAT (dihydrolipoamide S-acetyltransferase) (eg, pyruvate dehydrogenase E2 deficiency), full gene sequence

DLD (dihydrolipoamide dehydrogenase) (eg, maple syrup urine disease, type III), full gene sequence

DSC2 (desmocollin) (eg, arrhythmogenic right ventricular dysplasia/cardiomyopathy 11), full gene sequence

DSG2 (desmoglein 2) (eg, arrhythmogenic right ventricular dysplasia/cardiomyopathy 10), full gene sequence

DSP (desmoplakin) (eg, arrhythmogenic right ventricular dysplasia/cardiomyopathy 8), full gene sequence

EFHC1 (EF-hand domain [C-terminal] containing 1) (eg, juvenile myoclonic epilepsy), full gene sequence

EIF2B3 (eukaryotic translation initiation factor 2B, subunit 3 gamma, 58kDa) (eg, leukoencephalopathy with vanishing white matter), full gene sequence

EIF2B4 (eukaryotic translation initiation factor 2B, subunit 4 delta, 67kDa) (eg, leukoencephalopathy with vanishing white matter), full gene sequence

EIF2B5 (eukaryotic translation initiation factor 2B, subunit 5 epsilon, 82kDa) (eg, childhood ataxia with central nervous system hypomyelination/vanishing white matter), full gene sequence

ENG (endoglin) (eg, hereditary hemorrhagic telangiectasia, type 1), full gene sequence

EYA1 (eyes absent homolog 1 [Drosophila]) (eg, branchio-oto-renal [BOR] spectrum disorders), full gene sequence

F8 (coagulation factor VIII) (eg, hemophilia A), duplication/deletion analysis

FAH (fumarylacetoacetate hydrolase [fumarylacetoacetase]) (eg, tyrosinemia, type 1), full gene sequence

FASTKD2 (FAST kinase domains 2) (eg, mitochondrial respiratory chain complex IV deficiency), full gene sequence

FIG4 (FIG4 homolog, SAC1 lipid phosphatase domain containing [S. cerevisiae]) (eg, Charcot-Marie-Tooth disease), full gene sequence

FTSJ1 (FtsJ RNA methyltransferase homolog 1 [E. coli]) (eg, X-linked mental retardation 9), full gene sequence

FUS (fused in sarcoma) (eg, amyotrophic lateral sclerosis), full gene sequence

GAA (glucosidase, alpha; acid) (eg, glycogen storage disease type II [Pompe disease]), full gene sequence

GALC (galactosylceramidase) (eg, Krabbe disease), full gene sequence

GALT (galactose-1-phosphate uridylyltransferase) (eg, galactosemia), full gene sequence

GARS (glycyl-tRNA synthetase) (eg, Charcot-Marie-Tooth disease), full gene sequence

GCDH (glutaryl-CoA dehydrogenase) (eg, glutaricacidemia type 1), full gene sequence

GCK (glucokinase [hexokinase 4]) (eg, maturity-onset diabetes of the young [MODY]), full gene sequence

GLUD1 (glutamate dehydrogenase 1) (eg, familial hyperinsulinism), full gene sequence

GNE (glucosamine [UDP-N-acetyl]-2-epimerase/N-acetylmannosamine kinase) (eg, inclusion body myopathy 2 [IBM2], Nonaka myopathy), full gene sequence

GRN (granulin) (eg, frontotemporal dementia), full gene sequence

HADHA (hydroxyacyl-CoA dehydrogenase/3-ketoacyl-CoA thiolase/enoyl-CoA hydratase [trifunctional protein] alpha subunit) (eg, long chain acyl-coenzyme A dehydrogenase deficiency), full gene sequence

HADHB (hydroxyacyl-CoA dehydrogenase/3-ketoacyl-CoA thiolase/enoyl-CoA hydratase [trifunctional protein], beta subunit) (eg, trifunctional protein deficiency), full gene sequence

HEXA (hexosaminidase A, alpha polypeptide) (eg, Tay-Sachs disease), full gene sequence

HLCS (HLCS holocarboxylase synthetase) (eg, holocarboxylase synthetase deficiency), full gene sequence

HMBS (hydroxymethylbilane synthase) (eg, acute intermittent porphyria), full gene sequence

HNF4A (hepatocyte nuclear factor 4, alpha) (eg, maturity-onset diabetes of the young [MODY]), full gene sequence

IDUA (iduronidase, alpha-L-) (eg, mucopolysaccharidosis type I), full gene sequence

INF2 (inverted formin, FH2 and WH2 domain containing) (eg, focal segmental glomerulosclerosis), full gene sequence

IVD (isovaleryl-CoA dehydrogenase) (eg, isovaleric acidemia), full gene sequence

JAG1 (jagged 1) (eg, Alagille syndrome), duplication/deletion analysis

JUP (junction plakoglobin) (eg, arrhythmogenic right ventricular dysplasia/cardiomyopathy 11), full gene sequence

KCNH2 (potassium voltage-gated channel, subfamily H [eag-related], member 2) (eg, short QT syndrome, long QT syndrome), full gene sequence

KCNQ1 (potassium voltage-gated channel, KQT-like subfamily, member 1) (eg, short QT syndrome, long QT syndrome), full gene sequence

KCNQ2 (potassium voltage-gated channel, KQT-like subfamily, member 2) (eg, epileptic encephalopathy), full gene sequence

LDB3 (LIM domain binding 3) (eg, familial dilated cardiomyopathy, myofibrillar myopathy), full gene sequence

LDLR (low density lipoprotein receptor) (eg, familial hypercholesterolemia), full gene sequence

LEPR (leptin receptor) (eg, obesity with hypogonadism), full gene sequence

LHCGR (luteinizing hormone/choriogonadotropin receptor) (eg, precocious male puberty), full gene sequence

LMNA (lamin A/C) (eg, Emery-Dreifuss muscular dystrophy [EDMD1, 2 and 3] limb-girdle muscular dystrophy [LGMD] type 1B, dilated cardiomyopathy [CMD1A], familial partial lipodystrophy [FPLD2]), full gene sequence

LRP5 (low density lipoprotein receptor-related protein 5) (eg, osteopetrosis), full gene sequence

MAP2K1 (mitogen-activated protein kinase 1) (eg, cardiofaciocutaneous syndrome), full gene sequence

MAP2K2 (mitogen-activated protein kinase 2) (eg, cardiofaciocutaneous syndrome), full gene sequence

MAPT (microtubule-associated protein tau) (eg, frontotemporal dementia), full gene sequence

MCCC1 (methylcrotonoyl-CoA carboxylase 1 [alpha]) (eg, 3-methylcrotonyl-CoA carboxylase deficiency), full gene sequence

MCCC2 (methylcrotonoyl-CoA carboxylase 2 [beta]) (eg, 3-methylcrotonyl carboxylase deficiency), full gene sequence

MFN2 (mitofusin 2) (eg, Charcot-Marie-Tooth disease), full gene sequence

MTM1 (myotubularin 1) (eg, X-linked centronuclear myopathy), full gene sequence

MUT (methylmalonyl CoA mutase) (eg, methylmalonic acidemia), full gene sequence

MUTYH (mutY homolog [E. coli]) (eg, MYH-associated polyposis), full gene sequence

NDUFS1 (NADH dehydrogenase [ubiquinone] Fe-S protein 1, 75kDa [NADH-coenzyme Q reductase]) (eg, Leigh syndrome, mitochondrial complex I deficiency), full gene sequence

NF2 (neurofibromin 2 [merlin]) (eg, neurofibromatosis, type 2), full gene sequence

NOTCH3 (notch 3) (eg, cerebral autosomal dominant arteriopathy with subcortical infarcts and leukoencephalopathy [CADASIL]), targeted sequence analysis (eg, exons 1-23)

NPC1 (Niemann-Pick disease, type C1) (eg, Niemann-Pick disease), full gene sequence

NPHP1 (nephronophthisis 1 [juvenile]) (eg, Joubert syndrome), full gene sequence

NSD1 (nuclear receptor binding SET domain protein 1) (eg, Sotos syndrome), full gene sequence

OPA1 (optic atrophy 1) (eg, optic atrophy), duplication/deletion analysis

OPTN (optineurin) (eg, amyotrophic lateral sclerosis), full gene sequence

PAFAH1B1 (platelet-activating factor acetylhydrolase 1b, regulatory subunit 1 [45kDa]) (eg, lissencephaly, Miller-Dieker syndrome), full gene sequence

PAH (phenylalanine hydroxylase) (eg, phenylketonuria), full gene sequence

PARK2 (Parkinson protein 2, E3 ubiquitin protein ligase [parkin]) (eg, Parkinson disease), full gene sequence

PAX2 (paired box 2) (eg, renal coloboma syndrome), full gene sequence

PC (pyruvate carboxylase) (eg, pyruvate carboxylase deficiency), full gene sequence

PCCA (propionyl CoA carboxylase, alpha polypeptide) (eg, propionic acidemia, type 1), full gene sequence

PCCB (propionyl CoA carboxylase, beta polypeptide) (eg, propionic acidemia), full gene sequence

PCDH15 (protocadherin-related 15) (eg, Usher syndrome type 1F), duplication/deletion analysis

PCSK9 (proprotein convertase subtilisin/kexin type 9) (eg, familial hypercholesterolemia), full gene sequence

PDHA1 (pyruvate dehydrogenase [lipoamide] alpha 1) (eg, lactic acidosis), full gene sequence

PDHX (pyruvate dehydrogenase complex, component X) (eg, lactic acidosis), full gene sequence

PHEX (phosphate-regulating endopeptidase homolog, X-linked) (eg, hypophosphatemic rickets), full gene sequence

PKD2 (polycystic kidney disease 2 [autosomal dominant]) (eg, polycystic kidney disease), full gene sequence

PKP2 (plakophilin 2) (eg, arrhythmogenic right ventricular dysplasia/cardiomyopathy 9), full gene sequence

PNKD (paroxysmal nonkinesigenic dyskinesia) (eg, paroxysmal nonkinesigenic dyskinesia), full gene sequence

POLG (polymerase [DNA directed], gamma) (eg, Alpers-Huttenlocher syndrome, autosomal dominant progressive external ophthalmoplegia), full gene sequence

POMGNT1 (protein O-linked mannose beta1,2-N acetylglucosaminyltransferase) (eg, muscle-eye-brain disease, Walker-Warburg syndrome), full gene sequence

POMT1 (protein-O-mannosyltransferase 1) (eg, limb-girdle muscular dystrophy [LGMD] type 2K, Walker-Warburg syndrome), full gene sequence

POMT2 (protein-O-mannosyltransferase 2) (eg, limb-girdle muscular dystrophy [LGMD] type 2N, Walker-Warburg syndrome), full gene sequence

PPOX (protoporphyrinogen oxidase) (eg, variegate porphyria), full gene sequence

PRKAG2 (protein kinase, AMP-activated, gamma 2 non-catalytic subunit) (eg, familial hypertrophic cardiomyopathy with Wolff-Parkinson-White syndrome, lethal congenital glycogen storage disease of heart), full gene sequence

PRKCG (protein kinase C, gamma) (eg, spinocerebellar ataxia), full gene sequence

PSEN2 (presenilin 2 [Alzheimer disease 4]) (eg, Alzheimer disease), full gene sequence

PTPN11 (protein tyrosine phosphatase, non-receptor type 11) (eg, Noonan syndrome, LEOPARD syndrome), full gene sequence

PYGM (phosphorylase, glycogen, muscle) (eg, glycogen storage disease type V, McArdle disease), full gene sequence

RAF1 (v-raf-1 murine leukemia viral oncogene homolog 1) (eg, LEOPARD syndrome), full gene sequence

RET (ret proto-oncogene) (eg, Hirschsprung disease), full gene sequence

RPE65 (retinal pigment epithelium-specific protein 65kDa) (eg, retinitis pigmentosa, Leber congenital amaurosis), full gene sequence

RYR1 (ryanodine receptor 1, skeletal) (eg, malignant hyperthermia), targeted sequence analysis of exons with functionally-confirmed mutations

SCN4A (sodium channel, voltage-gated, type IV, alpha subunit) (eg, hyperkalemic periodic paralysis), full gene sequence

SCNN1A (sodium channel, nonvoltage-gated 1 alpha) (eg, pseudohypoaldosteronism), full gene sequence

SCNN1B (sodium channel, nonvoltage-gated 1, beta) (eg, Liddle syndrome, pseudohypoaldosteronism), full gene sequence

SCNN1G (sodium channel, nonvoltage-gated 1, gamma) (eg, Liddle syndrome, pseudohypoaldosteronism), full gene sequence

SDHA (succinate dehydrogenase complex, subunit A, flavoprotein [Fp]) (eg, Leigh syndrome, mitochondrial complex II deficiency), full gene sequence

SETX (senataxin) (eg, ataxia), full gene sequence

SGCE (sarcoglycan, epsilon) (eg, myoclonic dystonia), full gene sequence

SH3TC2 (SH3 domain and tetratricopeptide repeats 2) (eg, Charcot-Marie-Tooth disease), full gene sequence

SLC9A6 (solute carrier family 9 [sodium/hydrogen exchanger], member 6) (eg, Christianson syndrome), full gene sequence

SLC26A4 (solute carrier family 26, member 4) (eg, Pendred syndrome), full gene sequence

SLC37A4 (solute carrier family 37 [glucose-6-phosphate transporter], member 4) (eg, glycogen storage disease type Ib), full gene sequence

SMAD4 (SMAD family member 4) (eg, hemorrhagic telangiectasia syndrome, juvenile polyposis), full gene sequence

SOS1 (son of sevenless homolog 1) (eg, Noonan syndrome, gingival fibromatosis), full gene sequence

SPAST (spastin) (eg, spastic paraplegia), full gene sequence

SPG7 (spastic paraplegia 7 [pure and complicated autosomal recessive]) (eg, spastic paraplegia), full gene sequence

STXBP1 (syntaxin-binding protein 1) (eg, epileptic encephalopathy), full gene sequence

TAZ (tafazzin) (eg, methylglutaconic aciduria type 2, Barth syndrome), full gene sequence

TCF4 (transcription factor 4) (eg, Pitt-Hopkins syndrome), full gene sequence

TH (tyrosine hydroxylase) (eg, Segawa syndrome), full gene sequence

TMEM43 (transmembrane protein 43) (eg, arrhythmogenic right ventricular cardiomyopathy), full gene sequence

TNNT2 (troponin T, type 2 [cardiac]) (eg, familial hypertrophic cardiomyopathy), full gene sequence

TRPC6 (transient receptor potential cation channel, subfamily C, member 6) (eg, focal segmental glomerulosclerosis), full gene sequence

TSC1 (tuberous sclerosis 1) (eg, tuberous sclerosis), full gene sequence

TSC2 (tuberous sclerosis 2) (eg, tuberous sclerosis), duplication/deletion analysis

UBE3A (ubiquitin protein ligase E3A) (eg, Angelman syndrome), full gene sequence

UMOD (uromodulin) (eg, glomerulocystic kidney disease with hyperuricemia and isosthenuria), full gene sequence

VWF (von Willebrand factor) (von Willebrand disease type 2A), extended targeted sequence analysis (eg, exons 11-16, 24-26, 51, 52)

WAS (Wiskott-Aldrich syndrome [eczema-thrombocytopenia]) (eg, Wiskott-Aldrich syndrome), full gene sequence

Rationale

In accordance with the establishment of Tier 1 codes 81277, 81307, and 81308, the term "cytogenomic array analysis for neoplasia," two exclusionary parenthetical notes, and PALB2 gene test have been removed from code 81406.

Refer to the codebook and the Rationale for codes 81277, 81307, and 81308 for a full discussion of these changes.

▲ **81407** Molecular pathology procedure, Level 8 (eg, analysis of 26-50 exons by DNA sequence analysis, mutation scanning or duplication/deletion variants of >50 exons, sequence analysis of multiple genes on one platform)

ABCC8 (ATP-binding cassette, sub-family C [CFTR/MRP], member 8) (eg, familial hyperinsulinism), full gene sequence

AGL (amylo-alpha-1, 6-glucosidase, 4-alpha-glucanotransferase) (eg, glycogen storage disease type III), full gene sequence

AHI1 (Abelson helper integration site 1) (eg, Joubert syndrome), full gene sequence

▶ *APOB (apolipoprotein B)* (eg, familial hypercholesterolemia type B) full gene sequence ◀

ASPM (asp [abnormal spindle] homolog, microcephaly associated [Drosophila]) (eg, primary microcephaly), full gene sequence

CHD7 (chromodomain helicase DNA binding protein 7) (eg, CHARGE syndrome), full gene sequence

COL4A4 (collagen, type IV, alpha 4) (eg, Alport syndrome), full gene sequence

COL4A5 (collagen, type IV, alpha 5) (eg, Alport syndrome), duplication/deletion analysis

COL6A1 (collagen, type VI, alpha 1) (eg, collagen type VI-related disorders), full gene sequence

COL6A2 (collagen, type VI, alpha 2) (eg, collagen type VI-related disorders), full gene sequence

COL6A3 (collagen, type VI, alpha 3) (eg, collagen type VI-related disorders), full gene sequence

CREBBP (CREB binding protein) (eg, Rubinstein-Taybi syndrome), full gene sequence

F8 (coagulation factor VIII) (eg, hemophilia A), full gene sequence

JAG1 (jagged 1) (eg, Alagille syndrome), full gene sequence

KDM5C (lysine [K]-specific demethylase 5C) (eg, X-linked mental retardation), full gene sequence

KIAA0196 (KIAA0196) (eg, spastic paraplegia), full gene sequence

L1CAM (L1 cell adhesion molecule) (eg, MASA syndrome, X-linked hydrocephaly), full gene sequence

LAMB2 (laminin, beta 2 [laminin S]) (eg, Pierson syndrome), full gene sequence

MYBPC3 (myosin binding protein C, cardiac) (eg, familial hypertrophic cardiomyopathy), full gene sequence

MYH6 (myosin, heavy chain 6, cardiac muscle, alpha) (eg, familial dilated cardiomyopathy), full gene sequence

MYH7 (myosin, heavy chain 7, cardiac muscle, beta) (eg, familial hypertrophic cardiomyopathy, Liang distal myopathy), full gene sequence

MYO7A (myosin VIIA) (eg, Usher syndrome, type 1), full gene sequence

NOTCH1 (notch 1) (eg, aortic valve disease), full gene sequence

NPHS1 (nephrosis 1, congenital, Finnish type [nephrin]) (eg, congenital Finnish nephrosis), full gene sequence

OPA1 (optic atrophy 1) (eg, optic atrophy), full gene sequence

PCDH15 (protocadherin-related 15) (eg, Usher syndrome, type 1), full gene sequence

PKD1 (polycystic kidney disease 1 [autosomal dominant]) (eg, polycystic kidney disease), full gene sequence

PLCE1 (phospholipase C, epsilon 1) (eg, nephrotic syndrome type 3), full gene sequence

SCN1A (sodium channel, voltage-gated, type 1, alpha subunit) (eg, generalized epilepsy with febrile seizures), full gene sequence

SCN5A (sodium channel, voltage-gated, type V, alpha subunit) (eg, familial dilated cardiomyopathy), full gene sequence

SLC12A1 (solute carrier family 12 [sodium/potassium/chloride transporters], member 1) (eg, Bartter syndrome), full gene sequence

SLC12A3 (solute carrier family 12 [sodium/chloride transporters], member 3) (eg, Gitelman syndrome), full gene sequence

SPG11 (spastic paraplegia 11 [autosomal recessive]) (eg, spastic paraplegia), full gene sequence

SPTBN2 (spectrin, beta, non-erythrocytic 2) (eg, spinocerebellar ataxia), full gene sequence

TMEM67 (transmembrane protein 67) (eg, Joubert syndrome), full gene sequence

TSC2 (tuberous sclerosis 2) (eg, tuberous sclerosis), full gene sequence

USH1C (Usher syndrome 1C [autosomal recessive, severe]) (eg, Usher syndrome, type 1), full gene sequence

VPS13B (vacuolar protein sorting 13 homolog B [yeast]) (eg, Cohen syndrome), duplication/deletion analysis

WDR62 (WD repeat domain 62) (eg, primary autosomal recessive microcephaly), full gene sequence

Rationale

Tier 2 code 81407 has been revised to include full-gene sequencing of the APOB gene. This test is helpful in identifying the presence of familial hypercholesterolemia.

Multianalyte Assays with Algorithmic Analyses

81518   Oncology (breast), mRNA, gene expression profiling by real-time RT-PCR of 11 genes (7 content and 4 housekeeping), utilizing formalin-fixed paraffin-embedded tissue, algorithms reported as percentage risk for metastatic recurrence and likelihood of benefit from extended endocrine therapy

#● 81522   Oncology (breast), mRNA, gene expression profiling by RT-PCR of 12 genes (8 content and 4 housekeeping), utilizing formalin-fixed paraffin-embedded tissue, algorithm reported as recurrence risk score

81519   Oncology (breast), mRNA, gene expression profiling by real-time RT-PCR of 21 genes, utilizing formalin-fixed paraffin-embedded tissue, algorithm reported as recurrence score

81520   Oncology (breast), mRNA gene expression profiling by hybrid capture of 58 genes (50 content and 8 housekeeping), utilizing formalin-fixed paraffin-embedded tissue, algorithm reported as a recurrence risk score

81521   Oncology (breast), mRNA, microarray gene expression profiling of 70 content genes and 465 housekeeping genes, utilizing fresh frozen or formalin-fixed paraffin-embedded tissue, algorithm reported as index related to risk of distant metastasis

81522   Code is out of numerical sequence. See 81512-81520

Rationale

A new Category I multianalyte assay with algorithmic analysis (MAAA) code 81522 has been established to report risk-recurrence score reporting for breast oncology mRNA gene expression profiling.

This code is intended to identify a 12-gene RNA expression test, which measures gene expression, tumor size, and nodal status, and places them into a proprietary algorithm that generates a patient-specific score. This score allows estimation of the disease state and facilitates decisions regarding treatments, such as chemotherapy and endocrine therapy, by differentiating patients who are unlikely to experience recurrence and can use endocrine therapy alone versus those who will need both.

Clinical Example (81522)

During annual breast mammography, a 1-cm suspicious lesion is identified in a 63-year-old female. A biopsy reveals an ER positive, HER2 negative breast cancer. To determine whether the patient would benefit from addition of adjuvant chemotherapy to the postoperative standard of care that involves five years of endocrine therapy, an 8-gene ribonucleic acid (RNA) expression test is ordered.

Description of Procedure (81522)

Extract RNA from formalin-fixed paraffin-embedded tumor tissue. Perform RT-PCR to measure the expression levels of eight cancer-related genes and the four housekeeping genes. A proprietary algorithm produces a score related to risk of tumor recurrence. Analyze the data and compose a report.

81541   Oncology (prostate), mRNA gene expression profiling by real-time RT-PCR of 46 genes (31 content and 15 housekeeping), utilizing formalin-fixed paraffin-embedded tissue, algorithm reported as a disease-specific mortality risk score

● 81542   Oncology (prostate), mRNA, microarray gene expression profiling of 22 content genes, utilizing formalin-fixed paraffin-embedded tissue, algorithm reported as metastasis risk score

Rationale

A new Category I MAAA code 81542 has been established to report prostate cancer metastasis risk score. Unlisted code 81479 was previously used; however, it does not adequately address the reporting of the prostate cancer metastasis risk score. In addition, the usage volume and clinical importance of this test warrant its own code.

A separate listing of this code that includes the proprietary test name has been added to Appendix O.

Clinical Example (81542)

A 66-year-old male was recently diagnosed with localized prostate cancer. According to the National Comprehensive Cancer Network's (NCCN's) classifications, his cancer is considered low risk with a PSA of 6.6 ng/mL, clinical stage T1c and Gleason Score 3 + 3 =6 (Grade Group 1). A gene expression assay is ordered to assess the patient's risk of metastasis.

Description of Procedure (81542)

Extract RNA from formalin-fixed and paraffin-embedded biopsy specimens. Evaluate for gene expression of 22 targeted genes related to prostate cancer metastasis. Quantitate the results and, using a proprietary algorithm, calculate a genomic risk score ranging from 0 to 1.0. Provide a genomic risk category (low, average, or high) based on pre-specified cut points. Return a report to the patient's physician.

81545	Oncology (thyroid), gene expression analysis of 142 genes, utilizing fine needle aspirate, algorithm reported as a categorical result (eg, benign or suspicious)
81551	Oncology (prostate), promoter methylation profiling by real-time PCR of 3 genes (*GSTP1, APC, RASSF1*), utilizing formalin-fixed paraffin-embedded tissue, algorithm reported as a likelihood of prostate cancer detection on repeat biopsy
●81552	Oncology (uveal melanoma), mRNA, gene expression profiling by real-time RT-PCR of 15 genes (12 content and 3 housekeeping), utilizing fine needle aspirate or formalin-fixed paraffin-embedded tissue, algorithm reported as risk of metastasis

Rationale

A new Category I MAAA code 81552 has been established to report mRNA analysis of 15 genes using fine needle aspirate or formalin-fixed paraffin-embedded uveal melanoma tissue from a primary eye tumor. The risk score obtained from the test is used to determine the appropriate management of the disease following treatment of the tumor.

A separate listing of this code that includes the proprietary test name has been added to Appendix O.

Clinical Example (81552)

A 60-year-old male with a suspicious eye lesion presents to an ophthalmologist or retina specialist. The patient is clinically diagnosed with uveal melanoma. The ophthalmologist performs an intraocular tumor biopsy (fine needle aspiration) prior to definitive treatment of the primary tumor. An aliquot of the aspiration material biopsy is immediately frozen and submitted for gene expression profile testing to determine his five-year metastatic risk.

Description of Procedure (81552)

Isolate RNA from primary uveal melanoma tumor tissue. Determine expression levels of 15 content and housekeeping genes by quantitative RT-PCR. Normalize the expression of 12 prognostic genes relative to three control genes, then analyze with a proprietary predictive modeling algorithm that classifies the specimen with related risk of metastasis. Issue a report specifying the risk class with the estimated three- and five-year metastatic risks associated with each class.

Microbiology

87471	Infectious agent detection by nucleic acid (DNA or RNA); Bartonella henselae and Bartonella quintana, amplified probe technique
87472	Bartonella henselae and Bartonella quintana, quantification
87562	Mycobacteria avium-intracellulare, quantification
●87563	Mycoplasma genitalium, amplified probe technique

Rationale

A new code (87563) has been established to report Mycoplasma genitalium infectious agent detection. This amplified probe technique is used to distinguish Mycoplasma genitalium from other types of sexually transmitted infections. Unlisted code 87798 was previously used to report the detection of Mycoplasma genitalium; however, it is not specific for testing for M. genitalium by amplified probe technique.

Clinical Example (87563)

A 19-year-old female presents to her primary care physician with dysuria and vaginal discharge.

Description of Procedure (87563)

Collect a specimen from the patient (eg, vaginal swab, urethral swab). Submit the specimen to the laboratory for target capture, amplification, and detection. Qualitatively report the result.

Reproductive Medicine Procedures

89331 Sperm evaluation, for retrograde ejaculation, urine (sperm concentration, motility, and morphology, as indicated)

(For semen analysis on concurrent semen specimen, see 89300-89322 in conjunction with 89331)

(For detection of sperm in urine, use 81015)

89335 Cryopreservation, reproductive tissue, testicular

(For cryopreservation of embryo[s], use 89258. For cryopreservation of sperm, use 89259)

▶(For cryopreservation, ovarian tissue, oocytes, use 0058T; for mature oocytes, use 89337)◀

89337 Cryopreservation, mature oocyte(s)

Rationale

In accordance with the deletion of code 0357T, the parenthetical note following code 89335 has been revised with the removal of this code.

Refer to the codebook and the Rationale for code 0357T for a full discussion of these changes.

Proprietary Laboratory Analyses

Proprietary laboratory analyses (PLA) codes describe proprietary clinical laboratory analyses and can be either provided by a single ("sole-source") laboratory or licensed or marketed to multiple providing laboratories (eg, cleared or approved by the Food and Drug Administration [FDA]).

This subsection includes advanced diagnostic laboratory tests (ADLTs) and clinical diagnostic laboratory tests (CDLTs), as defined under the Protecting Access to Medicare Act (PAMA) of 2014. These analyses may include a range of medical laboratory tests including, but not limited to, multianalyte assays with algorithmic analyses (MAAA) and genomic sequencing procedures (GSP). The descriptor nomenclature follows, where possible, existing code conventions (eg, MAAA, GSP).

▶Unless specifically noted, even though the Proprietary Laboratory Analyses section of the code set is located at the end of the Pathology and Laboratory section of the code set, a PLA code does not fulfill Category I code criteria. PLA codes are not required to fulfill the Category I criteria. The standards for inclusion in the PLA section are:

- The test must be commercially available in the United States for use on human specimens and

- The clinical laboratory or manufacturer that offers the test must request the code.◀

For similar laboratory analyses that fulfill Category I criteria, see codes listed in the numeric 80000 series.

When a PLA code is available to report a given proprietary laboratory service, that PLA code takes precedence. The service should not be reported with any other CPT code(s) and other CPT code(s) should not be used to report services that may be reported with that specific PLA code. These codes encompass all analytical services required for the analysis (eg, cell lysis, nucleic acid stabilization, extraction, digestion, amplification, hybridization and detection). For molecular analyses, additional procedures that are required prior to cell lysis (eg, microdissection [codes 88380 and 88381]) may be reported separately.

Codes in this subsection are released on a quarterly basis to expedite dissemination for reporting. PLA codes will be published electronically on the AMA CPT website (ama-assn.org/cpt-pla-codes), distributed via CPT data files on a quarterly basis, and, at a minimum, made available in print annually in the CPT codebook. Go to https://www.ama-assn.org/systems/files/2019-06/cpt-pla-codes-long.pdf for the most current listing.

All codes that are included in this section are also included in Appendix O, with the procedure's proprietary name. In order to report a PLA code, the analysis performed must fulfill the code descriptor and must be the test represented by the proprietary name listed in Appendix O. In some instances, the descriptor language of PLA codes may be identical and the code may only be differentiated by the listed proprietary name in Appendix O. When more than one PLA has an identical descriptor, the codes will be denoted by the symbol "⌘."

▶All PLA tests will have assigned codes in the PLA section of the code set. Any PLA coded test(s) that satisfies Category I criteria and has been accepted by the CPT Editorial Panel will be designated by the addition of the symbol "↑↓" to the existing PLA code and will remain in the PLA section of the code set.

If a proprietary test has already been accepted for a Category I code and a code has not been published, subsequent application for a PLA code will take precedence. The code will only be placed in the PLA section.◀

Rationale

The guidelines in the Proprietary Laboratory Analyses subsection have been revised to explain the new PLA symbol ↕.

PLA codes describe proprietary clinical laboratory analyses, which can be provided either by a single ("sole source") laboratory or licensed or marketed to multiple providing laboratories (eg, cleared or approved by the Food and Drug Administration [FDA]).

This subsection includes advanced diagnostic laboratory tests (ADLTs) and clinical diagnostic laboratory tests (CDLTs), as defined under the Protecting Access to Medicare Act (PAMA) of 2014. These analyses may include a range of medical laboratory tests including, but not limited to, MAAAs and genomic sequencing procedures (GSPs). The descriptor nomenclature follows, where possible, existing code conventions (eg, MAAA, GSP). These codes are not required to fulfill the Category I criteria. The standards for inclusion in this section are:

- The test must be commercially available in the United States for use on human specimens; and
- The clinical laboratory or manufacturer that offers the test must request the code.

Even though PLA codes are not required to fulfill the Category I criteria, any PLA coded test that satisfies Category I criteria and has been accepted by the CPT Editorial Panel will be designated with the ↕ symbol to the existing PLA code and will remain in the PLA section of the code set.

▲ **0008U** Helicobacter pylori detection and antibiotic resistance, DNA, 16S and 23S rRNA, gyrA, pbp1, rdxA and rpoB, next generation sequencing, formalin-fixed paraffin-embedded or fresh tissue or fecal sample, predictive, reported as positive or negative for resistance to clarithromycin, fluoroquinolones, metronidazole, amoxicillin, tetracycline, and rifabutin

▶(0020U has been deleted)◀

▶(0028U has been deleted)◀

▶(0057U has been deleted)◀

● **0062U** Autoimmune (systemic lupus erythematosus), IgG and IgM analysis of 80 biomarkers, utilizing serum, algorithm reported with a risk score

● **0063U** Neurology (autism), 32 amines by LC-MS/MS, using plasma, algorithm reported as metabolic signature associated with autism spectrum disorder

● **0064U** Antibody, Treponema pallidum, total and rapid plasma reagin (RPR), immunoassay, qualitative

● **0065U** Syphilis test, non-treponemal antibody, immunoassay, qualitative (RPR)

● **0066U** Placental alpha-micro globulin-1 (PAMG-1), immunoassay with direct optical observation, cervico-vaginal fluid, each specimen

● **0067U** Oncology (breast), immunohistochemistry, protein expression profiling of 4 biomarkers (matrix metalloproteinase-1 [MMP-1], carcinoembryonic antigen-related cell adhesion molecule 6 [CEACAM6], hyaluronoglucosaminidase [HYAL1], highly expressed in cancer protein [HEC1]), formalin-fixed paraffin-embedded precancerous breast tissue, algorithm reported as carcinoma risk score

● **0068U** Candida species panel (*C. albicans, C. glabrata, C. parapsilosis, C. kruseii, C. tropicalis,* and *C. auris*), amplified probe technique with qualitative report of the presence or absence of each species

● **0069U** Oncology (colorectal), microRNA, RT-PCR expression profiling of miR-31-3p, formalin-fixed paraffin-embedded tissue, algorithm reported as an expression score

● **0070U** *CYP2D6 (cytochrome P450, family 2, subfamily D, polypeptide 6)* (eg, drug metabolism) gene analysis, common and select rare variants (ie, *2, *3, *4, *4N, *5, *6, *7, *8, *9, *10, *11, *12, *13, *14A, *14B, *15, *17, *29, *35, *36, *41, *57, *61, *63, *68, *83, *xN)

+● **0071U** *CYP2D6 (cytochrome P450, family 2, subfamily D, polypeptide 6)* (eg, drug metabolism) gene analysis, full gene sequence (List separately in addition to code for primary procedure)

▶(Use 0071U in conjunction with 0070U)◀

+● **0072U** *CYP2D6 (cytochrome P450, family 2, subfamily D, polypeptide 6)* (eg, drug metabolism) gene analysis, targeted sequence analysis (ie, *CYP2D6-2D7* hybrid gene) (List separately in addition to code for primary procedure)

▶(Use 0072U in conjunction with 0070U)◀

+● **0073U** *CYP2D6 (cytochrome P450, family 2, subfamily D, polypeptide 6)* (eg, drug metabolism) gene analysis, targeted sequence analysis (ie, *CYP2D7-2D6* hybrid gene) (List separately in addition to code for primary procedure)

▶(Use 0073U in conjunction with 0070U)◀

+● **0074U** *CYP2D6 (cytochrome P450, family 2, subfamily D, polypeptide 6)* (eg, drug metabolism) gene analysis, targeted sequence analysis (ie, non-duplicated gene when duplication/multiplication is trans) (List separately in addition to code for primary procedure)

▶(Use 0074U in conjunction with 0070U)◀

+● **0075U** *CYP2D6 (cytochrome P450, family 2, subfamily D, polypeptide 6)* (eg, drug metabolism) gene analysis, targeted sequence analysis (ie, 5' gene duplication/multiplication) (List separately in addition to code for primary procedure)

▶(Use 0075U in conjunction with 0070U)◀

▲ = Revised code   ● = New code   ▶◀ = Contains new or revised text   ✕ = Duplicate PLA test   ↕ = Category I PLA

Pathology and Laboratory

+● **0076U** CYP2D6 (cytochrome P450, family 2, subfamily D, polypeptide 6) (eg, drug metabolism) gene analysis, targeted sequence analysis (ie, 3' gene duplication/multiplication) (List separately in addition to code for primary procedure)

▶(Use 0076U in conjunction with 0070U)◀

● **0077U** Immunoglobulin paraprotein (M-protein), qualitative, immunoprecipitation and mass spectrometry, blood or urine, including isotype

● **0078U** Pain management (opioid-use disorder) genotyping panel, 16 common variants (ie, *ABCB1, COMT, DAT1, DBH, DOR, DRD1, DRD2, DRD4, GABA, GAL, HTR2A, HTTLPR, MTHFR, MUOR, OPRK1, OPRM1*), buccal swab or other germline tissue sample, algorithm reported as positive or negative risk of opioid-use disorder

● **0079U** Comparative DNA analysis using multiple selected single-nucleotide polymorphisms (SNPs), urine and buccal DNA, for specimen identity verification

● **0080U** Oncology (lung), mass spectrometric analysis of galectin-3-binding protein and scavenger receptor cysteine-rich type 1 protein M130, with five clinical risk factors (age, smoking status, nodule diameter, nodule-spiculation status and nodule location), utilizing plasma, algorithm reported as a categorical probability of malignancy

▶(0081U has been deleted. To report, use 81552)◀

● **0082U** Drug test(s), definitive, 90 or more drugs or substances, definitive chromatography with mass spectrometry, and presumptive, any number of drug classes, by instrument chemistry analyzer (utilizing immunoassay), urine, report of presence or absence of each drug, drug metabolite or substance with description and severity of significant interactions per date of service

● **0083U** Oncology, response to chemotherapy drugs using motility contrast tomography, fresh or frozen tissue, reported as likelihood of sensitivity or resistance to drugs or drug combinations

● **0084U** Red blood cell antigen typing, DNA, genotyping of 10 blood groups with phenotype prediction of 37 red blood cell antigens

● **0085U** Cytolethal distending toxin B (CdtB) and vinculin IgG antibodies by immunoassay (ie, ELISA)

● **0086U** Infectious disease (bacterial and fungal), organism identification, blood culture, using rRNA FISH, 6 or more organism targets, reported as positive or negative with phenotypic minimum inhibitory concentration (MIC)-based antimicrobial susceptibility

● **0087U** Cardiology (heart transplant), mRNA gene expression profiling by microarray of 1283 genes, transplant biopsy tissue, allograft rejection and injury algorithm reported as a probability score

● **0088U** Transplantation medicine (kidney allograft rejection), microarray gene expression profiling of 1494 genes, utilizing transplant biopsy tissue, algorithm reported as a probability score for rejection

● **0089U** Oncology (melanoma), gene expression profiling by RTqPCR, *PRAME* and *LINC00518*, superficial collection using adhesive patch(es)

● **0090U** Oncology (cutaneous melanoma), mRNA gene expression profiling by RT-PCR of 23 genes (14 content and 9 housekeeping), utilizing formalin-fixed paraffin-embedded tissue, algorithm reported as a categorical result (ie, benign, indeterminate, malignant)

● **0091U** Oncology (colorectal) screening, cell enumeration of circulating tumor cells, utilizing whole blood, algorithm, for the presence of adenoma or cancer, reported as a positive or negative result

● **0092U** Oncology (lung), three protein biomarkers, immunoassay using magnetic nanosensor technology, plasma, algorithm reported as risk score for likelihood of malignancy

● **0093U** Prescription drug monitoring, evaluation of 65 common drugs by LC-MS/MS, urine, each drug reported detected or not detected

● **0094U** Genome (eg, unexplained constitutional or heritable disorder or syndrome), rapid sequence analysis

● **0095U** Inflammation (eosinophilic esophagitis), ELISA analysis of eotaxin-3 *(CCL26 [C-C motif chemokine ligand 26])* and major basic protein *(PRG2 [proteoglycan 2, pro eosinophil major basic protein])*, specimen obtained by swallowed nylon string, algorithm reported as predictive probability index for active eosinophilic esophagitis

● **0096U** Human papillomavirus (HPV), high-risk types (ie, 16, 18, 31, 33, 35, 39, 45, 51, 52, 56, 58, 59, 66, 68), male urine

● **0097U** Gastrointestinal pathogen, multiplex reverse transcription and multiplex amplified probe technique, multiple types or subtypes, 22 targets (Campylobacter [C. jejuni/C. coli/C. upsaliensis], Clostridium difficile [C. difficile] toxin A/B, Plesiomonas shigelloides, Salmonella, Vibrio [V. parahaemolyticus/V. vulnificus/V. cholerae], including specific identification of Vibrio cholerae, Yersinia enterocolitica, Enteroaggregative Escherichia coli [EAEC], Enteropathogenic Escherichia coli [EPEC], Enterotoxigenic Escherichia coli [ETEC] lt/st, Shiga-like toxin-producing Escherichia coli [STEC] stx1/stx2 [including specific identification of the E. coli O157 serogroup within STEC], Shigella/Enteroinvasive Escherichia coli [EIEC], Cryptosporidium, Cyclospora cayetanensis, Entamoeba histolytica, Giardia lamblia [also known as G. intestinalis and G. duodenalis], adenovirus F 40/41, astrovirus, norovirus GI/GII, rotavirus A, sapovirus [Genogroups I, II, IV, and V])

CPT Changes 2020 — Pathology and Laboratory

● **0098U** Respiratory pathogen, multiplex reverse transcription and multiplex amplified probe technique, multiple types or subtypes, 14 targets (adenovirus, coronavirus, human metapneumovirus, influenza A, influenza A subtype H1, influenza A subtype H3, influenza A subtype H1-2009, influenza B, parainfluenza virus, human rhinovirus/enterovirus, respiratory syncytial virus, Bordetella pertussis, Chlamydophila pneumoniae, Mycoplasma pneumoniae)

● **0099U** Respiratory pathogen, multiplex reverse transcription and multiplex amplified probe technique, multiple types or subtypes, 20 targets (adenovirus, coronavirus 229E, coronavirus HKU1, coronavirus, coronavirus OC43, human metapneumovirus, influenza A, influenza A subtype, influenza A subtype H3, influenza A subtype H1-2009, influenza, parainfluenza virus, parainfluenza virus 2, parainfluenza virus 3, parainfluenza virus 4, human rhinovirus/enterovirus, respiratory syncytial virus, Bordetella pertussis, Chlamydophila pneumonia, Mycoplasma pneumoniae)

● **0100U** Respiratory pathogen, multiplex reverse transcription and multiplex amplified probe technique, multiple types or subtypes, 21 targets (adenovirus, coronavirus 229E, coronavirus HKU1, coronavirus NL63, coronavirus OC43, human metapneumovirus, human rhinovirus/enterovirus, influenza A, including subtypes H1, H1-2009, and H3, influenza B, parainfluenza virus 1, parainfluenza virus 2, parainfluenza virus 3, parainfluenza virus 4, respiratory syncytial virus, Bordetella parapertussis [IS1001], Bordetella pertussis [ptxP], Chlamydia pneumoniae, Mycoplasma pneumoniae)

● **0101U** Hereditary colon cancer disorders (eg, Lynch syndrome, PTEN hamartoma syndrome, Cowden syndrome, familial adenomatosis polyposis), genomic sequence analysis panel utilizing a combination of NGS, Sanger, MLPA, and array CGH, with mRNA analytics to resolve variants of unknown significance when indicated (15 genes [sequencing and deletion/duplication], EPCAM and GREM1 [deletion/duplication only])

● **0102U** Hereditary breast cancer-related disorders (eg, hereditary breast cancer, hereditary ovarian cancer, hereditary endometrial cancer), genomic sequence analysis panel utilizing a combination of NGS, Sanger, MLPA, and array CGH, with mRNA analytics to resolve variants of unknown significance when indicated (17 genes [sequencing and deletion/duplication])

● **0103U** Hereditary ovarian cancer (eg, hereditary ovarian cancer, hereditary endometrial cancer), genomic sequence analysis panel utilizing a combination of NGS, Sanger, MLPA, and array CGH, with mRNA analytics to resolve variants of unknown significance when indicated (24 genes [sequencing and deletion/duplication], EPCAM [deletion/duplication only])

▶(0104U has been deleted)◀

● **0105U** Nephrology (chronic kidney disease), multiplex electrochemiluminescent immunoassay (ECLIA) of tumor necrosis factor receptor 1A, receptor superfamily 2 (TNFR1, TNFR2), and kidney injury molecule-1 (KIM-1) combined with longitudinal clinical data, including APOL1 genotype if available, and plasma (isolated fresh or frozen), algorithm reported as probability score for rapid kidney function decline (RKFD)

● **0106U** Gastric emptying, serial collection of 7 timed breath specimens, non-radioisotope carbon-13 (^{13}C) spirulina substrate, analysis of each specimen by gas isotope ratio mass spectrometry, reported as rate of $^{13}CO_2$ excretion

● **0107U** Clostridium difficile toxin(s) antigen detection by immunoassay technique, stool, qualitative, multiple-step method

● **0108U** Gastroenterology (Barrett's esophagus), whole slide–digital imaging, including morphometric analysis, computer-assisted quantitative immunolabeling of 9 protein biomarkers (p16, AMACR, p53, CD68, COX-2, CD45RO, HIF1a, HER-2, K20) and morphology, formalin-fixed paraffin-embedded tissue, algorithm reported as risk of progression to high-grade dysplasia or cancer

● **0109U** Infectious disease (Aspergillus species), real-time PCR for detection of DNA from 4 species (A. fumigatus, A. terreus, A. niger, and A. flavus), blood, lavage fluid, or tissue, qualitative reporting of presence or absence of each species

● **0110U** Prescription drug monitoring, one or more oral oncology drug(s) and substances, definitive tandem mass spectrometry with chromatography, serum or plasma from capillary blood or venous blood, quantitative report with steady-state range for the prescribed drug(s) when detected

● **0111U** Oncology (colon cancer), targeted KRAS (codons 12, 13, and 61) and NRAS (codons 12, 13, and 61) gene analysis, utilizing formalin-fixed paraffin-embedded tissue

● **0112U** Infectious agent detection and identification, targeted sequence analysis (16S and 18S rRNA genes) with drug-resistance gene

● **0113U** Oncology (prostate), measurement of PCA3 and TMPRSS2-ERG in urine and PSA in serum following prostatic massage, by RNA amplification and fluorescence-based detection, algorithm reported as risk score

● **0114U** Gastroenterology (Barrett's esophagus), VIM and CCNA1 methylation analysis, esophageal cells, algorithm reported as likelihood for Barrett's esophagus

● **0115U** Respiratory infectious agent detection by nucleic acid (DNA and RNA), 18 viral types and subtypes and 2 bacterial targets, amplified probe technique, including multiplex reverse transcription for RNA targets, each analyte reported as detected or not detected

Pathology and Laboratory

● 0116U   Prescription drug monitoring, enzyme immunoassay of 35 or more drugs confirmed with LC-MS/MS, oral fluid, algorithm results reported as a patient-compliance measurement with risk of drug to drug interactions for prescribed medications

● 0117U   Pain management, analysis of 11 endogenous analytes (methylmalonic acid, xanthurenic acid, homocysteine, pyroglutamic acid, vanilmandelate, 5-hydroxyindoleacetic acid, hydroxymethylglutarate, ethylmalonate, 3-hydroxypropyl mercapturic acid (3-HPMA), quinolinic acid, kynurenic acid), LC-MS/MS, urine, algorithm reported as a pain-index score with likelihood of atypical biochemical function associated with pain

● 0118U   Transplantation medicine, quantification of donor-derived cell-free DNA using whole genome next-generation sequencing, plasma, reported as percentage of donor-derived cell-free DNA in the total cell-free DNA

● 0119U   Cardiology, ceramides by liquid chromatography–tandem mass spectrometry, plasma, quantitative report with risk score for major cardiovascular events

● 0120U   Oncology (B-cell lymphoma classification), mRNA, gene expression profiling by fluorescent probe hybridization of 58 genes (45 content and 13 housekeeping genes), formalin-fixed paraffin-embedded tissue, algorithm reported as likelihood for primary mediastinal B-cell lymphoma (PMBCL) and diffuse large B-cell lymphoma (DLBCL) with cell of origin subtyping in the latter

● 0121U   Sickle cell disease, microfluidic flow adhesion (VCAM-1), whole blood

● 0122U   Sickle cell disease, microfluidic flow adhesion (P-Selectin), whole blood

● 0123U   Mechanical fragility, RBC, shear stress and spectral analysis profiling

● 0124U   Fetal congenital abnormalities, biochemical assays of 3 analytes (free beta-hCG, PAPP-A, AFP), time-resolved fluorescence immunoassay, maternal dried-blood spot, algorithm reported as risk scores for fetal trisomies 13/18 and 21

● 0125U   Fetal congenital abnormalities and perinatal complications, biochemical assays of 5 analytes (free beta-hCG, PAPP-A, AFP, placental growth factor, and inhibin-A), time-resolved fluorescence immunoassay, maternal serum, algorithm reported as risk scores for fetal trisomies 13/18, 21, and preeclampsia

● 0126U   Fetal congenital abnormalities and perinatal complications, biochemical assays of 5 analytes (free beta-hCG, PAPP-A, AFP, placental growth factor, and inhibin-A), time-resolved fluorescence immunoassay, includes qualitative assessment of Y chromosome in cell-free fetal DNA, maternal serum and plasma, predictive algorithm reported as risk scores for fetal trisomies 13/18, 21, and preeclampsia

● 0127U   Obstetrics (preeclampsia), biochemical assays of 3 analytes (PAPP-A, AFP, and placental growth factor), time-resolved fluorescence immunoassay, maternal serum, predictive algorithm reported as a risk score for preeclampsia

● 0128U   Obstetrics (preeclampsia), biochemical assays of 3 analytes (PAPP-A, AFP, and placental growth factor), time-resolved fluorescence immunoassay, includes qualitative assessment of Y chromosome in cell-free fetal DNA, maternal serum and plasma, predictive algorithm reported as a risk score for preeclampsia

● 0129U   Hereditary breast cancer–related disorders (eg, hereditary breast cancer, hereditary ovarian cancer, hereditary endometrial cancer), genomic sequence analysis and deletion/duplication analysis panel *(ATM, BRCA1, BRCA2, CDH1, CHEK2, PALB2, PTEN,* and *TP53)*

+● 0130U   Hereditary colon cancer disorders (eg, Lynch syndrome, PTEN hamartoma syndrome, Cowden syndrome, familial adenomatosis polyposis), targeted mRNA sequence analysis panel *(APC, CDH1, CHEK2, MLH1, MSH2, MSH6, MUTYH, PMS2, PTEN,* and *TP53)* (List separately in addition to code for primary procedure)

▶(Use 0130U in conjunction with 81435, 0101U)◀

+● 0131U   Hereditary breast cancer–related disorders (eg, hereditary breast cancer, hereditary ovarian cancer, hereditary endometrial cancer), targeted mRNA sequence analysis panel (13 genes) (List separately in addition to code for primary procedure)

▶(Use 0131U in conjunction with 81162, 81432, 0102U)◀

+● 0132U   Hereditary ovarian cancer–related disorders (eg, hereditary breast cancer, hereditary ovarian cancer, hereditary endometrial cancer), targeted mRNA sequence analysis panel (17 genes) (List separately in addition to code for primary procedure)

▶(Use 0132U in conjunction with 81162, 81432, 0103U)◀

+● 0133U   Hereditary prostate cancer–related disorders, targeted mRNA sequence analysis panel (11 genes) (List separately in addition to code for primary procedure)

▶(Use 0133U in conjunction with 81162)◀

+● 0134U   Hereditary pan cancer (eg, hereditary breast and ovarian cancer, hereditary endometrial cancer, hereditary colorectal cancer), targeted mRNA sequence analysis panel (18 genes) (List separately in addition to code for primary procedure)

▶(Use 0134U in conjunction with 81162, 81432, 81435)◀

+● 0135U   Hereditary gynecological cancer (eg, hereditary breast and ovarian cancer, hereditary endometrial cancer, hereditary colorectal cancer), targeted mRNA sequence analysis panel (12 genes) (List separately in addition to code for primary procedure)

▶(Use 0135U in conjunction with 81162)◀

+● 0136U   ATM (ataxia telangiectasia mutated) (eg, ataxia telangiectasia) mRNA sequence analysis (List separately in addition to code for primary procedure)

▶(Use 0136U in conjunction with 81408)◀

+● 0137U   PALB2 (partner and localizer of BRCA2) (eg, breast and pancreatic cancer) mRNA sequence analysis (List separately in addition to code for primary procedure)

▶(Use 0137U in conjunction with 81307)◀

+● 0138U   BRCA1 (BRCA1, DNA repair associated), BRCA2 (BRCA2, DNA repair associated) (eg, hereditary breast and ovarian cancer) mRNA sequence analysis (List separately in addition to code for primary procedure)

▶(Use 0138U in conjunction with 81162)◀

Rationale

A total of 75 new PLA codes have been established for the 2020 CPT code set. PLA test codes will be released and posted online on a quarterly basis (fall, winter, spring, and summer), which are available online at https://www.ama-assn.org/practice-management/cpt-pla-codes. New codes are effective the quarter following their publication.

Other changes include the deletion of codes 0020U, 0028U, 0057U, 0081U, and 0104U, and the revision of code 0008U to report H. pylori and antibiotic resistance detection.

Clinical Example (0008U)

A 60-year-old male presents with gastrointestinal complaints following a 14-day standard treatment for H. pylori infection. A formalin-fixed paraffin-embedded gastric biopsy from a recent procedure is submitted for H. pylori-resistance panel testing.

Description of Procedure (0008U)

Subject DNA isolated from the tissue or fecal sample to H. pylori DNA enrichment and then examine for six genes that confer antibiotic resistance. A report is issued specifying DNA variant(s) and antibiotic resistance status.

Clinical Example (0062U)

A 45-year-old female with symptoms of joint pain, rash, mouth sores, numbness, and mild Raynauds disease has a positive ANA test but is unresponsive to treatment for presumed systemic lupus erythematosus (SLE). A serum specimen is submitted for biomarker analysis to determine the likelihood of SLE.

Description of Procedure (0062U)

Test serum by indirect ELISA using a microarray approach to semiquantitatively measure antibody levels. Then analyze using a validated algorithm, reported as likelihood of SLE.

Clinical Example (0063U)

An 18-month-old male presents to his physician with verbal delay and behavior concerns. The pediatrician submits a fasting plasma sample from the child to determine the risk for autism spectrum disorder.

Description of Procedure (0063U)

Subject a plasma sample to LC-MS/MS analysis to measure the level of amines. Enter the quantitative measurement of the individual amines and the presence of any metabolic imbalance identified through algorithmic analysis into the result report.

Clinical Example (0064U)

A 28-year-old male presents to his physician with a history of syphilis and high-risk behavior. He recently had a chancre sore. A serum or plasma sample is submitted to assess the patient's syphilis status.

Description of Procedure (0064U)

After a sample is isolated from the patient, load it onto the automated BioPlex 2200 immunoanalyzer that examines the sample for treponemal and nontreponemal reagin antibodies using the BioPlex 2200 Syphilis Total & RPR assay. Release the result (reactive or nonreactive) from the immunoanalyzer.

Clinical Example (0065U)

A 28-year-old female is undergoing routine prenatal screening which includes screening for syphilis infection. A serum or plasma sample is submitted to assess the patient's syphilis status.

Description of Procedure (0065U)

Load a patient sample and analyze using the automated BioPlex 2200 immunoanalyzer for nontreponemal reagin antibodies using the BioPlex 2200 RPR assay. Release the result (reactive or nonreactive) from the immunoanalyzer.

Clinical Example (0066U)

A 36-year-old pregnant female presents to her physician with signs and symptoms of preterm labor. The PartoSure™ test is ordered to assess the risk of spontaneous preterm delivery.

Description of Procedure (0066U)

Collect a vaginal sample of cervico-vaginal fluid using a sterile flocked swab. Place the swab into the solvent vial and rotate for 30 seconds. Remove the swab. Place the PartoSure™ test strip in the fluid.

Clinical Example (0067U)

A 45-year-old female was diagnosed with atypical ductal hyperplasia on breast biopsy. Her physician orders a four-protein expression panel with algorithmic analysis to determine her personal risk for developing breast cancer.

Description of Procedure (0067U)

Evaluate tissue sections of a breast biopsy sample with atypical ductal hyperplasia for the expression of four proteins by immunohistochemistry. Combine the protein expression scores using a validated algorithm to yield a "Cancer Risk Score" informative for the risk of developing breast cancer.

Clinical Example (0068U)

A 32-year-old male with acute myeloid leukemia (AML) on chemotherapy with pancytopenia develops a low-grade fever. The patient is admitted to rule out sepsis, possibly due to a Candida infection. A blood sample is submitted for Candida species evaluation.

Description of Procedure (0068U)

Extract high-quality DNA from whole blood samples. Subject to nested hydrolysis probe amplification for the presence of six Candida species. Analyze the data and compose a report specifying presence or absence of each Candida species.

Clinical Example (0069U)

A 65-year-old female presents to her oncologist with metastatic (Stage IV) colon cancer shown to be RAS nonmutated. The oncologist plans to initiate first-line biologic therapy in combination with chemotherapy. To determine which anti-EGFR (cetuximab or panitumumab) or anti-VEGF (bevacizumab) therapy may be more appropriate, the physician orders miR-31-3p expression evaluation.

Description of Procedure (0069U)

Extract total RNA from selected tumor samples. Perform two PCR reactions to quantify the expression of miR-31-3p, compared to housekeeping microRNA. Use an algorithm to calculate an expression score for miR-31-3p.

Clinical Example (0070U)

A 36-year-old postmenopausal female with newly diagnosed breast cancer undergoes CYP2D6 genotype testing prior to initiating tamoxifen therapy.

Description of Procedure (0070U)

Extract genomic DNA from EDTA whole blood. Amplify CYP2D6 gene sequence by conventional PCR and verify with gel electrophoresis. Perform targeted sequence variant analysis by sequence-specific hydrolysis probes. Determine copy number variations (including duplications, multiplications, and deletions) with CYP2D6-specific hydrolysis probes for the promoter, intron 6, and exon 9.

Clinical Example (0071U)

A 47-year-old postmenopausal female with newly diagnosed breast cancer undergoes CYP2D6 genotype testing to guide tamoxifen therapy. Initial genotyping result showed heterozygosity for the *9-defining variant and the presence of an incomplete *2A haplotype with CNV result of 2-2-2 (meaning 2 alleles present). Reflexive CYP2D6 full gene sequencing is indicated. [**Note:** This is an add-on code. Only consider the additional work related to the primary procedure.]

Description of Procedure (0071U)

Extract genomic DNA from EDTA whole blood and subject to full sequencing of the CYP2D6 gene. Analyze variations in the sequence of the exon and intron/exon boundaries of the exon and determine by a mutation detection software and visual inspection.

Clinical Example (0072U)

A 47-year-old postmenopausal female with newly diagnosed breast cancer undergoes CYP2D6 genotype testing to guide tamoxifen therapy. Initial genotyping result showed variants predicting *1/*4 and CNV results were 3-3-3, indicating presence of either a gene duplication or balanced CYP2D6-2D7 and CYP2D7-2D6 hybrids. Reflexive CYP2D6-2D7 hybrid gene sequencing is indicated. [**Note:** This is an add-on code. Only consider the additional work related to the primary procedure.]

Description of Procedure (0072U)

Extract genomic DNA from EDTA whole blood and subject to full sequencing of the CYP2D6-2D7 hybrid gene. Analyze variations in the sequence of the exon and intron/exon boundaries of the exon and determine by a mutation detection software and visual inspection.

Clinical Example (0073U)

A 47-year-old postmenopausal female with newly diagnosed breast cancer undergoes CYP2D6 genotype testing to guide tamoxifen therapy. Initial genotyping result showed variants predicting *1/*4 and CNV results were 3-3-3, indicating presence of either a gene duplication or balanced CYP2D6-2D7 and CYP2D7-2D6 hybrids. Reflexive CYP2D7-2D6 hybrid gene sequencing is indicated. [**Note:** This is an add-on code. Only consider the additional work related to the primary procedure.]

Description of Procedure (0073U)

Extract genomic DNA from EDTA whole blood and subject to full sequencing of the CYP2D7-2D6 hybrid gene. Analyze variations in the sequence of the exon and intron/exon boundaries of the exon and determine by a mutation detection software and visual inspection.

Clinical Example (0074U)

A 47-year-old postmenopausal female with newly diagnosed breast cancer undergoes CYP2D6 genotype testing to guide tamoxifen therapy. Initial genotyping result showed a *1/*9 with CNV 4-4-4 (four alleles present). Reflexive sequencing of the nonduplicated CYP2D6 gene is indicated to determine duplication of the *1 and *9 alleles or obtain sequence of the nonduplicated allele. [**Note:** This is an add-on code. Only consider the additional work related to the primary procedure.]

Description of Procedure (0074U)

Extract genomic DNA from EDTA whole blood and subject to full sequencing of the nonduplicated gene when CYP2D6 gene duplication or multiplication exists on the other chromosome. Analyze variations in the sequence of the exon and intron/exon boundaries of the exon and determine by a mutation detection software and visual inspection.

Clinical Example (0075U)

A 47-year-old postmenopausal female with newly diagnosed breast cancer undergoes CYP2D6 genotype testing to guide tamoxifen therapy. Initial genotyping result showed a *1/*9 with CNV 4-4-4 (four alleles present). Reflexive sequencing of the 5' gene of the CYP2D6 gene duplication or multiplication is indicated to determine sequence of the allele. [**Note:** This is an add-on code. Only consider the additional work related to the primary procedure.]

Description of Procedure (0075U)

Extract genomic DNA from EDTA whole blood and subject to full sequencing of the 5' gene of the CYP2D6 gene duplication or multiplication. Analyze variations in the sequence of the exon and intron/exon boundaries of the exon and determine by a mutation detection software and visual inspection.

Clinical Example (0076U)

A 47-year-old postmenopausal female with newly diagnosed breast cancer undergoes CYP2D6 genotype testing to guide tamoxifen therapy. Initial genotyping result showed a *1/*9 with CNV 4-4-4 (four alleles present). Reflexive sequencing of the 3' gene of the CYP2D6 gene duplication or multiplication is indicated to determine sequence of the allele. [**Note:** This is an add-on code. Only consider the additional work related to the primary procedure.]

Description of Procedure (0076U)

Extract genomic DNA from EDTA whole blood and subject to full sequencing of the 3' gene of the CYP2D6 gene duplication or multiplication. Analyze variations in the sequence of the exon and intron/exon boundaries of the exon and determine by a mutation detection software and visual inspection.

Clinical Example (0077U)

A 58-year-old male presents with chronic back pain, lethargy, anemia, and elevated free calcium in serum. Multiple lytic lesions are seen on bone scan, suggesting possible multiple myeloma. A serum specimen is submitted for monoclonal protein detection and isotyping.

Description of Procedure (0077U)

Concentrate a serum or urine sample by immunopreciptation, followed by MALDI-TOF mass spectrometry for detection and differentiation of M-protein and isotypes (eg, IgA, IgM, IgG, glycosylated and unglycosylated K and L light chains) based on interpretation of the characteristic spectra generated.

Clinical Example (0078U)

A 47-year-old male patient with chronic pain is being considered for opioid therapy. The physician is concerned that the patient might be a candidate for opioid use disorder (OUD) and orders the Neural Response Panel to determine the patient's risk of OUD. The test comes back positive, and the physician alters his treatment plan based on those results.

Description of Procedure (0078U)

Extract genomic DNA from buccal samples and subject to multiplex PCR, targeting 16 genetic loci associated with opioid dependency. Analyze PCR amplicons by analyte specific extension (ASPE) with microarray hybridization. Report specific genotypes along with an algorithmic analysis for risk of OUD.

Clinical Example (0079U)

A 31-year-old male presents to his physician for routine urinary drug testing (UDT). The patient has a history of aberrant opioid drug taking behavior and noncompliance with the agreed-upon treatment plan. To confidently verify the authenticity of the patient's urine sample for UDT, the physician submits a buccal scrape sample along with the urine sample to verify specimen authenticity prior to urine drug testing.

Description of Procedure (0079U)

Subject DNA isolated from patient's urine and buccal swab samples to SNP PCR, followed by MALDI-TOF analysis. Compare the genotyping results. Communicate a report to the appropriate caregiver.

Clinical Example (0080U)

A 45-year-old female smoker presents with a cough. A CT finds an 8-mm nodule on one lobe of the lung. A plasma proteomic test is ordered to determine if her tumor has a high probability of being benign prior to considering undergoing an invasive procedure.

Description of Procedure (0080U)

Isolate plasma from a blood sample. Subject to mass spectrometry for quantitative analysis of galectin-3-binding protein and soluble scavenger receptor cysteine-rich type 1 protein M130. Integrate protein measurements and five clinical factors using an algorithm to provide a revised probability of malignancy. Send a report to the ordering physician.

Clinical Example (0082U)

A 48-year-old female with a history of OUD presents to a physician because she has not been feeling well. The patient assures compliance with her current methadone maintenance treatment program. She states she is on no other medication but is seeing a psychiatrist. A urine sample is submitted for drug analysis, quantification, and drug-drug interaction analysis to identify potential undisclosed drug use based on patient historical use, risk, and community trend patient profiles, to identify and confirm adherence to prescribed drugs, and to identify significant drug-drug interactions.

Description of Procedure (0082U)

Analyze a urine sample utilizing definitive chromatography with mass spectrometry for 90 or more analytes in addition to a presumptive immunoassay by instrument chemistry analyzer for one or more analyte(s). Issue a report noting any potentially significant drug-drug interactions.

Clinical Example (0083U)

A 55-year-old female presents with breast cancer and a previous abnormal mammogram and undergoes needle biopsy. A sample of tissue is submitted to assess the tumor's ex-vivo response to three common chemotherapy regimens.

Description of Procedure (0083U)

Divide specimen into fragments of approximately 1 cubic mm and subject to motility contrast tomography (MCT). After a baseline period, apply challenge drugs and continue MCT for several hours. A proprietary algorithm compares the drug response phenotypes to baseline profiles, control specimens, and a training set of known therapeutic outcomes. Prepare a written report indicating the likelihood of response to each drug or drug combination.

Clinical Example (0084U)

A five-year-old female with sickle cell disease presents with anemia, requiring transfusion. A whole blood sample is referred to the molecular laboratory for red cell antigen genotyping to maximize red blood cell antigen matching.

Description of Procedure (0084U)

Extract genomic DNA from EDTA-anticoagulated whole blood. Amplify and biotinylate in a multiplex PCR. Denature and hybridize PCR products to microbead-bound oligonucleotide probes. Label hybridized DNA with a fluorescent conjugate and detect on a Luminex 200 flow cytometer. Process data to determine blood group genotypes and predict red blood cell antigen phenotype.

Clinical Example (0085U)

A 30-year-old female presents with complaint of bloating, diarrhea, and abdominal pain, but no blood in stool. Symptom-based criteria are indicative of irritable bowel syndrome (IBS). Cytolethal distending toxin B (CdtB) and vinculin IgG antibody testing is ordered to evaluate for IBS.

Description of Procedure (0085U)

Use EDTA plasma or serum to perform an ELISA-based analysis to detect anti-CdtB and anti-vinculin IgG antibodies. Report the semiquantitative result as positive or negative for a diagnosis of IBS-D or IBS-M if either or both antibodies are above the clinical cutoffs.

Clinical Example (0086U)

A 67-year-old male, who is a recent liver transplant patient, develops fever and hypotension. Blood is submitted for culture, and the patient is empirically treated with antibiotics. Blood cultures become positive for gram-negative rods. A sample of culture fluid is submitted for automated rRNA FISH testing for microbial identification and phenotypic MIC-based antimicrobial susceptibility testing.

Description of Procedure (0086U)

Dispense an aliquot of a positive blood culture sample into a sample cassette and place on the Accelerate Pheno™ system. The system automatically performs sample preparation, identification by FISH, and phenotypic MIC-based antimicrobial susceptibility and resistance detection. A report is automatically generated and returned to the ordering physician.

Clinical Example (0087U)

A 53-year-old female heart transplant patient, two years posttransplant, presents with shortness of breath, an elevated B-type natriuretic peptide, and a reduced left ventricular ejection fraction by echocardiography. Endomyocardial biopsy was sent for intragraft mRNA transcript analysis via Molecular Microscope® Diagnostic System (MMDx) to evaluate likelihood of rejection.

Description of Procedure (0087U)

Extract total RNA from allograft biopsies. Prepare complementary RNA (cRNA) for gene expression profiling and analyze on a microarray chip. Analyze the resulting data file using proprietary software to assign probabilistic diagnoses, including injury and rejection scores.

Clinical Example (0088U)

A 43-year-old male living unrelated kidney transplant patient, one year posttransplant, presents with rising creatinine level and proteinuria. The initial transplant biopsy did not show rejection, but kidney function continued to worsen. The MMDx test was ordered to determine active antibody mediated rejection (ABMR).

Description of Procedure (0088U)

Extract total RNA from allograft biopsies. Prepare complementary RNA (cRNA) for gene expression profiling and analyze on a microarray chip. Analyze the resulting data file using proprietary software to assign probabilistic diagnoses, including injury and rejection scores.

Clinical Example (0089U)

A 50-year-old female patient presents with a large pigmented nasal lesion that she believes has recently changed. To obtain more information to determine the need for biopsy, a noninvasively collected sample using an adhesive patch-based skin sample collection kit is used to assess the lesion's PRAME and LINC00518 gene expression.

Description of Procedure (0089U)

Macro-dissect an adhesive patch-collected skin sample to select the pigmented lesion. Lyse the tissue, then extract RNA and analyze for PRAME and LINC00518 gene expression. Prepare a report describing the gene expression status and risk.

Clinical Example (0090U)

A 72-year-old female has a suspicious "mole" biopsied. Histological evaluation shows atypical features suspicious but not diagnostic for malignancy. A gene expression profiling test is ordered.

Description of Procedure (0090U)

Extract the RNA from a biopsy. Use qRT-PCR to determine the expression levels of 14 genes known to be overexpressed in malignant melanomas and 9 reference genes. Compare the expression levels of the 14 genes to the baseline expression of the 9 reference genes using a proprietary algorithm to produce a clinically reportable numeric score.

Clinical Example (0091U)

A 50-year-old female is due for colorectal cancer screening; she has no elevated risk factors. Blood is submitted to detect circulating precancer and cancer cells and to determine the possible need for colonoscopy

Description of Procedure (0091U)

Collect EDTA whole blood for circulating tumor cell (CTC) isolation and enumeration using a proprietary film-based cell capture system with high-affinity antibodies, selection against leukocytes, and a special air-foam release technology. Count positive cells. Analyze results using an algorithm.

Clinical Example (0092U)

A 56-year-old male smoker presents after a low dose helical CT scan showed a 16-mm lung nodule suspicious for lung cancer. To assist in deciding whether to pursue biopsy or surgery, or put the patient on active surveillance, the physician orders the REVEAL test to better assess the patient's risk of malignancy.

Description of Procedure (0092U)

Evaluate patient plasma by the MagArray system, using immunoassay reactions to quantitatively measure protein concentrations. Algorithmically combine protein measurements and other clinical factors to produce a patient risk score that is reported to the ordering physician.

Clinical Example (0093U)

An 86-year-old female presents with a history of hyperlipidemia and multiple comorbidities. She was recently prescribed a new statin to control her hyperlipidemia. Because her cholesterol and blood glucose levels are not improving, the physician requests a ComplyRX test to make sure she is taking her medications.

Description of Procedure (0093U)

Analyze urine using high-pressure LC-MS/MS. Generate a report that includes a list of the patient's prescribed medications and the presence or absence of 65 commonly prescribed medications.

Clinical Example (0094U)

A full-term neonate was immediately admitted to the neonatal intensive care unit (NICU) for tonic-myoclonic seizures. While seizures were largely controlled medically, she was too sedated to tolerate oral feedings. But on dose reduction, seizures returned. Electroencephalogram (EEG) revealed multifocal, epileptiform abnormalities and burst suppression. A specimen was collected on the first day of life and analyzed using rapid (ie, <7 days) whole-genome sequencing (WGS) that returned a result supporting a diagnosis of early infantile epileptic encephalopathy type seven.

Description of Procedure (0094U)

Extract genomic DNA from peripheral blood. Fragment and use to prepare NGS libraries. Perform and analyze PCR-free rapid WGS. Clinical genomic analysts triage and curate data for review by a board-certified laboratory director. Once reviewed, results are communicated to the ordering physicians.

Clinical Example (0095U)

A 17-year-old male with eosinophilic esophagitis presents after 12 weeks of dietary treatment with symptom resolution. An esophageal string test (EST) is performed and the esophageal sample submitted to analyze for eosinophilic inflammation.

Description of Procedure (0095U)

Collect human esophageal mucosal sample by a nylon string. Elute the supernatant and subject to ELISA for two eosinophil-associated protein biomarkers, Eotaxin-3 and major basic protein-1 (MBP-1). The laboratory issues a report that provides a quantitative result and the probability of the patient having active eosinophilic esophagitis.

Clinical Example (0096U)

A 24-year-old male approaches his physician with concerns about sexually transmitted infections after having unprotected sex with a group of men at a party several weeks ago. A urine specimen is submitted for high-risk HPV testing.

Description of Procedure (0096U)

This test uses amplification of target DNA by PCR for the detection of 14 high-risk HPV types in a single analysis. The test specifically identifies genotypes 16 and 18, and detects genotypes 31, 33, 35, 39, 45, 51, 52, 56, 58, 59, 66, and 68.

Clinical Example (0097U)

A 3-year-old previously healthy male presents to the emergency department with a two-day history of diarrhea of increasing severity, abdominal pain, fever, vomiting, and irritability. One sibling (age 12) also had experienced one day of diarrhea but of much less severity and is now well. A stool specimen is submitted for gastrointestinal pathogen testing.

Description of Procedure (0097U)

Transfer a sample of a stool specimen submitted in Cary Blair transport media to a FilmArray® GI Panel reagent pouch and place on a FilmArray® instrument. Within the reagent pouch, the sample is subjected to fully automated nucleic acid extraction, nested multiplex PCR, and DNA melt curve analysis. A report listing each pathogen as "detected" or "not detected" is automatically generated. Review and report the results to the clinician.

Clinical Example (0098U)

An 81-year-old female presents with four-day history of a congestion, cough, and difficulty breathing but is afebrile. The patient has asthma that is well controlled using inhalers. The patient lives with her husband who is currently recovering from respiratory symptoms. Vaccinations, including influenza, are up to date. A nasopharyngeal swab sample (NPS) is collected and submitted for respiratory pathogen testing.

Description of Procedure (0098U)

Transfer a sample of an NPS specimen into the FilmArray® RP EZ reagent pouch and place into the FilmArray® 2.0 instrument (configured to run the RP EZ test). Within the reagent pouch, the sample is subjected to fully automated nucleic acid extraction, nested multiplex PCR, and DNA melt curve analysis. In approximately one hour, a single page report listing each pathogen as "detected" or "not detected" is automatically generated. Review and report the results to the ordering clinician.

Clinical Example (0099U)

An 81-year-old female presents with four-day history of congestion, cough, and difficulty breathing but is afebrile. The patient has asthma that is well controlled using inhalers. The patient lives with her husband who is currently recovering from respiratory symptoms. Vaccinations, including influenza, are up to date. An NPS is collected and submitted for respiratory pathogen testing.

Description of Procedure (0099U)

Transfer a sample of an NPS specimen into the FilmArray® RP 2 reagent pouch and place into the FilmArray® instrument. Within the reagent pouch, the sample is subjected to fully automated nucleic acid extraction, nested multiplex PCR, and DNA melt curve analysis. In approximately one hour, a single page report listing each pathogen as "detected" or "not detected" is automatically generated. Review and report the results to the ordering clinician.

Clinical Example (0100U)

An 81-year-old female presents with four-day history of congestion, cough, and difficulty breathing but is afebrile. The patient has asthma that is well controlled using inhalers. The patient lives with her husband who is currently recovering from respiratory symptoms. Vaccinations, including influenza, are up to date. An NPS is collected and submitted for respiratory pathogen testing.

Description of Procedure (0100U)

Transfer a sample of an NPS specimen into the FilmArray® Respiratory Panel 2 (RP2) reagent pouch and place into the FilmArray® instrument. Within the reagent pouch, the sample is subjected to fully automated nucleic acid extraction, nested multiplex PCR, and DNA melt curve analysis. In approximately one hour, a single page report listing each pathogen as "detected" or "not detected" is automatically generated. Review and report the results to the ordering clinician.

Clinical Example (0101U)

A 58-year-old male with a family history of colon cancer presents with a history of two primary colon cancers, diagnosed at ages 55 and 58. A blood specimen is submitted for germline hereditary colon cancer gene testing.

Description of Procedure (0101U)

Isolate high-quality genomic DNA from whole blood, saliva, or cells. Subject to NGS and Sanger sequencing to detect single nucleotide variants in APC, BMPR1A, CDH1, CHEK2, MLH1, MSH2, MSH6, MUTYH, PMS2, POLD1, POLE, PTEN, SMAD4, STK11, and TP53 (sequencing and deletion or duplication). Perform EPCAM and GREM1 (deletion or duplication only) by NGS, MLPA, array CGH, or qPCR for detection of copy number variants. Use mRNA analysis for variant resolution. Analyze the data and compose a report.

Clinical Example (0102U)

A 30-year-old female presents to her physician with a history of breast cancer. The patient has a family history of breast and ovarian cancer. A blood specimen is submitted for germline hereditary breast and ovarian cancer gene testing.

Description of Procedure (0102U)

Isolate high-quality genomic DNA from whole blood, saliva, or cells. Subject to NGS and Sanger sequencing to detect single nucleotide variants in ATM, BARD1, BRCA1, BRCA2, BRIP1, CDH1, CHEK2, MRE11A, MUTYH, NBN, NF1, PALB2, PTEN, RAD50, RAD51C, RAD51D, and TP53 (sequencing and deletion or duplication). Perform deletion or duplication by NGS, MLPA, array CGH, or qPCR for detection of copy number variants. Use mRNA analysis for variant resolution. Analyze the data and compose a report.

Clinical Example (0103U)

A 60-year-old female presents with a history of epithelial ovarian cancer. The patient also has a family history of breast cancer and colon cancer. Her physician recommends evaluation of germline hereditary breast, ovarian, and uterine cancer genes and submits a blood specimen for evaluation.

Description of Procedure (0103U)

Isolate high-quality genomic DNA from whole blood, saliva, or cells. Subject to NGS and Sanger sequencing to detect single nucleotide variants in ATM, BARD1, BRCA1, BRCA2, BRIP1, CDH1, CHEK2, DICER1, MLH1, MRE11A, MSH2, MSH6, MUTYH, NBN, NF1, PALB2, PMS2, PTEN, RAD50, RAD51C, RAD51D, SMARCA4, STK11, and TP53 (sequencing and deletion or duplication); and EPCAM (deletion or duplication only). Perform deletion or duplication by NGS, MLPA, array CGH, or qPCR for detection of copy number variants. Use mRNA analysis for variant resolution. Analyze the data and composes a report.

Clinical Example (0105U)

A 40-year-old male with type 2 diabetes on antidiabetic medication presents with an eGFR of 50 ml/min/1.73 m^2 and urine albumin creatinine ratio of 20 mg/g. Plasma is submitted to evaluate the risk for developing rapid kidney function decline with a decrease in eGFR of >5 ml/min/year over the next five years.

Description of Procedure (0105U)

Subject plasma to electrochemiluminescent immunoassay (ECLIA) for the simultaneous detection of tumor necrosis factor receptor 1A and 2 (TNFR1 and TNFR2) and the kidney injury molecule 1 (KIM-1). Combine quantitative results of the three plasma protein markers with clinical data to predict the probability of experiencing rapid kidney function decline over the next five years. Confirm all test results and release a report.

Clinical Example (0106U)

A 36-year-old male with a 20-year history of diabetes and other comorbidities presents with several months of recurrent nausea and vomiting and has fluctuating glucose levels that had previously been well controlled. The patient complains of frequent halitosis, especially in the morning. A gastric emptying study is performed.

Description of Procedure (0106U)

Isolate CO_2 in breath samples. Ionize CO_2 molecules and separate by gas isotope ratio mass spectrometry to determine the $13CO_2/12CO_2$ ratio in each of seven breath specimens. Calculate the rate of $13CO_2$ excretion (kPCD metric) for each time point.

Clinical Example (0107U)

A 74-year-old female presents with two-day history of diarrhea (>8 loose stools per 24 hour) and abdominal pain. The patient recently used antibiotics (clindamycin) to treat a severe skin infection. A stool sample is sent to the lab for C. difficile toxin testing.

Description of Procedure (0107U)

Subject stool to high-sensitivity digital single molecule counting testing for qualitative detection of C. difficile toxins A and B. Report a qualitative result.

Clinical Example (0108U)

A 65-year-old male presents with chronic gastroesophageal reflux disease (GERD). Endoscopy indicates probable Barrett's esophagus, and biopsy reveals Barrett's esophagus, negative for dysplasia. A protein-based test is ordered to determine risk for progression to high-grade dysplasia or esophageal cancer that is used to guide therapeutic intervention.

Description of Procedure (0108U)

Subject formalin-fixed paraffin-embedded tissue obtained during an upper endoscopy to multiplexed immunolabeling. Analyze protein-based biomarker and morphometric data and integrate using an algorithm to generate a risk score indicating patient risk of progression to high-grade dysplasia or cancer.

Clinical Example (0109U)

A 32-year-old AML pancytopenic patient on chemotherapy develops a low-grade fever. The physician admits the patient to rule out infection, including PCR for Aspergillus, using blood culture and analysis.

Description of Procedure (0109U)

Subject high-quality DNA from an appropriate patient sample to nested hydrolysis probe amplification for the presence of four Aspergillus species (A. fumigatus, A. terreus, A. niger, and A. flavus) using real-time PCR. Analyze the data and compose a report specifying presence or absence of each Aspergillus species.

Clinical Example (0110U)

A 57-year-old postmenopausal female with grade II/III HR+ HER2- breast cancer was prescribed ribociclib 600 mg daily and letrozole 2.5 mg daily. She complains of headache and nausea and informed the physician that the medications are not helping her cancer. The physician ordered a blood test for ribociclib and letrozole to verify patient adherence and adequate dosing.

Description of Procedure (0110U)

Process a plasma sample by protein precipitation and solid-phase extraction. Analyze by LC-MS/MS in positive ion multiple reaction mode (MRM). Return a quantitative report for the drugs and metabolites to the ordering clinician.

Clinical Example (0111U)

A 67-year-old is found to have metastatic colon cancer on routine endoscopy. A sample of formalin-fixed paraffin-embedded tissue is submitted for expanded KRAS and NRAS mutation testing to determine the patient's eligibility for targeted therapies.

Description of Procedure (0111U)

Extract DNA from selected tumor areas from formalin-fixed paraffin-embedded tissue. After quality verification, prepare a library by selective oligo hybridization to genomic tumor DNA, with enzymatic extension and amplification of targets, and then sequence. Bioinformatic analysis is provided via FDA-approved software incorporated in the platform. Analyze the data and compose a report.

Clinical Example (0112U)

A 60-year-old male with chronic prostatitis remains symptomatic after a course of ciprofloxacin. A sample of prostatic secretion is submitted for microbial detection and identification by rRNA gene sequence analysis and drug-resistant gene detection to inform an optimal therapy.

Description of Procedure (0112U)

Isolate DNA from the sample. Subject to targeted DNA sequence analysis of microbial 16S and 18S rRNA genes to detect and identify bacterial and fungal infectious agents present, and drug resistance genes, using a curated database. Compose a report and return to the ordering physician

Clinical Example (0113U)

A 65-year-old asymptomatic male presents to his urologist with a PSA of 9.3 ng/mL detected by his primary care physician. Urine is submitted for testing to evaluate the risk of prostate cancer.

Description of Procedure (0113U)

Collect urine following prostatic massage. Isolate RNA. Fluorescence monitoring of RNA-amplification quantifies levels of PCA3, TMPRSS2-ERG, and KLK3. Use these values and serum PSA in logistic regression models to generate a risk score for having prostate cancer and high-grade prostate cancer.

Clinical Example (0114U)

A 50-year-old obese male smoker with a five-year history of GERD and no prior endoscopic evaluation meets American College of Gastroenterology criteria for risk of Barrett's esophagus. His physician recommends testing for evaluation for Barrett's esophagus and esophageal adenocarcinoma.

Description of Procedure (0114U)

Isolate high-quality genomic DNA from a cellular specimen. Subject to bisulfite conversion of methylated sites, PCR amplification, and targeted next-generation sequencing of 31 methylation sites on the VIM and CCNA1 genes. Apply an algorithm. Return a report indicating the likelihood of Barrett's esophagus to the ordering physician.

Clinical Example (0115U)

A 66-year-old male with chronic obstructive pulmonary disease (COPD) was admitted with several days of dyspnea. He was febrile, tachycardic, tachypneic, and hypoxemic. Chest radiography was concerning for multifocal pneumonia. An NPS is submitted for the respiratory pathogen panel.

Description of Procedure (0115U)

Load an NPS received in universal transport medium (UTM) or viral transport medium (VTM) into the ePlex RP Panel cartridge. Insert into the ePlex instrument for processing (nucleic acid extraction, through PCR and electrochemical detection), which generates a result of "detected" or "not detected" for each of the analytes.

Clinical Example (0116U)

A 58-year-old female presents with a history of chronic pain, depression, and long-term opioid use. Her pain recently increased, and she requests a higher dose of oxycodone. She is currently prescribed oxycodone for her chronic pain, a benzodiazepine to treat her depression, and hydrocodone for breakthrough pain episodes. An oral fluid sample is submitted for toxicology analysis to assess her compliance with her current medication treatment plan.

Description of Procedure (0116U)

Split an oral fluid sample and subject to analysis on enzyme immunoassay (EIA) and LC-MS/MS for 35 or more prescription drugs. Input the results into an algorithm that compares the test results with the reported medication list to determine compliance. Review and report the results.

Clinical Example (0117U)

A 65-year-old male presents with chronic pain and long-term opioid use. His pain has increased, and he requests a higher oxycodone dose. A urine sample is submitted for Foundation PI[SM] test to determine the likelihood of atypical biochemistry function as a pain determinant.

Description of Procedure (0117U)

Analyze a urine sample by EIA and LC-MS/MS. Combine results for algorithmic analysis, producing a numeric score of likelihood of biochemistry as a pain determinant.

Clinical Example (0118U)

A 39-year-old male presents with elevated creatinine to his physician eight months following kidney transplant. To evaluate his risk for rejection prior to deciding on an invasive biopsy, the physician submits a whole-blood sample for testing.

Description of Procedure (0118U)

Isolate high-quality genomic cell free DNA from plasma and subject to whole-genome NGS. Analyze the data and compose a report specifying percentage donor DNA.

Clinical Example (0119U)

A 58-year-old male with hypertension, diabetes, obesity, and sedentary lifestyle is evaluated for risk of major cardiovascular events. Clinical risk factors and serum lipid levels indicate a 10-year atherosclerosis cardiovascular disease risk of 7.4%. A test is requested to determine his risk for major cardiovascular events in the next five years.

Description of Procedure (0119U)

Extract ceramides from plasma, then quantify by high-pressure LC-MS/MS for ceramide 16:0 (Cer16:0), ceramide 18:0 (Cer18:0), ceramide 24:1 (Cer24:1), and ceramide 24:0 (Cer24:0) levels. Calculate ratios of Cer16:0/Cer24:0, Cer18:0/Cer24:0, and Cer24:1/Cer24:0. Score each of the individual ceramide levels and the ratios for 0, 1, or 2 points, and calculate a total risk score.

Clinical Example (0120U)

A 79-year-old female presents with lethargy, 20-lb weight loss, anemia, and generalized lymphadenopathy. Histopathology of clavicular lymph–node biopsy showed large B-cell lymphoma. This test was requested to determine the specific type of B-cell lymphoma to provide prognosis and guide chemotherapy.

Description of Procedure (0120U)

Macro-dissect formalin-fixed paraffin-embedded sections. Extract total RNA for quantification by spectrophotometry. Hybridize RNA to 58 fluorescently labeled probes. Purify probe-RNA complexes for quantification with proprietary single-molecule imaging analysis. Process data using an algorithm program for QC and B-cell subtype analyses. Report results as probability scores for primary mediastinal and diffuse large B-cell lymphoma, with cell of origin subtype in the latter type.

Clinical Example (0121U)

A 10-year-old male with sickle cell disease (SCD) treated by exchange transfusion therapy (ExTx) presents with complaint of increasingly frequent pain episodes. His hematologist orders a cell-adhesion test to evaluate the effectiveness of the current ExTx schedule.

Description of Procedure (0121U)

Analyze peripheral blood by microfluidic flow across an immobilized VCAM substrate. VCAM-1 selectively captures erythrocytes from the whole-blood sample. Quantify adhered erythrocytes and report an adhesion index (AI) as cells per millimeter squared.

Clinical Example (0122U)

A 10-year-old male with SCD treated by ExTx presents with complaint of increasingly frequent pain episodes. His hematologist orders a cell-adhesion test to evaluate the effectiveness of the current ExTx schedule.

Description of Procedure (0122U)

Draw a peripheral-blood sample in a sodium citrate tube and flow through a microfluidic channel across an immobilized P-Selectin substrate. P-Selectin selectively captures white blood cells (WBCs). Quantify adhered WBCs and report an AI as the number of cells per millimeter squared. Document and report the AI.

Clinical Example (0123U)

A 10-year-old male with SCD on ExTx every four weeks presents for his next exchange with elevated serum iron and LDH levels. A mechanical fragility profile is ordered to evaluate the hemolysis risks to determine if the patient's exchange frequency can be decreased.

Description of Procedure (0123U)

Analyze peripheral blood. Construct a mechanical fragility profile based on the percent induced hemolysis as a function of stress duration.

Clinical Example (0124U)

A 28-year-old female at 12-weeks gestation presents for routine prenatal screening. A maternal dried–blood sample is submitted to measure free beta-hCG, PAPP-A, and AFP to assess the fetal risks for Down syndrome and trisomy 13/18.

Description of Procedure (0124U)

Analyze maternal dried–blood specimens for free beta-hCG, PAPP-A, and AFP using sandwich immunoassays. Calculate risks for Down syndrome and trisomy 13/18 based on demographic factors, ultrasound information, and analyte concentrations.

Clinical Example (0125U)

A 32-year-old female at 12-weeks gestation presents for routine prenatal care. A maternal-serum sample is submitted to measure free beta-hCG, PAPP-A, AFP, PlGF, and inhibin to assess the patient's risks for Down syndrome, trisomy 13/18, and preeclampsia.

Description of Procedure (0125U)

Analyze maternal serum for free beta-hCG, PAPP-A, AFP, inhibin, and PlGF using sandwich immunoassays. Calculate risks for Down syndrome, trisomy 13/18, and optionally early onset preeclampsia based on demographic factors, serum analyte concentrations, and ultrasound information.

Clinical Example (0126U)

A 24-year-old female at 12-weeks gestation presents for routine prenatal care. A maternal-serum sample is collected to measure free beta-hCG, PAPP-A, AFP, PlGF, and inhibin. A cell-free DNA tube is collected (plasma) to determine presence of Y chromosome.

Description of Procedure (0126U)

Analyze maternal serum for free beta-hCG, PAPP-A, AFP, inhibin, and PlGF using sandwich immunoassays. Analyze cell-free DNA collected in plasma using a Y chromosome–specific probe. Use the Y-chromosome result in serum-analyte adjustment for risk assessment. Calculate risks for Down syndrome, trisomy 13/18, and optionally preeclampsia based on demographic factors, ultrasound information, and serum-analyte concentration.

Clinical Example (0127U)

A 30-year-old female at 13-weeks gestation with a family history of preeclampsia presents for routine prenatal care. A maternal-serum sample is submitted to measure PAPP-A, AFP, and PlGF.

Description of Procedure (0127U)

Analyze maternal serum for PAPP-A, AFP, and PlGF using sandwich immunoassays. Calculate risk for early onset preeclampsia based on demographic factors, mean arterial pressure, uterine artery Doppler pulsatility index (UtAD-PI), and serum-analyte levels.

Clinical Example (0128U)

A 33-year-old female at 11.5-weeks gestation presents for routine prenatal care. A maternal-serum sample is collected to measure PAPP-A, AFP, and PlGF. A cell-free DNA tube (plasma) is collected for the determination of presence of Y chromosome.

Description of Procedure (0128U)

Analyze maternal serum for PAPP-A, AFP, and PlGF using sandwich immunoassays. Analyze cell-free DNA using a Y chromosome–specific probe collected in plasma. Use the Y-chromosome result in serum-analytes adjustment for risk assessment. Calculate risk for preeclampsia based on demographic factors, ultrasound information, and serum-analyte concentrations.

Clinical Example (0129U)

A 55-year-old female presents with a history of breast cancer diagnosed at age 52. The patient also has a family history of ovarian cancer (mother diagnosed at 50). Her physician recommends a targeted hereditary breast ovarian cancer germline gene panel because her personal and family history could be suggestive of several different hereditary cancer syndromes.

Description of Procedure (0129U)

Isolate high-quality genomic DNA from whole blood, saliva, or cells. Subject to NGS and Sanger sequencing to detect single nucleotide variants in ATM, BRCA1, BRCA2, CDH1, CHEK2, PALB2, PTEN, and TP53 (sequencing and deletion or duplication). Analyze the data and compose a report.

Clinical Example (0130U)

A 53-year-old female has a personal history of basal cell carcinoma and a tubular adenoma with a family history of endometrial adenocarcinoma. Her physician recommends an additional targeted mRNA hereditary cancer germline gene panel. [**Note:** This is an add-on code. Only consider the additional work related to the primary procedure.]

Description of Procedure (0130U)

Isolate high-quality RNA from whole blood. Subject to NGS to screen for abnormal RNA transcripts in the following genes associated with colorectal carcinoma: APC, CDH1, CHEK2, MLH1, MSH2, MSH6, MUTYH, PMS2, PTEN, and TP53. Use mRNA analysis to screen for abnormal RNA transcripts (even in absence of DNA variant) and for variant resolution. Analyze the data and include results on report.

Clinical Example (0131U)

A 41-year-old female has breast cancer and a family history consistent with hereditary breast and ovarian cancer syndrome. Her physician orders an additional targeted mRNA hereditary cancer germline gene panel. [**Note:** This is an add-on code. Only consider the additional work related to the primary procedure.]

Description of Procedure (0131U)

Isolate high-quality RNA from whole blood. Subject to NGS to screen for abnormal RNA transcripts in the following hereditary breast cancer genes: ATM, BRCA1, BRCA2, BRIP1, CDH1, CHEK2, MUTYH, NF1, PALB2, PTEN, RAD51C, RAD51D, and TP53. Use mRNA analysis to screen for abnormal RNA transcription (even in absence of DNA variant) and for variant resolution. Analyze the data and include results on report.

Clinical Example (0132U)

A 44-year-old female is diagnosed with papillary serous carcinoma of the right fallopian tube and both ovaries and has a family history of ovarian cancer. Her physician orders an additional targeted mRNA targeted hereditary cancer germline gene panel. [**Note:** This is an add-on code. Only consider the additional work related to the primary procedure.]

Description of Procedure (0132U)

Isolate high-quality RNA from whole blood. Subject to NGS to screen for abnormal RNA transcripts in the following hereditary cancer genes: ATM, BRCA1, BRCA2, BRIP1, CDH1, CHEK2, MLH1, MSH2, MSH6, MUTYH, NF1, PALB2, PMS2, PTEN, RAD51C, RAD51D, and TP53. Use mRNA analysis to screen for abnormal RNA transcription (even in absence DNA variant) and for variant resolution. Analyze the data and include results on report.

Clinical Example (0133U)

A 49-year-old male has prostate cancer and a family history of breast and ovarian cancer. His physician orders an additional targeted mRNA targeted hereditary cancer germline gene panel. [**Note:** This is an add-on code. Only consider the additional work related to the primary procedure.]

Description of Procedure (0133U)

Isolate high-quality RNA from whole blood. Subject to NGS to screen for abnormal RNA transcripts in the following hereditary cancer genes: ATM, BRCA1, BRCA2, CHEK2, MLH1, MSH2, MSH6, PALB2, PMS2, RAD51D, and TP53. Use mRNA analysis for variant resolution and to screen for abnormal RNA transcription (even in absence of DNA variant). Analyze the data and include results on report.

Clinical Example (0134U)

A 40-year-old female has a personal and family history of colon and ovarian cancer. Her physician orders an additional targeted mRNA targeted pan hereditary cancer germline gene panel. [**Note:** This is an add-on code. Only consider the additional work related to the primary procedure.]

Description of Procedure (0134U)

Isolate high-quality RNA from whole blood. Subject to NGS to screen for abnormal transcripts in the following hereditary cancer genes: APC, ATM, BRCA1, BRCA2, BRIP1, CDH1, CHEK2, MLH1, MSH2, MSH6, MUTYH, NF1, PALB2, PMS2, PTEN, RAD51C, RAD51D, and TP53. Use mRNA analysis for variant resolution and to screen for abnormal RNA transcription (even in absence of DNA variant). Analyze the data and include results on report.

Clinical Example (0135U)

A 55-year-old female has endometrial cancer (loss of PMS2 on IHC) and a family history of colon cancer. Her physician orders an additional targeted mRNA hereditary cancer germline gene panel. [**Note:** This is an add-on code. Only consider the additional work related to the primary procedure.]

Description of Procedure (0135U)

Isolate high-quality RNA from whole blood. Subject to NGS to screen for abnormal RNA transcripts in the following hereditary cancer genes: BRCA1, BRCA2, BRIP1, MLH1, MSH2, MSH6, PALB2, PMS2, PTEN, RAD51C, RAD51D, and TP53. Use mRNA analysis for variant resolution and to screen for abnormal RNA transcription (even in absence of DNA variant). Analyze the data and include results on report.

Clinical Example (0136U)

A 35-year-old female presents with a family history of breast cancer in maternal relatives in their 40s. Her physician orders an additional mRNA sequence analysis for the ATM gene. [**Note:** This is an add-on code. Only consider the additional work related to the primary procedure.]

Description of Procedure (0136U)

Isolate high-quality RNA from whole blood. Subject to NGS to screen for abnormal RNA transcripts in the ATM gene associated with ATM-related hereditary breast cancer. Use mRNA analysis for variant resolution and to screen for abnormal RNA transcription (even in absence of DNA variant). Analyze the data and include results on report.

Clinical Example (0137U)

A 37-year-old female presents with a family history of breast cancer in many paternal relatives. Her physician orders an additional mRNA sequence analysis for the PALB2 gene. [**Note:** This is an add-on code. Only consider the additional work related to the primary procedure.]

Description of Procedure (0137U)

Isolate high-quality RNA from whole blood. Subject to NGS to screen for abnormal RNA transcripts in the PALB2 gene associated with PALB2-related hereditary breast cancer. Use mRNA analysis to screen for abnormal RNA transcription (even in absence of DNA variant) and for variant resolution. Analyze the data and include results on report.

Clinical Example (0138U)

A 41-year-old female presents with breast cancer and a family history consistent with hereditary breast and ovarian cancer syndrome. Her physician orders an additional targeted mRNA sequence analysis for BRCA1 and BRCA2. [**Note:** This is an add-on code. Only consider the additional work related to the primary procedure.]

Description of Procedure (0138U)

Isolate high-quality RNA from whole blood. Subject to NGS to screen for abnormal RNA transcripts in the BRCA1 and BRCA2 genes associated with hereditary breast and ovarian cancer syndromes. Use mRNA analysis to screen for abnormal RNA transcription (even in absence of DNA variant) and for variant resolution. Analyze the data and include results on report.

Notes

Medicine

Summary of Additions, Deletions, and Revisions

The summary of changes shows the actual changes that have been made to the code descriptors.

New codes appear with a bullet (●) and are indicated as "Code added." Revised codes are preceded with a triangle (▲). Within revised codes, or if a code symbol has been deleted, the deleted language and code symbol appear with a ~~strikethrough~~ (⊖), while new text appears underlined.

The ⩗ symbol is used to identify codes for vaccines that are pending FDA approval. The # symbol is used to identify codes that have been resequenced. CPT add-on codes are annotated by the + symbol. The ⊘ symbol is used to identify codes that are exempt from the use of modifier 51. The ★ symbol is used to identify codes that may be used for reporting telemedicine services. The ⩕ is used to identify proprietary laboratory analyses (PLA) test that has an identical descriptor as another PLA test. A PLA code that satisfies Category I code criteria and has been accepted by the CPT Editorial Panel is annotated with the ↑↓ symbol.

Code	Description
#⩗●90619	Code added
#⩗●90694	Code added
▲90734	Meningococcal conjugate vaccine, serogroups A, C, W, Y ~~and W-135, quadrivalent (MCV4~~, quadrivalent, diphtheria toxoid carrier (MenACWY-D) or ~~MenACWY~~CRM197 carrier (MenACWY-CRM), for intramuscular use
90911	~~Biofeedback training, perineal muscles, anorectal or urethral sphincter, including EMG and/or manometry~~
●90912	Code added
+●90913	Code added
●92201	Code added
●92202	Code added
92225	~~Ophthalmoscopy, extended, with retinal drawing (eg, for retinal detachment, melanoma), with interpretation and report; initial~~
92226	~~subsequent~~
▲92548	Computerized dynamic posturography sensory organization test (CDP-SOT), 6 conditions (ie, eyes open, eyes closed, visual sway, platform sway, eyes closed platform sway, platform and visual sway), including interpretation and report;
●92549	Code added
▲92626	Evaluation of auditory ~~rehabilitation~~function for surgically implanted device(s) candidacy or postoperative status of a surgically implanted device(s); first hour
+▲92627	each additional 15 minutes (List separately in addition to code for primary procedure)
93299	~~implantable cardiovascular physiologic monitor system or subcutaneous cardiac rhythm monitor system, remote data acquisition(s), receipt of transmissions and technician review, technical support and distribution of results~~
#+●93356	Code added

Medicine

Code	Description
▲93784	Ambulatory blood pressure monitoring, utilizing ~~a system such as magnetic tape and/or computer disk,~~ <u>report-generating software, automated, worn continuously</u> for 24 hours or longer; including recording, scanning analysis, interpretation and report
▲93786	recording only
▲93788	scanning analysis with report
▲93790	review with interpretation and report
●93985	Code added
●93986	Code added
▲94728	Airway resistance by ~~impulse~~ oscillometry
▲95813	~~greater than 1 hour~~<u>61-119 minutes</u>
95827	~~all night recording~~
95831	~~Muscle testing, manual (separate procedure) with report; extremity (excluding hand) or trunk~~
95832	~~hand, with or without comparison with normal side~~
95833	~~total evaluation of body, excluding hands~~
95834	~~total evaluation of body, including hands~~
95950	~~Monitoring for identification and lateralization of cerebral seizure focus, electroencephalographic (eg, 8 channel EEG) recording and interpretation, each 24 hours~~
95951	~~Monitoring for localization of cerebral seizure focus by cable or radio, 16 or more channel telemetry, combined electroencephalographic (EEG) and video recording and interpretation (eg, for presurgical localization), each 24 hours~~
95953	~~Monitoring for localization of cerebral seizure focus by computerized portable 16 or more channel EEG, electroencephalographic (EEG) recording and interpretation, each 24 hours, unattended~~
95956	~~Monitoring for localization of cerebral seizure focus by cable or radio, 16 or more channel telemetry, electroencephalographic (EEG) recording and interpretation, each 24 hours, attended by a technologist or nurse~~
#●95700	Code added
#●95705	Code added
#●95706	Code added
#●95707	Code added
#●95708	Code added
#●95709	Code added
#●95710	Code added
#●95711	Code added
#●95712	Code added
#●95713	Code added
#●95714	Code added

CPT Changes 2020 — Medicine

Code	Description
#●95715	Code added
#●95716	Code added
#●95717	Code added
#●95718	Code added
#●95719	Code added
#●95720	Code added
#●95721	Code added
#●95722	Code added
#●95723	Code added
#●95724	Code added
#●95725	Code added
#●95726	Code added
96150	~~Health and behavior assessment (eg, health-focused clinical interview, behavioral observations, psychophysiological monitoring, health-oriented questionnaires), each 15 minutes face-to-face with the patient; initial assessment~~
96151	~~re-assessment~~
96152	~~Health and behavior intervention, each 15 minutes, face-to-face; individual~~
96153	~~group (2 or more patients)~~
96154	~~family (with the patient present)~~
96155	~~family (without the patient present)~~
●96156	Code added
●96158	Code added
+●96159	Code added
#●96164	Code added
#+●96165	Code added
#●96167	Code added
#+●96168	Code added
#●96170	Code added
#+●96171	Code added
97127	~~Therapeutic interventions that focus on cognitive function (eg, attention, memory, reasoning, executive function, problem solving, and/or pragmatic functioning) and compensatory strategies to manage the performance of an activity (eg, managing time or schedules, initiating, organizing and sequencing tasks), direct (one-on-one) patient contact~~
●97129	Code added
+●97130	Code added

▲ = Revised code   ● = New code   ▶◀ = Contains new or revised text   ✕ = Duplicate PLA test   ↕ = Category I PLA

Medicine

CPT Changes 2020

Code	Description
98969	~~Online assessment and management service provided by a qualified nonphysician health care professional to an established patient or guardian, not originating from a related assessment and management service provided within the previous 7 days, using the Internet or similar electronic communications network~~
●98970	Code added
●98971	Code added
●98972	Code added

Medicine

Vaccines, Toxoids

✠ **90587** Dengue vaccine, quadrivalent, live, 3 dose schedule, for subcutaneous use

90619 Code is out of numerical sequence. See 90733-90739

✠ **90689** Influenza virus vaccine, quadrivalent (IIV4), inactivated, adjuvanted, preservative free, 0.25 mL dosage, for intramuscular use

#✠● **90694** Influenza virus vaccine, quadrivalent (aIIV4), inactivated, adjuvanted, preservative free, 0.5 mL dosage, for intramuscular use

90690 Typhoid vaccine, live, oral

90691 Typhoid vaccine, Vi capsular polysaccharide (ViCPs), for intramuscular use

90694 Code is out of numerical sequence. See 90688-90691

▲ **90734** Meningococcal conjugate vaccine, serogroups A, C, W, Y, quadrivalent, diphtheria toxoid carrier (MenACWY-D) or CRM197 carrier (MenACWY-CRM), for intramuscular use

#✠● **90619** Meningococcal conjugate vaccine, serogroups A, C, W, Y, quadrivalent, tetanus toxoid carrier (MenACWY-TT), for intramuscular use

90620 Meningococcal recombinant protein and outer membrane vesicle vaccine, serogroup B (MenB-4C), 2 dose schedule, for intramuscular use

Rationale

New code 90694 has been established in the Vaccines, Toxoids subsection to report a new quadrivalent influenza vaccine. Code 90694 describes an adjuvanted, inactivated, and preservative-free, quadrivalent flu vaccine for the 0.5 mL dosage. Administration of the vaccine is reported separately using codes 90460-90472 (immunization administration for vaccines/toxoids). Code 90694 carries the US Food and Drug Administration (FDA) approval pending symbol (✠); therefore, interim updates on the FDA status of this code will be reflected on the AMA CPT website at www.ama-assn.org/go/cpt-vaccine, under the CPT Category I Vaccine codes on a semiannual basis (July 1 and January 1).

Clinical Example (90694)

A 65-year-old male presents to his physician's office for a preventive care visit. The provider recommends influenza vaccination to decrease the patient's risk of influenza according to Advisory Committee on Immunization Practice (ACIP) recommendations.

Description of Procedure (90694)

Review the patient's chart to confirm that vaccination to decrease the risk of influenza is indicated. Counsel patient on the risks and benefits of influenza vaccination. Obtain consent for vaccination. Aseptically administer influenza vaccine by intramuscular injection.

Rationale

Code 90619 has been added to identify a meningococcal conjugate vaccine using a tetanus-toxoid carrier. Code 90734 has been revised to make the language consistent with code 90619 and to distinguish the type of meningococcal vaccine and carrier it describes from that of code 90619. Reporting requirements of immunization registries, vaccine distribution programs, and reporting systems (eg, Vaccine Adverse Event Reporting System) indicate that the exact vaccine product administered should be identified. To accommodate this, code 90619 specifies the exact vaccine (MenACWY-TT) used. Code 90619 also specifies the carrier used for the vaccine, which is a tetanus-toxoid carrier, and the serogroups (A, C, W, and Y) that the vaccine protects against.

Originally, code 90734 used more generic language to describe the meningococcal vaccine (MCV4 or MenACWY), did not specify the carrier used, and listed serogroups A, C, Y, and W-135. For 2020, code 90734 has been revised to reflect the appropriate ACIP vaccine abbreviations (MenACWY-D or MenACWY-CRM), the carrier used for each vaccine (diphtheria-toxoid carrier for MenACWY-D, and CRM197 carrier for MenACWY-CRM), and the serogroups that the vaccines protect against (A, C, W, Y).

Clinical Example (90619)

A 17-year-old is seen in a physician or other qualified health care professional (QHP) office for a preventive care visit. The physician/QHP reviews the patient's immunization record and determines that vaccination to decrease the risk of meningitis is indicated.

Description of Procedure (90619)

Review the patient's chart to confirm that vaccination to decrease the risk of meningitis is indicated. Counsel patient on the benefits and risks of vaccination to decrease the risk of meningitis and obtain consent. Administer quadrivalent meningococcal conjugate vaccine tetanus toxoid carrier by intramuscular injection.

Medicine | CPT Changes 2020

Clinical Example (90734)

A 17-year-old is seen in a physician or other QHP office for a preventive care visit. The physician or other QHP reviews the patient's immunization record and determines that vaccination to decrease the risk of meningitis is indicated.

Description of Procedure (90734)

Review the patient's chart to confirm that vaccination to decrease the risk of meningitis is indicated. Counsel patient on the benefits and risks of vaccination to decrease the risk of meningitis and obtain consent. Administer quadrivalent meningococcal conjugate vaccine diptheria toxoid carrier by intramuscular injection.

Psychiatry

Psychiatric Diagnostic Procedures

★ **90792** Psychiatric diagnostic evaluation with medical services

▶(Do not report 90791 or 90792 in conjunction with 99201-99337, 99341-99350, 99366-99368, 99401-99443, 97151, 97152, 97153, 97154, 97155, 97156, 97157, 97158, 0362T, 0373T)◀

(Use 90785 in conjunction with 90791, 90792 when the diagnostic evaluation includes interactive complexity services)

Rationale

In accordance with the deletion of online evaluation and management (E/M) code 99444, the parenthetical note following code 90792 has been revised with the removal of code 99444.

Refer to the codebook and the Rationale for code 99444 for a full discussion of these changes.

Biofeedback

▶(90911 has been deleted. To report, see 90912, 90913)◀

● **90912** Biofeedback training, perineal muscles, anorectal or urethral sphincter, including EMG and/or manometry, when performed; initial 15 minutes of one-on-one physician or other qualified health care professional contact with the patient

+● **90913** each additional 15 minutes of one-on-one physician or other qualified health care professional contact with the patient (List separately in addition to code for primary procedure)

▶(Use 90913 in conjunction with 90912)◀

(For testing of rectal sensation, tone and compliance, use 91120)

(For incontinence treatment by pulsed magnetic neuromodulation, use 53899)

Rationale

Code 90911 has been deleted and codes 90912 and 90913 have been added to report biofeedback training. Parenthetical notes have been added regarding the proper reporting of the new codes. Prior to 2020, code 90911 described biofeedback training of the perineal muscles, anorectal sphincter, or urethral sphincter, including electromyography (EMG) and/or manometry. The AMA/Specialty Society Relative Value Scale (RVS) Update Committee (RUC) Relativity Assessment Workgroup (RAW) identified code 90911 as potentially misvalued. Since 1994, when code 90911 was added to the code set, biofeedback training for pelvic floor weakness has evolved and different patients need disparate amounts of time for each session. For this reason, it was determined that reporting biofeedback training for pelvic floor weakness should be time-based. Therefore, code 90911 has been deleted and new codes have been added because the inclusion of time for these services represents a significant change in how these services are reported. Codes 90912 and 90913 describe 15-minute increments of one-on-one physician or other qualified health care professional contact with the patient for biofeedback training of the perineal muscles, anorectal sphincter, or urethral sphincter. EMG and/or manometry is included, when performed. Code 90912 describes the first 15 minutes and add-on code 90913 describes each additional 15 minutes.

Clinical Example (90912)

A 67-year-old female has an overactive bladder with symptoms consisting of urgency, frequency, and occasional urge incontinence. The patient has responded inadequately to medical therapy now and presents for biofeedback training.

Description of Procedure (90912)

Instruct the patient as to what muscles to contract to help with their symptoms and the goal of treatment. Active, minute-by-minute interaction with the patient helps them identify muscles and increase attention to the specific muscles of interest in the perineum. The patient views their real-time progress on the feedback monitor. After adequate recognition and exercise of the muscles, terminate the treatment and remove electrodes.

Clinical Example (90913)

A 67-year-old female has an overactive bladder with symptoms consisting of urgency, frequency, and occasional urge incontinence. The patient has undergone the first 15 minutes of biofeedback training, and the clinician determines she requires additional biofeedback training. [**Note:** This is an add-on service. Only consider the additional work related to an additional 15 minutes of biofeedback training.]

Description of Procedure (90913)

Continued active, minute-by-minute interaction with the patient helps them identify muscles and increase attention to the specific muscles of interest in the perineum. The patient views their real-time progress on the feedback monitor. Treatment continues until the physician or other QHP determines that adequate recognition and exercise of the muscle has been accomplished.

Gastroenterology

91120   Rectal sensation, tone, and compliance test (ie, response to graded balloon distention)

▶(For biofeedback training, see 90912, 90913)◀

(For anorectal manometry, use 91122)

91122   Anorectal manometry

(Do not report 91120, 91122 in conjunction with 91117)

Rationale

In accordance with the deletion of code 90911 and the addition of codes 90912 and 90913, the cross-reference parenthetical note following code 91120 has been revised to reflect these changes.

Refer to the codebook and the Rationale for codes 90911, 90912, and 90913, for a full discussion of these changes.

Ophthalmology

Special Ophthalmological Services

Ophthalmoscopy

Routine ophthalmoscopy is part of general and special ophthalmologic services whenever indicated. It is a non-itemized service and is not reported separately.

● **92201**   Ophthalmoscopy, extended; with retinal drawing and scleral depression of peripheral retinal disease (eg, for retinal tear, retinal detachment, retinal tumor) with interpretation and report, unilateral or bilateral

● **92202**   with drawing of optic nerve or macula (eg, for glaucoma, macular pathology, tumor) with interpretation and report, unilateral or bilateral

▶(Do not report 92201, 92202 in conjunction with 92250)◀

▶(92225, 92226 have been deleted. To report, see 92201, 92202)◀

Rationale

Codes 92225 and 92226 have been deleted and codes 92201 and 92202 have been added to the Ophthalmoscopy subsection. Two parenthetical notes have been added to provide instruction on the appropriate use of the new codes.

Prior to 2020, codes 92225 and 92226 described initial and subsequent extended ophthalmoscopy with retinal drawing, respectively. However, since these two codes' (92225, 92226) establishment, it has been determined that initial and subsequent reviews involve the same work. Therefore, there is no need to distinguish between initial and subsequent reviews in the code set, which is why new codes (92201, 92202) do not make this distinction. Peripheral retinal disease and the optic nerve are typically evaluated in this examination.

Code 92201 describes retinal drawing and scleral depression of peripheral retinal disease, and code 92202 describes drawing of the optic nerve or macula. Interpretation and report are included and must be performed in order to report codes 92201 and 92202.

Codes 92201 and 92202 should not be reported if fundus photography (92250) is performed. An exclusionary parenthetical note has been added following code 92202 instructing users not to report codes 92201 and 92202 with code 92250.

Medicine   CPT Changes 2020

Extended Ophthalmoscopy
92201, 92202

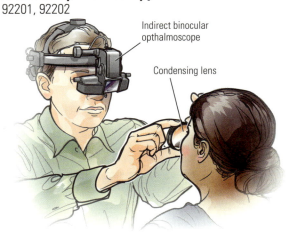

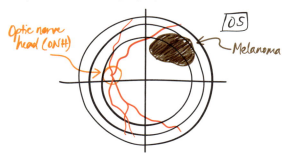

Example of clinical drawing of peripheral retinal disease

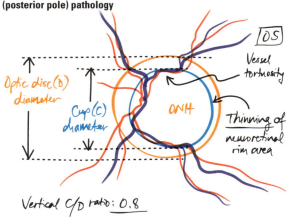

Example of clinical drawing of optic nerve or macular (posterior pole) pathology

Clinical Example (92201)

A 66-year-old female had a posterior vitreous detachment evaluated two months ago. At the time, no retinal tear was found. She returns with increased floaters in the same eye.

Description of Procedure (92201)

In a darkened room, position the patient in a reclining position for examination with indirect ophthalmoscopy and scleral depression and, when necessary, at the slit lamp biomicroscope for examination with a three-mirror contact lens. Carefully view the entire retinal periphery for 360° to detect a retinal break(s) or other retinal abnormalities. Transfer findings to a multicolored retinal drawing.

Clinical Example (92202)

A 54-year-old male presents with ocular hypertension and an enlarged optic nerve cup with a thin rim suspicious of glaucoma.

Description of Procedure (92202)

In a darkened room, position the patient at the slit lamp biomicroscope. Carefully examine the optic nerves of both eyes with indirect ophthalmoscopy using a noncontact 78D lens, paying attention to contours, rims, ratios, asymmetry, notches, and other findings. Transfer findings to a multicolored optic nerve drawing.

Other Specialized Services

92270   Electro-oculography with interpretation and report

(For vestibular function tests with recording, see 92537, 92538, 92540, 92541, 92542, 92544, 92545, 92546, 92547, 92548)

▶(Do not report 92270 in conjunction with 92537, 92538, 92540, 92541, 92542, 92544, 92545, 92546, 92547, 92548, 92549)◀

(To report saccadic eye movement testing with recording, use 92700)

Rationale

In accordance with the addition of code 92549, the exclusionary parenthetical note following code 92270 has been revised with the addition of code 92549 and to instruct users not to report code 92270 with code 92549.

Refer to the codebook and the Rationale for code 92549 for a full discussion of these changes.

Special Otorhinolaryngologic Services

Vestibular Function Tests, With Recording (eg, ENG)

▲ **92548** Computerized dynamic posturography sensory organization test (CDP-SOT), 6 conditions (ie, eyes open, eyes closed, visual sway, platform sway, eyes closed platform sway, platform and visual sway), including interpretation and report;

● **92549** with motor control test (MCT) and adaptation test (ADT)

▶(Do not report 92548, 92549 in conjunction with 92270)◀

Rationale

Code 92548 has been revised to describe computerized dynamic posturography (CDP) with greater specificity, and code 92549 has been added to describe CDP with motor control testing (MCT) and adaptation testing (ADT).

Prior to 2020, code 92548 described CDP with no additional description of the work performed in this service. The AMA/RVS RUC RAW identified code 92548 as having negative intraservice work per unit of time (IWPUT). A survey of medical specialties that perform CDP indicated that there is variation among providers in the use of equipment in this procedure. To more accurately describe the work performed in CDP, code 92548 has been revised to describe CDP sensory organization test (CDP-SOT) for six conditions with interpretation and report, which are listed in parentheses. Code 92549 has been added for CDP-SOT performed with a motor control test (MCT) and an adaptation test (ADT).

Codes 92548 and 92549 should not be reported with code 92270, which is reflected in the exclusionary parenthetical note below code 92549.

Clinical Example (92548)

A 65-year-old female presents with complaints of constant unsteadiness when standing or walking. Symptoms are made worse when walking in the dark or on uneven surfaces. Walking with head movement also exacerbates the symptoms.

Description of Procedure (92548)

Prepare the patient for the computerized dynamic posturography (CDP) testing, which includes a forceplate to measure sway and a visual surround that can be stationary, move in response to the forceplate, or move independent of the forceplate. The QHP performs testing under the following six distinct conditions: (1) eyes open, (2) eyes closed, (3) visual sway, (4) platform sway, (5) eyes closed platform sway, and (6) platform and visual sway. Before each of the six trials, the QHP informs the patient regarding what to expect (eg, both the visual surround and the force platform will move). Instruct the patient to stand with their eyes open or closed and to stand as still as possible. The QHP reviews the computer-generated results of the CDP sensory organization test (CDP-SOT) and develops a report of their impressions and recommendations. The report includes the patient's balance complaints and symptoms, the pattern of results, and the QHP's recommendations.

Clinical Example (92549)

A 77-year-old male presents with complaints of constant severe unsteadiness when standing or walking and a history of falls. Symptoms are made worse when standing or walking in the dark or on uneven surfaces, as well as on soft and/or moving surfaces. Rapid movements and walking with head movement also exacerbate the symptoms.

Description of Procedure (92549)

Prepare the patient for the CDP testing, which includes a forceplate to measure sway and a visual surround that can be stationary, move in response to the forceplate, or move independent of the forceplate. The QHP performs testing under the following six distinct conditions: (1) eyes open, (2) eyes closed, (3) visual sway, (4) platform sway, (5) eyes closed platform sway, and (6) platform and visual sway. Before each of the six trials, the QHP informs the patient regarding what to expect (eg, both the visual surround and the force platform will move). Instruct the patient to stand with their eyes open or closed and to stand as still as possible. After the six CDP-SOT conditions are performed, rapidly shift the platform horizontally (CDP-MCT [motor control test]), at least three different set distances and multiple times. Following the horizontal shifts, rapidly rotate the platform multiple times around the ankle axis (CDP-ADT [adaptation test]). The QHP reviews the computer-generated results of the CDP-SOT, -MCT, and -ADT and develops a report of their impressions and recommendations. The report includes the patient's balance complaints and symptoms, the pattern of results, and the QHP's recommendations.

Evaluative and Therapeutic Services

92625 Assessment of tinnitus (includes pitch, loudness matching, and masking)

(Do not report 92625 in conjunction with 92562)

(For unilateral assessment, use modifier 52)

| Medicine | CPT Changes 2020 |

▲ **92626** Evaluation of auditory function for surgically implanted device(s) candidacy or postoperative status of a surgically implanted device(s); first hour

+▲ **92627** each additional 15 minutes (List separately in addition to code for primary procedure)

(Use 92627 in conjunction with 92626)

(When reporting 92626, 92627, use the face-to-face time with the patient or family)

►(Do not report 92626, 92627 in conjunction with 92590, 92591, 92592, 92593, 92594, 92595 for hearing aid evaluation, fitting, follow-up, or selection)◄

Rationale

Codes 92626 and 92627 have been revised to describe evaluation of auditory function for surgically implanted device candidacy or postoperative status of a surgically implanted device. Code 92626 was identified for high-volume growth by the AMA/RVS RUC RAW. There was concern that this high-volume growth was due to a misinterpretation of code 92626's intended use. A recommendation was made to revise code 92626 to more clearly define the intended use and the work involved in the evaluation, and to ensure the descriptor reflects current practice. Code 92626 described evaluation of auditory rehabilitation status; however, the intent of the evaluation is to determine if a patient is a suitable candidate for a surgically implanted device such as a cochlear implant. If the evaluation indicates a patient is not a suitable candidate, then the patient may be considered for auditory rehabilitation therapy. To clarify the intent of the evaluation, codes 92626 and 92627 have been revised by replacing "evaluation of auditory rehabilitation status" with "evaluation of auditory function for surgically implanted device(s) candidacy or postoperative status of a surgically implanted device(s)." Code 92626 describes the first hour of evaluation. Add-on code 92627 describes each additional 15 minutes of evaluation.

Codes 92626 and 92627 do not describe hearing-aid evaluation, fitting, follow-up, or selection as described by codes 92590, 92591, 92592, 92593, 92594, and 92595. An exclusionary parenthetical note has been added following code 92627 instructing users not to report codes 92626 and 92627 with codes 92590, 92591, 92592, 92593, 92594, and 92595.

Clinical Example (92626)

A 60-year-old female, who is a hearing-aid user with progressive hearing loss, is no longer receiving benefit from amplification. This is demonstrated by a reduced ability to understand speech in all listening environments, even with adjustments and optimization of the patient's amplification system. The patient is referred for an assessment of candidacy for an implanted hearing device.

Description of Procedure (92626)

The QHP takes a detailed case history with attention to history of hearing loss, incidence of familial hearing loss, and use of amplification. Verify the electroacoustic integrity of existing hearing aids prior to subsequent aided testing. The patient is seated in a sound-controlled environment with loudspeakers located at defined azimuths for controlled signal presentation and sound intensity. Determine speech perception of word and sentence intelligibility in a quiet environment independently at varying sound intensity levels at one or more loudspeaker locations. Then repeat testing in varying levels of background noise. Quantify the performance of each aided ear separately and then together in the binaural mode. Score results of the examination and interpret based on available performance standards to determine implantation candidacy or prognosis for success. Prepare a report.

Clinical Example (92627)

A 60-year-old female, who is a hearing-aid user with progressive hearing loss, is no longer receiving benefit from amplification. This is demonstrated by a reduced ability to understand speech in all listening environments, even with adjustments and optimization of the patient's amplification system. The patient is referred for an assessment of candidacy for an implanted hearing device. The patient requires an additional 15 minutes of testing beyond the first hour.

Description of Procedure (92627)

The patient is seated in a sound-controlled environment with loudspeakers located at defined azimuths for controlled signal presentation and sound intensity. Determine speech perception of word and sentence intelligibility in a quiet environment independently at varying sound intensity levels at one or more loudspeaker locations. Then repeat testing in varying levels of background noise. Quantify the performance of each aided ear separately and then together in the binaural mode.

Cardiovascular

Cardiography

93040   Rhythm ECG, 1-3 leads; with interpretation and report

93041   tracing only without interpretation and report

93042   interpretation and report only

--- *Coding Tip* ---

Instructions for Reporting Electrocardiographic Recording

Do not report 93268-93272 when performing 93260, 93261, 93279-93289, 93291-93296, or 93298. *Do not report 93040-93042 when performing 93260, 93261, 93279-93289, 93291-93296, or 93298.*

CPT Coding Guidelines, Cardiovascular, Implantable, Insertable, and Wearable Cardiac Device Evaluations

Rationale

In accordance with the deletion of code 93299, the Instructions for Reporting Electrocardiographic Recording coding tip has been updated with the removal of code 93299.

Refer to the codebook and the Rationale for code 93299 for a full discussion of these changes.

Cardiovascular Monitoring Services

★ **93268**   External patient and, when performed, auto activated electrocardiographic rhythm derived event recording with symptom-related memory loop with remote download capability up to 30 days, 24-hour attended monitoring; includes transmission, review and interpretation by a physician or other qualified health care professional

★ **93270**   recording (includes connection, recording, and disconnection)

★ **93271**   transmission and analysis

★ **93272**   review and interpretation by a physician or other qualified health care professional

▶(For subcutaneous cardiac rhythm monitoring, see 33285, 93285, 93291, 93298)◀

Rationale

In accordance with the deletion of code 93299, the cross-reference parenthetical note following code 93272 has been revised to reflect this change.

Refer to the codebook and the Rationale for code 93299 for a full discussion of these changes.

Implantable, Insertable, and Wearable Cardiac Device Evaluations

▶Cardiac device evaluation services are diagnostic medical procedures using in-person and remote technology to assess device therapy and cardiovascular physiologic data. Codes 93260, 93261, 93279-93298 describe this technology and technical/professional and service center practice. Codes 93260, 93261, 93279-93292 are reported per procedure. Codes 93293, 93294, 93295, 93296 are reported no more than **once** every 90 days. Do not report 93293, 93294, 93295, 93296, if the monitoring period is less than 30 days. Codes 93297, 93298 are reported no more than **once** up to every 30 days, per patient. Do not report 93297, 93298, if the monitoring period is less than 10 days. Do not report 93264 if the monitoring period is less than 30 days. Code 93264 is reported no more than once up to every 30 days, per patient.

A service center may report 93296 during a period in which a physician or other qualified health care professional performs an in-person interrogation device evaluation. The same individual may not report an in-person and remote interrogation of the same device during the same period. Report only remote services when an in-person interrogation device evaluation is performed during a period of remote interrogation device evaluation. A period is established by the initiation of the remote monitoring or the 91st day of a pacemaker or implantable defibrillator monitoring or the 31st day of monitoring a subcutaneous cardiac rhythm monitor or implantable cardiovascular physiologic monitor, and extends for the subsequent 90 or 30 days respectively, for which remote monitoring is occurring. Programming device evaluations and in-person interrogation device evaluations may not be reported on the same date by the same individual. Programming device evaluations and remote interrogation device evaluations may both be reported during the remote interrogation device evaluation period.◀

For monitoring by wearable devices, see 93224-93272.

ECG rhythm derived elements are distinct from physiologic data, even when the same device is capable of producing both. Implantable cardiovascular physiologic

Medicine

monitor services are always separately reported from implantable defibrillator services. When cardiac rhythm data are derived from an implantable defibrillator or pacemaker, do not report subcutaneous cardiac rhythm monitor services with pacemaker or implantable defibrillator services.

▶Do not report 93268-93272 when performing 93260, 93261, 93279-93289, 93291-93296, or 93298. Do not report 93040, 93041, 93042 when performing 93260, 93261, 93279-93289, 93291-93296, or 93298.◀

The pacemaker and implantable defibrillator interrogation device evaluations, peri-procedural device evaluations and programming, and programming device evaluations may not be reported in conjunction with pacemaker or implantable defibrillator device and/or lead insertion or revision services by the same individual.

▶The following definitions and instructions apply to codes 93260, 93261, 93279-93298.◀

Attended surveillance: the immediate availability of a remote technician to respond to rhythm or device alert transmissions from a patient, either from an implanted, inserted, or wearable monitoring or therapy device, as they are generated and transmitted to the remote surveillance location or center.

Rationale

In accordance with the deletion of code 93299, the Implantable, Insertable, and Wearable Cardiac Device Evaluations guidelines have been revised to reflect this change.

Refer to the codebook and the Rationale for code 93299 for a full discussion of these changes.

93288 Interrogation device evaluation (in person) with analysis, review and report by a physician or other qualified health care professional, includes connection, recording and disconnection per patient encounter; single, dual, or multiple lead pacemaker system, or leadless pacemaker system

(Do not report 93288 in conjunction with 93279-93281, 93286, 93294, 93296)

93289 single, dual, or multiple lead transvenous implantable defibrillator system, including analysis of heart rhythm derived data elements

(For monitoring physiologic cardiovascular data elements derived from an implantable defibrillator, use 93290)

(Do not report 93289 in conjunction with 93261, 93282, 93283, 93284, 93287, 93295, 93296)

 # 93261 implantable subcutaneous lead defibrillator system

(Do not report 93261 in conjunction with 93260, 93287, 93289)

(Do not report 93261 in conjunction with pulse generator and lead insertion or repositioning codes 33240, 33241, 33262, 33270, 33271, 33272, 33273)

93290 implantable cardiovascular physiologic monitor system, including analysis of 1 or more recorded physiologic cardiovascular data elements from all internal and external sensors

(For heart rhythm derived data elements, use 93289)

▶(Do not report 93290 in conjunction with 93297)◀

93291 subcutaneous cardiac rhythm monitor system, including heart rhythm derived data analysis

▶(Do not report 93291 in conjunction with 33285, 93288-93290, 93298)◀

Rationale

In accordance with the deletion of code 93299, the exclusionary parenthetical notes following codes 93290 and 93291 have been revised to reflect this change.

Refer to the codebook and the Rationale for code 93299 for a full discussion of these changes.

93292 wearable defibrillator system

(Do not report 93292 in conjunction with 93745)

93294 Interrogation device evaluation(s) (remote), up to 90 days; single, dual, or multiple lead pacemaker system, or leadless pacemaker system with interim analysis, review(s) and report(s) by a physician or other qualified health care professional

(Do not report 93294 in conjunction with 93288, 93293)

(Report 93294 only once per 90 days)

93295 single, dual, or multiple lead implantable defibrillator system with interim analysis, review(s) and report(s) by a physician or other qualified health care professional

(For remote monitoring of physiologic cardiovascular data elements derived from an ICD, use 93297)

(Do not report 93295 in conjunction with 93289)

(Report 93295 only once per 90 days)

▶(For remote interrogation device evaluation[s] of implantable cardioverter-defibrillator with substernal lead, see 0578T, 0579T)◀

Rationale

In accordance with the addition of Category III codes 0578T and 0579T, a cross-reference parenthetical note has been added following code 93295 to direct users to codes 0578T and 0579T for remote interrogation device evaluation(s) of implantable cardioverter-defibrillator with substernal lead.

Refer to the codebook and the Rationale for codes 0578T and 0579T for a full discussion of these changes.

93296 single, dual, or multiple lead pacemaker system, leadless pacemaker system, or implantable defibrillator system, remote data acquisition(s), receipt of transmissions and technician review, technical support and distribution of results

▶(Do not report 93296 in conjunction with 93288, 93289)◀

Rationale

In accordance with the deletion of code 93299, the exclusionary parenthetical note following code 93296 has been revised to reflect this change.

Refer to the codebook and the Rationale for code 93299 for a full discussion of these changes.

(Report 93296 only once per 90 days)

▶(For remote interrogation device evaluation[s] of implantable cardioverter-defibrillator with substernal lead, see 0578T, 0579T)◀

Rationale

In accordance with the addition of Category III codes 0578T and 0579T, a parenthetical note has been added following code 93296 to direct users to codes 0578T and 0579T for remote interrogation device evaluation(s) of implantable cardioverter-defibrillator with substernal lead.

Refer to the codebook and the Rationale for codes 0578T and 0579T for a full discussion of these changes.

93297 Interrogation device evaluation(s), (remote) up to 30 days; implantable cardiovascular physiologic monitor system, including analysis of 1 or more recorded physiologic cardiovascular data elements from all internal and external sensors, analysis, review(s) and report(s) by a physician or other qualified health care professional

(For heart rhythm derived data elements, use 93295)

▶(Do not report 93297 in conjunction with 93264, 93290, 93298, 99091, 99454)◀

(Report 93297 only once per 30 days)

93298 subcutaneous cardiac rhythm monitor system, including analysis of recorded heart rhythm data, analysis, review(s) and report(s) by a physician or other qualified health care professional

▶(Do not report 93298 in conjunction with 33285, 93291, 93297, 99091, 99454)◀

(Report 93298 only once per 30 days)

Rationale

The exclusionary parenthetical notes following codes 93297 and 93298 have been revised with the addition of codes 99091 and 99454.

The exclusionary parenthetical notes have been revised to clarify that codes 93297 and 93298 should not be reported with other remote monitoring services and collection and interpretation of physiologic data as described by codes 99091 and 99454. In addition, the Telemedicine symbol has been removed from code 93298 as it does not qualify as a synchronous type of procedure as described in the guidelines of Appendix P.

▶(93299 has been deleted. To report, see 93297, 93298)◀

(For remote monitoring of an implantable wireless pulmonary artery pressure sensor, use 93264)

Rationale

Code 93299 has been deleted. A parenthetical note has been added directing users to codes 93297 and 93298.

The AMA/RVS RUC RAW identified code 93299 as a high-volume, carrier-priced code. Code 93299 described the technical component associated with codes 93297 and 93298. The level of clinical staff work varies significantly between codes 93297 and 93298, which makes a single, separate code for reporting the technical component of these services inadequate. To address this discrepancy, code 93299 has been deleted and practice expense (PE) inputs that accurately reflect the clinical staff work associated were recommended for codes 93297 and 93298. A separate code to report the PE associated with codes 93297 and 93298 is no longer necessary.

Medicine | CPT Changes 2020

Echocardiography

93350 Echocardiography, transthoracic, real-time with image documentation (2D), includes M-mode recording, when performed, during rest and cardiovascular stress test using treadmill, bicycle exercise and/or pharmacologically induced stress, with interpretation and report;

(Stress testing codes 93016-93018 should be reported, when appropriate, in conjunction with 93350 to capture the cardiovascular stress portion of the study)

(Do not report 93350 in conjunction with 93015)

93351 including performance of continuous electrocardiographic monitoring, with supervision by a physician or other qualified health care professional

(Do not report 93351 in conjunction with 93015-93018, 93350. Do not report 93351-26 in conjunction with 93016, 93018, 93350-26)

#+● **93356** Myocardial strain imaging using speckle tracking-derived assessment of myocardial mechanics (List separately in addition to codes for echocardiography imaging)

▶(Use 93356 in conjunction with 93303, 93304, 93306, 93307, 93308, 93350, 93351)◀

▶(Report 93356 once per session)◀

93356 Code is out of numerical sequence. See 93350-93355

Rationale

Category III code 0399T has been converted to Category I add-on code 93356 for reporting myocardial strain imaging using speckle tracking-derived assessment of myocardial mechanics. Two parenthetical notes have been added to provide instruction on the proper use of this code.

Since the establishment of code 0399T in 2016, the performance of myocardial strain imaging using speckle tracking-derived assessment of myocardial mechanics has increased to a level that warranted conversion to Category I. This procedure is an adjunct procedure performed with transthoracic echocardiography. Therefore, code 93356 is designated as an add-on code, and an inclusionary parenthetical note has been added instructing users to report code 93356 with transthoracic echocardiography codes (93303, 93304, 93306, 93307, 93308, 93350, 93351), as appropriate.

Code 93356 is reported only once per session and an instructional parenthetical note has been added to clarify this.

Clinical Example (93356)

A 68-year-old female is receiving trastuzumab in treatment of HER2-positive breast cancer. She presents for an echocardiogram to exclude chemotherapy-related cardiotoxicity. A complete echocardiogram is performed with myocardial strain imaging.

Description of Procedure (93356)

The physician reviews request for service to clarify the indications for the procedure and determine the clinical questions that need to be answered by the myocardial strain echo examination. Analyze images of the acquired myocardial strain data (static and real time) on an appropriate software program to determine regional and global longitudinal, radial, and/or circumferential strain and/or strain rates. Compare these data to previous studies, when available. Dictate a report and review the findings in detail with the referring physician.

Cardiac Catheterization

93451 Right heart catheterization including measurement(s) of oxygen saturation and cardiac output, when performed

(Do not report 93451 in conjunction with 33289, 93453, 93456, 93457, 93460, 93461)

▶(Do not report 93451 in conjunction with 33418, 0345T, 0483T, 0484T, 0544T, 0545T for diagnostic right heart catheterization procedures intrinsic to the valve repair or annulus reconstruction procedure)◀

93452 Left heart catheterization including intraprocedural injection(s) for left ventriculography, imaging supervision and interpretation, when performed

(Do not report 93452 in conjunction with 93453, 93458-93461, 0408T, 0409T, 0410T, 0411T, 0414T, 0415T)

▶(Do not report 93452 in conjunction with 33418, 0345T, 0483T, 0484T, 0544T, 0545T for diagnostic left heart catheterization procedures intrinsic to the valve repair or annulus reconstruction procedure)◀

93453 Combined right and left heart catheterization including intraprocedural injection(s) for left ventriculography, imaging supervision and interpretation, when performed

(Do not report 93453 in conjunction with 93451, 93452, 93456-93461, 0408T, 0409T, 0410T, 0411T, 0414T, 0415T)

▶(Do not report 93453 in conjunction with 33418, 0345T, 0483T, 0484T, 0544T, 0545T for diagnostic left and right heart catheterization procedures intrinsic to the valve repair or annulus reconstruction procedure)◀

93454 Catheter placement in coronary artery(s) for coronary angiography, including intraprocedural injection(s) for coronary angiography, imaging supervision and interpretation;

▶(Do not report 93454 in conjunction with 33418, 0345T, 0483T, 0484T, 0544T, 0545T for coronary angiography intrinsic to the valve repair or annulus reconstruction procedure)◀

93455 with catheter placement(s) in bypass graft(s) (internal mammary, free arterial, venous grafts) including intraprocedural injection(s) for bypass graft angiography

▶(Do not report 93455 in conjunction with 33418, 0345T, 0483T, 0484T, 0544T, 0545T for coronary angiography intrinsic to the valve repair or annulus reconstruction procedure)◀

93456 with right heart catheterization

▶(Do not report 93456 in conjunction with 33418, 0345T, 0483T, 0484T, 0544T, 0545T for diagnostic coronary angiography or right heart catheterization procedures intrinsic to the valve repair or annulus reconstruction procedure)◀

93457 with catheter placement(s) in bypass graft(s) (internal mammary, free arterial, venous grafts) including intraprocedural injection(s) for bypass graft angiography and right heart catheterization

▶(Do not report 93457 in conjunction with 33418, 0345T, 0483T, 0484T, 0544T, 0545T for diagnostic coronary angiography or right heart catheterization procedures intrinsic to the valve repair or annulus reconstruction procedure)◀

93458 with left heart catheterization including intraprocedural injection(s) for left ventriculography, when performed

▶(Do not report 93458 in conjunction with 33418, 0345T, 0483T, 0484T, 0544T, 0545T for diagnostic coronary angiography or left heart catheterization procedures intrinsic to the valve repair or annulus reconstruction procedure)◀

(Do not report 93458 in conjunction with 0408T, 0409T, 0410T, 0411T, 0414T, 0415T)

93459 with left heart catheterization including intraprocedural injection(s) for left ventriculography, when performed, catheter placement(s) in bypass graft(s) (internal mammary, free arterial, venous grafts) with bypass graft angiography

▶(Do not report 93459 in conjunction with 33418, 0345T, 0483T, 0484T, 0544T, 0545T for diagnostic coronary angiography or left heart catheterization procedures intrinsic to the valve repair or annulus reconstruction procedure)◀

(Do not report 93459 in conjunction with 0408T, 0409T, 0410T, 0411T, 0414T, 0415T)

93460 with right and left heart catheterization including intraprocedural injection(s) for left ventriculography, when performed

▶(Do not report 93460 in conjunction with 33418, 0345T, 0483T, 0484T, 0544T, 0545T for diagnostic coronary angiography or left and right heart catheterization procedures intrinsic to the valve repair or annulus reconstruction procedure)◀

(Do not report 93460 in conjunction with 0408T, 0409T, 0410T, 0411T, 0414T, 0415T)

93461 with right and left heart catheterization including intraprocedural injection(s) for left ventriculography, when performed, catheter placement(s) in bypass graft(s) (internal mammary, free arterial, venous grafts) with bypass graft angiography

▶(Do not report 93461 in conjunction with 33418, 0345T, 0483T, 0484T, 0544T, 0545T for diagnostic coronary angiography or left and right heart catheterization procedures intrinsic to the valve repair or annulus reconstruction procedure)◀

(Do not report 93461 in conjunction with 0408T, 0409T, 0410T, 0411T, 0414T, 0415T)

+ 93462 Left heart catheterization by transseptal puncture through intact septum or by transapical puncture (List separately in addition to code for primary procedure)

(Use 93462 in conjunction with 33477, 93452, 93453, 93458, 93459, 93460, 93461, 93582, 93653, 93654)

(Use 93462 in conjunction with 93590, 93591 for transapical puncture performed for left heart catheterization and percutaneous transcatheter closure of paravalvular leak)

(Do not report 93462 in conjunction with 93590 for transseptal puncture through intact septum performed for left heart catheterization and percutaneous transcatheter closure of paravalvular leak)

(Do not report 93462 in conjunction with 93656)

▶(Do not report 93462 in conjunction with 0345T, 0544T unless transapical puncture is performed)◀

Rationale

Several exclusionary parenthetical notes have been revised and added throughout the Cardiac Catheterization subsection to instruct users not to report cardiac catheterization codes with codes 33418, 0345T, 0483T, and 0484T and new codes 0544T and 0545T for diagnostic catheterization procedures that are intrinsic to transcatheter valve repair or annulus reconstruction procedures (33418, 0345T, 0483T, 0484T, 0544T, 0545T).

Refer to the codebook and the Rationale for codes 0544T and 0545T for a full discussion of these changes.

Medicine

Injection Procedures

+ 93563 Injection procedure during cardiac catheterization including imaging supervision, interpretation, and report; for selective coronary angiography during congenital heart catheterization (List separately in addition to code for primary procedure)

+ 93564 for selective opacification of aortocoronary venous or arterial bypass graft(s) (eg, aortocoronary saphenous vein, free radial artery, or free mammary artery graft) to one or more coronary arteries and in situ arterial conduits (eg, internal mammary), whether native or used for bypass to one or more coronary arteries during congenital heart catheterization, when performed (List separately in addition to code for primary procedure)

▶(Do not report 93563, 93564 in conjunction with 33418, 0345T, 0483T, 0484T, 0544T, 0545T for coronary angiography intrinsic to the valve repair or annulus reconstruction procedure)◀

+ 93565 for selective left ventricular or left atrial angiography (List separately in addition to code for primary procedure)

(Do not report 93563-93565 in conjunction with 93452-93461)

(Use 93563-93565 in conjunction with 93530-93533)

+ 93566 for selective right ventricular or right atrial angiography (List separately in addition to code for primary procedure)

(Use 93566 in conjunction with 93451, 93453, 93456, 93457, 93460, 93461, 93530-93533)

(Do not report 93566 in conjunction with 33274 for right ventriculography performed during leadless pacemaker insertion)

▶(Do not report 93566 in conjunction with 0545T for right ventricular or right atrial angiography procedures intrinsic to the annulus reconstruction procedure)◀

Rationale

Several exclusionary parenthetical notes have been revised and added throughout the Cardiac Catheterization/Injection Procedures subsection to indicate selective injection procedure codes (eg, 93563, 93564, 93566) and transcatheter valve repair or annulus reconstruction codes (eg, 33418, 0483T, 0484T, 0544T, 0545T) that should not be reported together for coronary angiography procedures performed intrinsic to transcatheter valve repair or annulus reconstruction procedures.

Refer to the codebook and the Rationale for codes 0544T and 0545T for a full discussion of these changes.

Intracardiac Electrophysiological Procedures/Studies

Intracardiac electrophysiologic studies (EPS) are invasive diagnostic medical procedures which include the insertion and repositioning of electrode catheters, recording of electrograms before and during pacing, programmed stimulation of multiple locations in the heart, analysis of recorded information, and report of the procedure. In many circumstances, patients with arrhythmias are evaluated and treated at the same encounter. In this situation, a diagnostic electrophysiologic study is performed, induced tachycardia(s) are mapped, and on the basis of the diagnostic and mapping information, the tissue is ablated.

Definitions

Arrhythmia Induction: In most electrophysiologic studies, an attempt is made to induce arrhythmia(s) from single or multiple sites within the heart. Arrhythmia induction may be achieved by multiple techniques, eg, by performing pacing at different rates or programmed stimulation (introduction of critically timed electrical impulses). Because arrhythmia induction occurs via the same catheter(s) inserted for the electrophysiologic study(ies), catheter insertion and temporary pacemaker codes are not additionally reported. Codes 93600-93603, 93610, 93612, and 93618 are used to describe unusual situations where there may be recording, pacing, or an attempt at arrhythmia induction from only one site in the heart. Code 93619 describes only evaluation of the sinus node, atrioventricular node, and His-Purkinje conduction system, without arrhythmia induction. Codes 93620-93624, 93640-93642, 93653, 93654, and 93656 all include recording, pacing, and attempted arrhythmia induction from one or more site(s) in the heart.

Mapping: When a tachycardia is induced, the site of tachycardia origination or its electrical path through the heart is often defined by mapping. Mapping creates a multidimensional depiction of a tachycardia by recording multiple electrograms obtained sequentially or simultaneously from multiple catheter sites in the heart. Depending upon the technique, certain types of mapping catheters may be repositioned from point-to-point within the heart, allowing sequential recording from the various sites to construct maps. Other types of mapping catheters allow mapping without a point-to-point technique by allowing simultaneous recording from many electrodes on the same catheter and computer-assisted three-dimensional reconstruction of the tachycardia activation sequence.

Mapping is a distinct procedure performed in addition to a diagnostic electrophysiologic study or ablation procedure and may be separately reported using 93609 or 93613. Do not report standard mapping (93609) in addition to 3-dimensional mapping (93613).

Ablation: Once the part of the heart involved in the tachycardia is localized, the tachycardia may be treated by ablation (the delivery of a radiofrequency or cryo-energy to the area to selectively destroy cardiac tissue). Ablation procedures (93653-93657) are performed at the same session as electrophysiology studies and therefore represent a combined code description. When reporting ablation therapy codes (93653-93657), the single site electrophysiology studies (93600-93603, 93610, 93612, 93618) and the comprehensive electrophysiology studies (93619, 93620) may not be reported separately. Code 93622 may be reported separately with 93653 and 93656. Code 93623 may be reported separately with 93653, 93654, and 93656. However, 93621 for left atrial pacing and recording from coronary sinus or left atrium should not be reported in conjunction with 93656, as this procedure is a component of 93656. Codes 93653 and 93654 include right ventricular pacing and recording and His bundle recording when clinically indicated. When performance of one or more components is not possible or indicated, document the reason for not performing. Code 93656 includes each of left atrial pacing/recording, right ventricular pacing/recording, and His bundle recording when clinically indicated. When performance of one or more components is not possible or indicated, document the reason for not performing.

The differences in the techniques involved for ablation of supraventricular arrhythmias, ventricular arrhythmias, and atrial fibrillation are reflected within the descriptions for 93653-93657. Code 93653 is a primary code for catheter ablation for treatment of supraventricular tachycardia caused by dual atrioventricular nodal pathways, accessory atrioventricular connections, or other atrial foci. Code 93654 describes catheter ablation for treatment of ventricular tachycardia or focus of ventricular ectopy. Code 93656 is a primary code for reporting treatment of atrial fibrillation by ablation to achieve complete pulmonary vein electrical isolation. Codes 93653, 93654, and 93656 are distinct primary procedure codes and may not be reported together.

Codes 93655 and 93657 are add-on codes listed in addition to the primary ablation code to report ablation of sites distinct from the primary ablation site. After ablation of the primary target site, post-ablation electrophysiologic evaluation is performed as part of those ablation services (93653, 93654, 93656) and additional mechanisms of tachycardia may be identified. For example, if the primary tachycardia ablated was atrioventricular nodal reentrant tachycardia and during post-ablation testing an atrial tachycardia, atrial flutter, or accessory pathway with orthodromic reentry tachycardia was identified, this would be considered a separate mechanism of tachycardia. Pacing maneuvers are performed to define the mechanism(s) of the new tachycardia(s). Catheter ablation of this distinct mechanism of tachycardia is then performed at the newly discovered atrial or ventricular origin. Appropriate post-ablation attempts at re-induction and observation are again performed. Code 93655 is listed in conjunction with 93653 when repeat ablation is for treatment of an additional supraventricular tachycardia mechanism and with 93654 when the repeat ablation is for treatment of an additional ventricular tachycardia mechanism. Code 93655 may be reported with 93656 when an additional non-atrial fibrillation tachycardia is separately diagnosed after pulmonary vein isolation. Code 93657 is reported in conjunction with 93656 when successful pulmonary vein isolation is achieved, attempts at re-induction of atrial fibrillation identify an additional left or right atrial focus for atrial fibrillation, and further ablation of this new focus is performed.

In certain circumstances, depending on the chamber of origin, a catheter or catheters may be maneuvered into the left ventricle to facilitate arrhythmia diagnosis. This may be accomplished via a retrograde aortic approach by means of the arterial access or through a transseptal puncture. For ablation treatment of supraventricular tachycardia (93653) and ventricular tachycardia (93654), the left heart catheterization by transseptal puncture through intact septum (93462) may be reported separately as an add-on code. However, for ablation treatment of atrial fibrillation (93656), the transseptal puncture (93462) is a standard component of the procedure and may not be reported separately. Do not report 93462 in conjunction with 93656.

▶Modifier 51 should not be appended to 93600-93603, 93610, 93612, 93615-93618.◀

Rationale

In accordance with the removal of modifier 51-exempt designation from code 93631, the Intracardiac Electrophysiological Procedures/Studies guidelines have been revised to reflect this change.

Medicine

⊘ **93600** Bundle of His recording

(Do not report 93600 in conjunction with 93619, 93620, 93653, 93654, 93656)

93620 Comprehensive electrophysiologic evaluation including insertion and repositioning of multiple electrode catheters with induction or attempted induction of arrhythmia; with right atrial pacing and recording, right ventricular pacing and recording, His bundle recording

(Do not report 93620 in conjunction with 93600, 93602, 93603, 93610, 93612, 93618, 93619, 93653, 93654, 93655, 93656, 93657)

+ **93621** with left atrial pacing and recording from coronary sinus or left atrium (List separately in addition to code for primary procedure)

(Use 93621 in conjunction with 93620, 93653, 93654)

(Do not report 93621 in conjunction with 93656)

+ **93623** Programmed stimulation and pacing after intravenous drug infusion (List separately in addition to code for primary procedure)

(Use 93623 in conjunction with 93610, 93612, 93619, 93620, 93653, 93654, 93656)

▶(Do not report 93623 more than once per day)◀

Rationale

An instructional parenthetical note has been added following add-on code 93623. Code 93623 describes programmed stimulation and pacing after a drug is infused intravenously to create an arrhythmia, which is performed in conjunction with intracardiac electrophysiological studies (93610, 93612, 93619, 93620, 93653, 93654, 93656). The drug may be infused more than once per day; however, code 93623 should be reported only once per day. Therefore, a new instructional parenthetical note has been added to clarify that code 93623 should not be reported more than once per day.

93624 Electrophysiologic follow-up study with pacing and recording to test effectiveness of therapy, including induction or attempted induction of arrhythmia

93644 Electrophysiologic evaluation of subcutaneous implantable defibrillator (includes defibrillation threshold evaluation, induction of arrhythmia, evaluation of sensing for arrhythmia termination, and programming or reprogramming of sensing or therapeutic parameters)

(Do not report 93644 in conjunction with 33270 at the time of subcutaneous implantable defibrillator device insertion)

(For subsequent or periodic electrophysiologic evaluation of a subcutaneous implantable defibrillator device, see 93260, 93261)

▶(For electrophysiological evaluation of subcutaneous implantable defibrillator system, with substernal electrode, use 0577T)◀

Rationale

In accordance with the addition of Category III code 0577T, a cross-reference parenthetical note has been added following code 93644 directing users to code 0577T for electrophysiological evaluation of subcutaneous implantable defibrillator system with substernal electrode.

Refer to the codebook and the Rationale for code 0577T for full discussion of these changes.

+ **93662** Intracardiac echocardiography during therapeutic/diagnostic intervention, including imaging supervision and interpretation (List separately in addition to code for primary procedure)

(Use 93662 in conjunction with 92987, 93453, 93460-93462, 93532, 93580, 93581, 93620, 93621, 93622, 93653, 93654, 93656 as appropriate)

▶(Do not report 93662 in conjunction with 92961, 0569T, 0570T)◀

Rationale

In accordance with the establishment of Category III codes 0569T and 0570T (transcatheter tricuspid valve repair), the exclusionary parenthetical note following code 93662 has been revised to reflect the new codes.

Refer to the codebook and the Rationale for codes 0569T and 0570T for a full discussion of these changes.

Noninvasive Physiologic Studies and Procedures

▲ **93784** Ambulatory blood pressure monitoring, utilizing report-generating software, automated, worn continuously for 24 hours or longer; including recording, scanning analysis, interpretation and report

▲ **93786** recording only

▲ **93788** scanning analysis with report

▲ **93790** review with interpretation and report

▶(For self-measured blood pressure monitoring, see 99473, 99474)◀

Rationale

In accordance with the establishment of codes 99473 and 99474, codes 93784-93790 have been revised to include report-generating software that is automated and worn continuously. A cross-reference parenthetical note has also been added following code 93790 to direct users to codes 99473 and 99474 for self-measured blood pressure (BP) monitoring.

Refer to the codebook and the Rationale for codes 99473 and 99474 for a full discussion of these changes.

Clinical Example (93784)

An elderly female has elevated blood pressure (BP) readings on several consecutive visits to her physician, but reports BP measurements taken with her home BP cuff or at the local pharmacy are consistently normal. The physician suspects "white coat" hypertension and refers the patient for ambulatory BP monitoring (ABPM).

Description of Procedure (93784)

N/A

Clinical Example (93786)

An elderly female has elevated BP readings on several consecutive visits to her physician, but reports that BPs taken with her home BP cuff or at the local pharmacy are consistently normal. The physician suspects "white coat" hypertension and refers the patient for ABPM.

Description of Procedure (93786)

N/A

Clinical Example (93788)

An elderly female has elevated BP readings on several consecutive visits to her physician, but reports that BPs taken with her home BP cuff or at the local pharmacy are consistently normal. The physician suspects "white coat" hypertension and refers the patient for ABPM.

Description of Procedure (93788)

N/A

Clinical Example (93790)

An elderly female has elevated BP readings on several consecutive visits to her physician, but reports that BPs taken with her home BP cuff or at the local pharmacy are consistently normal. The physician suspects "white coat" hypertension and refers the patient for ABPM.

Description of Procedure (93790)

Scan the report for spurious values (eg, BP of 140/130). Analyze report in conjunction with patient's medical history and in relationship to reported activities.

Home and Outpatient International Normalized Ratio (INR) Monitoring Services

Home and outpatient international normalized ratio (INR) monitoring services describe the management of warfarin therapy, including ordering, review, and interpretation of new INR test result(s), patient instructions, and dosage adjustments as needed.

If a significantly, separately identifiable evaluation and management (E/M) service is performed on the same day as 93792, the appropriate E/M service may be reported using modifier 25.

Do not report 93793 on the same day as an E/M service.

▶Do not report 93792, 93793 in conjunction with 98966, 98967, 98968, 99421, 99422, 99423, 99441, 99442, 99443, when telephone or online digital evaluation and management services address home and outpatient INR monitoring.◀

Do not report 93792, 93793 when performed during the service time of 99487, 99489, 99490, 99495, 99496.

93792 Patient/caregiver training for initiation of home international normalized ratio (INR) monitoring under the direction of a physician or other qualified health care professional, face-to-face, including use and care of the INR monitor, obtaining blood sample, instructions for reporting home INR test results, and documentation of patient's/caregiver's ability to perform testing and report results

(For provision of test materials and equipment for home INR monitoring, see 99070 or the appropriate supply code)

Rationale

In accordance with the deletion of codes 98969 and 99444, and the addition of codes 99421, 99422, and 99423, the Home and Outpatient International Normalized Ratio (INR) Monitoring Services guidelines have been revised to reflect these changes.

Refer to the codebook and the Rationale for codes 99421, 99422, and 99423 for a full discussion of these changes.

Medicine | CPT Changes 2020

Noninvasive Vascular Diagnostic Studies

Extremity Arterial Studies (Including Digits)

93925 Duplex scan of lower extremity arteries or arterial bypass grafts; complete bilateral study

▶(Do not report 93925 in conjunction with 93985 for the same extremities)◀

93926 unilateral or limited study

▶(Do not report 93926 in conjunction with 93986 for the same extremity)◀

93930 Duplex scan of upper extremity arteries or arterial bypass grafts; complete bilateral study

▶(Do not report 93930 in conjunction with 93985, 93986 for the same extremity[ies])◀

93931 unilateral or limited study

▶(Do not report 93931 in conjunction with 93985, 93986 for the same extremity)◀

Rationale

In accordance with the establishment of codes 93985 and 93986, exclusionary parenthetical notes have been added following codes 93925, 93926, 93930, and 93931 to instruct users on the proper reporting of these codes when duplex scan is performed for the same extremity(ies).

Refer to the codebook and the Rationale for codes 93985 and 93986 for a full discussion of these changes.

Extremity Venous Studies (Including Digits)

(93965 has been deleted)

93970 Duplex scan of extremity veins including responses to compression and other maneuvers; complete bilateral study

▶(Do not report 93970 in conjunction with 93985, 93986 for the same extremity[ies])◀

93971 unilateral or limited study

(Do not report 93970, 93971 in conjunction with 36475, 36476, 36478, 36479)

▶(Do not report 93971 in conjunction with 93985, 93986 for the same extremity)◀

Rationale

In accordance with the establishment of codes 93985 and 93986, exclusionary parenthetical notes have been added following codes 93970 and 93971 instructing users not to report codes 93970 and 93971 with the new codes for the same extremity(ies).

Refer to the codebook and the Rationale for codes 93985 and 93986 for a full discussion of these changes.

Extremity Arterial-Venous Studies

▶A complete extremity duplex scan (93985, 93986) includes evaluation of both arterial inflow and venous outflow for preoperative vessel assessment prior to creation of hemodialysis access. If only an arterial extremity duplex scan is performed, see 93925, 93926, 93930, 93931. If only a venous extremity duplex scan is performed, see 93970, 93971. If a physiologic arterial evaluation of extremities is performed, see 93922, 93923, 93924.◀

● **93985** Duplex scan of arterial inflow and venous outflow for preoperative vessel assessment prior to creation of hemodialysis access; complete bilateral study

▶(Do not report 93985 in conjunction with 93925, 93930, 93970 for the same extremity[ies])◀

▶(Do not report 93985 in conjunction with 93990 for the same extremity)◀

● **93986** complete unilateral study

▶(Do not report 93986 in conjunction with 93926, 93931, 93971, 93990 for the same extremity)◀

93990 Duplex scan of hemodialysis access (including arterial inflow, body of access and venous outflow)

(For measurement of hemodialysis access flow using indicator dilution methods, use 90940)

Rationale

Codes 93985 and 93986 have been added to report complete bilateral and unilateral duplex scan study of arterial inflow and venous outflow for preoperative vessel assessment prior to creation of hemodialysis access. Guidelines and parenthetical notes have been added to provide instruction on the proper reporting of these codes.

The AMA/RVS RUC RAW identified HCPCS Level II code G0365 in a screen of CMS codes with Medicare utilization of 30,000 or more. RUC recommended that code G0365 be deleted and CPT codes be established to report this duplex scan study. Code 93985 describes a complete bilateral study, and code 93986 describes a complete unilateral study.

New guidelines have been added to provide instructions for appropriate reporting of codes 93985 and 93986; 93925, 93926, 93930, and 93931 (arterial extremity duplex scanning); 93970 and 93971 (venous extremity duplex scan); and 93922, 93923, and 93924 (physiologic arterial evaluation).

Clinical Example (93985)

A 65-year-old male presents for evaluation for an autogenous arteriovenous fistula for hemodialysis. Complete bilateral duplex scans of arterial inflow and venous outflow are performed.

Description of Procedure (93985)

Supervise the technologist's image acquisition and evaluation of the bilateral upper extremity arterial inflow and venous outflow structures for the potential creation of a new hemodialysis access. This includes assessment of the anatomy, internal vessel diameters, patency and flow dynamics of the bilateral subclavian, axillary, brachial, median cubital, basilic and cephalic veins, as well as the axillary, brachial, ulnar and/or radial arteries. Special attention must be paid to the superficial veins regarding their suitability for use as arterial venous fistula. Analyze images, velocities, and data. Summarize findings regarding all evaluated vessels and make final recommendation regarding best fistula options. Dictate a report.

Clinical Example (93986)

A 65-year-old male presents for evaluation for an autogenous arteriovenous fistula for hemodialysis. Complete unilateral duplex scans of arterial inflow and venous outflow are performed.

Description of Procedure (93986)

Supervise the technologist's image acquisition and evaluation of the selected upper extremity arterial inflow and venous outflow structures for the potential creation of a new hemodialysis access. This includes assessment of the anatomy, internal vessel diameters, patency and flow dynamics of the subclavian, axillary, brachial, median cubital, basilic and cephalic veins, as well as the axillary, brachial, ulnar and/or radial arteries. Special attention must be paid to the superficial veins regarding their suitability for use as arterial venous fistula. Analyze all images, velocities, and data. Summarize findings regarding all evaluated vessels and make final recommendation regarding best fistula options. Dictate a report.

Pulmonary

Pulmonary Diagnostic Testing and Therapies

Codes 94010-94799 include laboratory procedure(s) and interpretation of test results. If a separate identifiable evaluation and management service is performed, the appropriate E/M service code including new or established patient office or other outpatient services (99201-99215), office or other outpatient consultations (99241-99245), emergency department services (99281-99285), nursing facility services (99304-99318), domiciliary, rest home, or custodial care services (99324-99337), and home services (99341-99350) may be reported in addition to 94010-94799.

Spirometry (94010) measures expiratory airflow and volumes and forms the basis of most pulmonary function testing. When spirometry is performed before and after administration of a bronchodilator, report 94060. Measurement of vital capacity (94150) is a component of spirometry and is only reported when performed alone. The flow-volume loop (94375) is used to identify patterns of inspiratory and/or expiratory obstruction in central or peripheral airways. Spirometry (94010, 94060) includes maximal breathing capacity (94200) and flow-volume loop (94375), when performed.

▶Measurement of lung volumes may be performed using plethysmography, helium dilution or nitrogen washout. Plethysmography (94726) is utilized to determine total lung capacity, residual volume, functional residual capacity, and airway resistance. Nitrogen washout or helium dilution (94727) may be used to measure lung volumes, distribution of ventilation and closing volume. Oscillometry (94728) assesses airway resistance and may be reported in addition to gas dilution techniques. Spirometry (94010, 94060) and bronchial provocation (94070) are not included in 94726 and 94727 and may be reported separately.◀

Diffusing capacity (94729) is most commonly performed in conjunction with lung volumes or spirometry and is an add-on code to 94726-94728, 94010, 94060, 94070, and 94375.

Pulmonary function tests (94011-94013) are reported for measurements in infants and young children through 2 years of age.

Pulmonary function testing measurements are reported as actual values and as a percent of predicted values by age, gender, height, and race.

Chest wall manipulation for the mobilization of secretions and improvement in lung function can be performed using manual (94667, 94668) or mechanical (94669) methods. Manual techniques include cupping,

Medicine

percussing, and use of a hand-held vibration device. A mechanical technique is the application of an external vest or wrap that delivers mechanical oscillation.

▲ **94728** Airway resistance by oscillometry

(Do not report 94728 in conjunction with 94010, 94060, 94070, 94375, 94726)

Rationale

Code 94728 and the Pulmonary Diagnostic Testing and Therapies guidelines have been revised with the removal of the term "impulse." The term "impulse" has been removed to enable code 94728 to be used for any device that performs airway resistance by oscillometry.

Neurology and Neuromuscular Procedures

Neurologic services are typically consultative, and any of the levels of consultation (99241-99255) may be appropriate.

In addition, services and skills outlined under **Evaluation and Management** levels of service appropriate to neurologic illnesses should be reported similarly.

►The electroencephalogram (EEG), video electroencephalogram (VEEG), autonomic function, evoked potential, reflex tests, electromyography (EMG), nerve conduction velocity (NCV), and magnetoencephalography (MEG) services (95700-95726, 95812-95829, and 95860-95967) include recording, interpretation, and report by a physician or other qualified health care professional. For interpretation only, use modifier 26 with 95812-95829, 95860-95967. For interpretation only for long-term EEG services, report 95717, 95718, 95719, 95720, 95721, 95722, 95723, 95724, 95725, 95726.

Codes 95700-95726 and 95812-95822 use EEG/VEEG recording time as a basis for code use. Recording time is when the recording is underway and diagnostic EEG data is being collected. Recording time excludes set up and take down time. If diagnostic EEG recording is disrupted, recording time stops until diagnostic EEG recording is resumed. Codes 95961-95962 use physician or other qualified health care professional attendance time as a basis for code use.◄

(Do not report codes 95860-95875 in addition to 96000-96004)

Rationale

In accordance with the deletion of codes 95950, 95951, 95953, and 95956 and the establishment of codes 95700-95726, the electroencephalogram (EEG) guidelines in the Neurology and Neuromuscular Procedures subsection have been revised to reflect these changes.

Refer to the codebook and the Rationale for codes 95950, 95951, 95953, 95956, and 95700-95726 for a full discussion of these changes.

Sleep Medicine Testing

95700	Code is out of numerical sequence. See 95966-95971
95705	Code is out of numerical sequence. See 95966-95971
95706	Code is out of numerical sequence. See 95966-95971
95707	Code is out of numerical sequence. See 95966-95971
95708	Code is out of numerical sequence. See 95966-95971
95709	Code is out of numerical sequence. See 95966-95971
95710	Code is out of numerical sequence. See 95966-95971
95711	Code is out of numerical sequence. See 95966-95971
95712	Code is out of numerical sequence. See 95966-95971
95713	Code is out of numerical sequence. See 95966-95971
95714	Code is out of numerical sequence. See 95966-95971
95715	Code is out of numerical sequence. See 95966-95971
95716	Code is out of numerical sequence. See 95966-95971
95717	Code is out of numerical sequence. See 95966-95971
95718	Code is out of numerical sequence. See 95966-95971
95719	Code is out of numerical sequence. See 95966-95971
95720	Code is out of numerical sequence. See 95966-95971
95721	Code is out of numerical sequence. See 95966-95971
95722	Code is out of numerical sequence. See 95966-95971
95723	Code is out of numerical sequence. See 95966-95971
95724	Code is out of numerical sequence. See 95966-95971
95725	Code is out of numerical sequence. See 95966-95971
95726	Code is out of numerical sequence. See 95966-95971

Routine Electroencephalography (EEG)

EEG codes 95812-95822 include hyperventilation and/or photic stimulation when appropriate. Routine EEG codes 95816-95822 include 20 to 40 minutes of recording. Extended EEG codes 95812-95813 include reporting times longer than 40 minutes.

95812	Electroencephalogram (EEG) extended monitoring; 41-60 minutes	95852	hand, with or without comparison with normal side

▶(Do not report 95812 in conjunction with 95700-95726)◀

▲ **95813** 61-119 minutes

▶(Do not report 95813 in conjunction with 95700-95726)◀

▶(For long-term EEG services [2 hours or more], see 95700-95726)◀

95816 Electroencephalogram (EEG); including recording awake and drowsy

▶(Do not report 95816 in conjunction with 95700-95726)◀

95819 including recording awake and asleep

▶(Do not report 95819 in conjunction with 95700-95726)◀

95822 recording in coma or sleep only

▶(Do not report 95822 in conjunction with 95700-95726)◀

95824 cerebral death evaluation only

▶(95827 has been deleted. To report all night EEG recording, see 95705, 95706, 95707, 95711, 95712, 95713, 95717, 95718)◀

▶(For long-term EEG monitoring, see 95700-95726)◀

(For EEG during nonintracranial surgery, use 95955)

(For Wada test, use 95958)

Rationale

EEG code 95813 has been editorially revised to make the language consistent with code 95812. Code 95812 describes unit of time in minutes; however, code 95813 described unit of time in hours. For consistency, code 95813 has been revised to describe the time in minutes rather than hours. In accordance with the establishment of codes 95700-95726, code 95827 has been deleted and parenthetical notes have been revised and added throughout the Routine Electroencephalography (EEG) subsection to reflect these changes.

Refer to the codebook and the Rationale for codes 95700-95726 for a full discussion of these changes.

▶Range of Motion Testing◀

▶(95831, 95832, 95833, 95834 have been deleted. To report manual muscle testing, see Physical Medicine and Rehabilitation services 97161-97172)◀

95836 Code is out of numerical sequence. See 95824-95852

95851 Range of motion measurements and report (separate procedure); each extremity (excluding hand) or each trunk section (spine)

Rationale

Codes 95831, 95832, 95833, and 95834 (manual muscle testing) have been deleted. The heading of the Muscle and Range of Motion Testing subsection has been revised with the removal of the reference to muscle testing. A parenthetical note has been added directing users to codes 97161-97172 (physical medicine and rehabilitation services).

Code 95831 was identified by the AMA/RVS RUC RAW screen for Medicare with utilization of 30,000 or more. RAW requested a review of all four manual muscle testing codes (95831-95834). It was revealed that manual muscle testing is typically performed as a part of an E/M service, or an evaluation or re-evaluation as described by codes 97161-97172.

Ischemic Muscle Testing and Guidance for Chemodenervation

+ **95873** Electrical stimulation for guidance in conjunction with chemodenervation (List separately in addition to code for primary procedure)

▶(Do not report 95873 in conjunction with 64451, 64617, 64625, 95860-95870, 95874)◀

+ **95874** Needle electromyography for guidance in conjunction with chemodenervation (List separately in addition to code for primary procedure)

(Use 95873, 95874 in conjunction with 64612, 64615, 64616, 64642, 64643, 64644, 64645, 64646, 64647)

(Do not report more than one guidance code for each corresponding chemodenervation code)

▶(Do not report 95874 in conjunction with 64451, 64617, 64625, 95860-95870, 95873)◀

Rationale

In accordance with the establishment of codes 64451 and 64625, the exclusionary parenthetical notes following codes 95873 and 95874 have been revised to reflect these changes.

Refer to the codebook and the Rationale for codes 64451 and 64625 for a full discussion of the changes.

Special EEG Tests

▶Codes 95961 and 95962 use physician or other qualified health care professional time as a basis for unit of service. Report 95961 for the first hour of attendance. Use modifier 52 with 95961 for 30 minutes or less. Report 95962 for each additional hour of attendance. Codes 95961, 95962 may be reported with 95700-95726 when functional cortical or subcortical mapping is performed with long-term EEG monitoring.

Codes 95700-95726 describe long-term continuous recording services for electroencephalography (EEG), which are performed to differentiate seizures from other abnormalities, determine type or location of seizures, monitor treatment of seizures and status epilepticus, establish if the patient is a candidate for epilepsy surgery, and/or screen for adverse change in critically ill patients.

The set of codes that describe long-term continuous recording EEG services (95700-95726) is divided into two major groups: (1) technical services, and (2) professional services. Codes 95700-95726 may be reported for any site of service. The technical component of the services is reported with 95700-95716. The professional component of the services is reported with 95717, 95718, 95719, 95720, 95721, 95722, 95723, 95724, 95725, 95726. Diagnostic EEG recording time of less than 2 hours (ie, 1 minute, up to 1 hour and 59 minutes) is not reported separately as a long-term EEG service.

Long-term continuous recording EEG services (95700-95726) are different than routine EEGs (95812, 95813, 95816, 95819, 95822). Routine EEGs capture brain-wave activity within a short duration of testing, defined as less than 2 hours. Long-term continuous recording EEGs capture brain-wave activity for durations of time equal to or greater than 2 hours. The length of recording is based on a number of factors, including the clinical indication for the test and the frequency of seizures.

Use of automated spike and seizure detection and trending software is included in 95700-95726, when performed. Do not report 95957 for use of automated software.

Definitions

EEG technologist: An individual who is qualified by education, training, licensure/certification/regulation (when applicable) in seizure recognition. An EEG technologist(s) performs EEG setup, takedown when performed, patient education, technical description, maintenance, and seizure recognition when within his or her scope of practice and as allowed by law, regulation, and facility policy (when applicable).

Unmonitored: Services that have no real-time monitoring by an EEG technologist(s) during the continuous recording. If the criteria for intermittent or continuous monitoring are not met, then the study is an unmonitored study.

Intermittent monitoring (remote or on-site): Requires an EEG technologist(s) to perform and document real-time review of data at least every 2 hours during the entire recording period to assure the integrity and quality of the recording (ie, EEG, VEEG), identify the need for maintenance, and, when necessary, notify the physician or other qualified health care professional of clinical issues. For intermittent monitoring, a single EEG technologist may monitor a maximum of 12 patients concurrently. If the number of intermittently monitored patients exceeds 12, then all of the studies are reported as unmonitored.

Continuous real-time monitoring (may be provided remotely): Requires all elements of intermittent monitoring. In addition, the EEG technologist(s) performs and documents real-time concurrent monitoring of the EEG data and video (when performed) during the entire recording period. The EEG technologist(s) identifies when events occur and notifies, as instructed, the physician or other qualified health care professional. For continuous monitoring, a single EEG technologist may monitor a maximum of four patients concurrently. If the number of concurrently monitored patients exceeds four, then all of the studies are reported as either unmonitored or intermittent studies. If there is a break in the real-time monitoring of the EEG recording, the study is an intermittent study.

Technical description: The EEG technologist(s)'s written documentation of the reviewed EEG/VEEG data, including technical interventions. The technical description is based on the EEG technologist(s)'s review of data and includes the following required elements: uploading and/or transferring EEG/VEEG data from EEG equipment to a server or storage device; reviewing raw EEG/VEEG data and events and automated detection, as well as patient activations; and annotating, editing, and archiving EEG/VEEG data for review by the physician or other qualified health care professional. For unmonitored services, the EEG technologist(s) annotates the recording for review by the physician or other qualified health care professional and creates a single summary.

Maintenance of long-term EEG equipment: Performed by the EEG technologist(s) and involves ensuring the integrity and quality of the recording(s) (eg, camera position, electrode placement, and impedances).

Setup: Performed in person by the EEG technologist(s) and includes preparing supplies and equipment and securing electrodes using the 10/20 system. Code 95700 is reported only once per recording period on the date the setup was performed. "In person" means that the EEG technologist(s) must be physically present with the patient.

Technical Component Services

Code 95700 describes any long-term continuous EEG/VEEG recording, setup, takedown when performed, and patient/caregiver education by the EEG technologist(s). To report 95700, the setup must include a minimum of eight channels of EEG. Services with fewer than eight channels may be reported using 95999. Eight to 15 channels are typically used for neonates and when electrodes cannot be placed on certain regions of the scalp that are sterile. Twenty or more channels are typically used for children and adults. If setup is performed by someone who does not meet the definition of an EEG technologist(s), report 95999.

Codes 95705-95716 describe monitoring, maintenance, review of data, and creating a summary technical description. These codes are divided into four groups based on duration and whether video is utilized. Key elements in determining the appropriate technical code (95705-95716) for long-term EEG continuous recording are: (1) whether diagnostic video recording is captured in conjunction and simultaneously with the EEG service, which is referred to as video-EEG (VEEG), and (2) technologist monitoring for the study (ie, unmonitored, intermittently monitored, or continuously monitored). Codes 95711, 95712, 95713, 95714, 95715, 95716 are reported if diagnostic video of the patient is recorded a minimum of 80% of the time of the entire long-term VEEG service, concurrent with diagnostic EEG recording (ie, the entire study is reported as an EEG without video if concurrent diagnostic video occurs less than 80% of the entire study). Diagnostic EEG recording is an essential component of all long-term EEG services. If diagnostic EEG recording stops, timing stops until the diagnostic EEG is resumed.

Codes 95705, 95706, 95707, 95711, 95712, 95713 are reported when total diagnostic recording time is between 2 and 12 hours, or to capture the final increment of a multiple-day service when the final increment extends 2 to 12 hours beyond the time reported by the appropriate greater-than-12-hour-up-to-26-hour code(s) (95708, 95709, 95710, 95714, 95715, 95716). A maximum of one 2-12 hour code may be reported for an entire long-term EEG service. For example, if the testing lasts 48 hours, but diagnostic recording occurs only in the initial 11 hours and the final 11 hours of the testing period, a single greater-than-12-hour-up-to-26-hour technical code is reported, rather than two 2-12 hour code for the 48-hour service (see the Long-Term EEG Monitoring Table).

Professional Component Services

Codes 95717, 95718, 95719, 95720, 95721, 95722, 95723, 95724, 95725, 95726 describe the professional services performed by a physician or other qualified health care professional for reviewing, analyzing, interpreting, and reporting the results of the continuous recording EEG/VEEG with recommendations based on the findings of the studies. These codes do not include E/M services, which may be reported separately.

Codes 95719, 95720 are used for greater than 12 hours (ie, 12 hours and 1 minute) up to 26 hours of recording. Code selection for professional interpretation for long-term EEG is based on: (1) length of the recording being interpreted, and (2) when the physician or other qualified health care professional reports are generated (ie, whether diagnostic interpretations and reports are made daily during the study, or whether the entire professional interpretation is performed after the entire study is completed). Codes 95717, 95718, 95719, 95720 are reported when: (1) daily professional reports are generated during the long-term recording, even if the entire study extends over multiple days or (2) the time of recording for the entire study is between 2 hours and 36 hours. Codes 95717, 95718 are reported once for each 2-12 hour recording and reported a maximum of once for an entire long-term EEG service. Codes 95719, 95720 are reported once for each greater-than-12-hours-up-to-26-hours recording period. Studies lasting 26 to 36 hours or longer are reported using building blocks and reported using one or more of the greater-than-12-hours-up-to-26-hour code with one 2-12 hour code. The recorded data are reviewed, interpreted, and reported daily by the physician or other qualified health care professional, and summary reports are made for the entire multiple-day study. The summary reports are included in each code (95717, 95718, 95719, 95720, 95721, 95722, 95723, 95724, 95725, 95726) and not reported separately (see the Long-Term EEG Monitoring Table).

For 95721, 95722, 95723, 95724, 95725, 95726, the entire professional interpretation (including retrospective daily reports and a summary report) is made after the entire study is recorded and downloaded at the completion of the study. When the entire professional interpretation is provided for a multiple-day study that is greater than 36 hours, 95721, 95722, 95723, 95724, 95725, 95726 are used to report the entire professional service with the appropriate code determined by the span of diagnostic recording time, as defined by the codes. A single code (95721, 95722, 95723, 95724, 95725, 95726) is reported for the multiple-day study. For example, a long-term EEG recording that spans three days with a total of 50 hours of VEEG recording would be reported with 95722. Sixty hours and one minute of diagnostic VEEG recording is reported with 95724 (see the Long-Term EEG Monitoring Table).◄

▶(95950, 95951, 95953 have been deleted. To report, see 95700-95726. See Long-Term EEG Monitoring Table for guidance)◄

▶ Long-Term EEG Monitoring Table

Duration of Long-Term EEG/VEEG Recording	Professional Services — With report each 24 hours	Professional Services — With report at conclusion of entire recording period	Technical Services — Unmonitored	Technical Services — Intermittent	Technical Services — Continuous
Less than 120 minutes (w/video or w/out video)	Not reported separately	See 95812/95813	Not reported separately	Not reported separately	Not reported separately
2 to 12 hours (w/out video)	95717 x 1	95717 x 1	95705 x 1	95706 x 1	95707 x 1
2 to 12 hours (w/video)	95718 x 1	95718 x 1	95711 x 1	95712 x 1	95713 x 1
12 hours and 1 minute to 26 hours (w/out video)	95719 x 1	95719 x 1	95708 x 1	95709 x 1	95710 x 1
12 hours and 1 minute to 26 hours (w/video)	95720 x 1	95720 x 1	95714 x 1	95715 x 1	95716 x 1
26 hours and 1 minute to 36 hours (w/out video)	95719 x 1 and 95717 x 1	95719 x 1 and 95717 x 1	95708 x 1 and 95705 x 1	95709 x 1 and 95706 x 1	95710 x 1 and 95707 x 1
26 hours and 1 minute to 36 hours (w/video)	95720 x 1 and 95718 x 1	95720 x 1 and 95718 x 1	95714 x 1 and 95711 x 1	95715 x 1 and 95712 x 1	95716 x 1 and 95713 x 1
36 hours and 1 minute to 50 hours (w/out video)	95719 x 2	95721 x 1	95708 x 2	95709 x 2	95710 x 2
36 hours and 1 minute to 50 hours (w/video)	95720 x 2	95722 x 1	95714 x 2	95715 x 2	95716 x 2
50 hours and 1 minute to 60 hours (w/out video)	95719 x 2 and 95717 x 1	95721 x 1	95708 x 1 and 95705 x 1	95709 x 2 and 95706 x 1	95710 x 2 and 95707 x 1
50 hours and 1 minute to 60 hours (w/video)	95720 x 2 and 95718 x 1	95722 x 1	95714 x 2 and 95711 x 1	95715 x 2 and 95712 x 1	95716 x 2 and 95713 x 1
60 hours and 1 minute to 74 hours (w/out video)	95719 x 3	95723 x 1	95708 x 3	95709 x 3	95710 x 3
60 hours and 1 minute to 74 hours (w/video)	95720 x 3	95724 x 1	95714 x 3	95715 x 3	95716 x 3
74 hours and 1 minute to 84 hours (w/out video)	95719 x 3 and 95717 x 1	95723 x 1	95708 x 3 and 95705 x 1	95709 x 3 and 95706 x 1	95710 x 3 and 95707 x 1
74 hours and 1 minute to 84 hours (w/video)	95720 x 3 and 95718 x 1	95724 x 1	95714 x 3 and 95711 x 1	95715 x 3 and 95712 x 1	95716 x 3 and 95713 x 1
84 hours and 1 minute to 98 hours (w/out video)	95719 x 4	95725 x 1	95708 x 4	95709 x 4	95710 x 4
84 hours and 1 minute to 98 hours (w/video)	95720 x 4	95726 x 1	95714 x 4	95715 x 4	95716 x 4 ◀

95954	Pharmacological or physical activation requiring physician or other qualified health care professional attendance during EEG recording of activation phase (eg, thiopental activation test)
95955	Electroencephalogram (EEG) during nonintracranial surgery (eg, carotid surgery)

►(95956 has been deleted. To report, see 95700-95726. See Long-Term EEG Monitoring Table for guidance)◄

95957	Digital analysis of electroencephalogram (EEG) (eg, for epileptic spike analysis)

►(Do not report 95957 for use of automated software. For use of automated spike and seizure detection and trending software when performed with long-term EEG, see 95700-95726)◄

95965	Magnetoencephalography (MEG), recording and analysis; for spontaneous brain magnetic activity (eg, epileptic cerebral cortex localization)
95966	for evoked magnetic fields, single modality (eg, sensory, motor, language, or visual cortex localization)
+ 95967	for evoked magnetic fields, each additional modality (eg, sensory, motor, language, or visual cortex localization) (List separately in addition to code for primary procedure)

(Use 95967 in conjunction with 95966)

►(For electroencephalography performed in addition to magnetoencephalography, see 95812-95824)◄

(For somatosensory evoked potentials, auditory evoked potentials, and visual evoked potentials performed in addition to magnetic evoked field responses, see 92585, 95925, 95926, and/or 95930)

(For computerized tomography performed in addition to magnetoencephalography, see 70450-70470, 70496)

(For magnetic resonance imaging performed in addition to magnetoencephalography, see 70551-70553)

►Long-term EEG Setup◄

#● 95700	Electroencephalogram (EEG) continuous recording, with video when performed, setup, patient education, and takedown when performed, administered in person by EEG technologist, minimum of 8 channels

►(95700 should be reported once per recording period)◄

►(For EEG using patient-placed electrode sets, use 95999)◄

►(For setup performed by non-EEG technologist or remotely supervised by an EEG technologist, use 95999)◄

►Monitoring◄

#● 95705	Electroencephalogram (EEG), without video, review of data, technical description by EEG technologist, 2-12 hours; unmonitored
#● 95706	with intermittent monitoring and maintenance
#● 95707	with continuous, real-time monitoring and maintenance
#● 95708	Electroencephalogram (EEG), without video, review of data, technical description by EEG technologist, each increment of 12-26 hours; unmonitored
#● 95709	with intermittent monitoring and maintenance
#● 95710	with continuous, real-time monitoring and maintenance
#● 95711	Electroencephalogram with video (VEEG), review of data, technical description by EEG technologist, 2-12 hours; unmonitored
#● 95712	with intermittent monitoring and maintenance
#● 95713	with continuous, real-time monitoring and maintenance
#● 95714	Electroencephalogram with video (VEEG), review of data, technical description by EEG technologist, each increment of 12-26 hours; unmonitored
#● 95715	with intermittent monitoring and maintenance
#● 95716	with continuous, real-time monitoring and maintenance

►(95705, 95706, 95707, 95711, 95712, 95713 may be reported a maximum of once for an entire longer-term EEG service to capture either the entire time of service or the final 2-12 hour increment of a service extending beyond 26 hours)◄

#● 95717	Electroencephalogram (EEG), continuous recording, physician or other qualified health care professional review of recorded events, analysis of spike and seizure detection, interpretation and report, 2-12 hours of EEG recording; without video
#● 95718	with video (VEEG)

►(For recording greater than 12 hours, see 95719, 95720, 95721, 95722, 95723, 95724, 95725, 95726)◄

►(95717, 95718 may be reported a maximum of once for an entire long-term EEG service to capture either the entire time of service or the final 2-12 hour increment of a service extending beyond 24 hours)◄

#● 95719	Electroencephalogram (EEG), continuous recording, physician or other qualified health care professional review of recorded events, analysis of spike and seizure detection, each increment of greater than 12 hours, up to 26 hours of EEG recording, interpretation and report after each 24-hour period; without video
#● 95720	with video (VEEG)

Medicine

▶(95719, 95720 may be reported only once for a recording period greater than 12 hours up to 26 hours. For multiple-day studies, 95719, 95720 may be reported after each 24-hour period during the extended recording period. 95719, 95720 describe reporting for a 26-hour recording period, whether done as a single report or as multiple reports during the same time)◀

▶(95717, 95718 may be reported in conjunction with 95719, 95720 for studies lasting greater than 26 hours)◀

▶(Do not report 95717, 95718, 95719, 95720 for professional interpretation of long-term EEG studies when the recording is greater than 36 hours and the entire professional report is retroactively generated, even if separate daily reports are rendered after the completion of recording)◀

▶(When the entire study includes recording greater than 36 hours, and the professional interpretation is performed after the entire recording is completed, see 95721, 95722, 95723, 95724, 95725, 95726)◀

#● **95721** Electroencephalogram (EEG), continuous recording, physician or other qualified health care professional review of recorded events, analysis of spike and seizure detection, interpretation, and summary report, complete study; greater than 36 hours, up to 60 hours of EEG recording, without video

#● **95722** greater than 36 hours, up to 60 hours of EEG recording, with video (VEEG)

#● **95723** greater than 60 hours, up to 84 hours of EEG recording, without video

#● **95724** greater than 60 hours, up to 84 hours of EEG recording, with video (VEEG)

#● **95725** greater than 84 hours of EEG recording, without video

#● **95726** greater than 84 hours of EEG recording, with video (VEEG)

▶(When the entire study includes recording greater than 36 hours, and the professional interpretation is performed after the entire recording is completed, see 95721, 95722, 95723, 95724, 95725, 95726)◀

▶(Do not report 95721, 95722, 95723, 95724, 95725, 95726 in conjunction with 95717, 95718, 95719, 95720)◀

Rationale

Extensive changes have been made to long-term EEG monitoring services codes to reflect current clinical practice. Codes 95950, 95951, 95953, and 95956 have been deleted. Twenty-three new codes (95700-95726) have been added, two new subsections within the Special EEG Tests subsection have been added, and guidelines have been revised and added including new definitions

and a long-term EEG monitoring table to educate users about long-term EEG monitoring and provide instructions on the proper use of the new codes.

Long-term EEG captures brain-wave activity for a duration of two or more hours. Prior to 2020, long-term EEG could only be reported for each 24-hour period of monitoring with code 95950, 95951, 95953, or 95956, depending on the type of EEG service performed. Long-term EEG services involve several variables (eg, type of monitoring, duration of testing, type of report generated), which were not described by codes 95950, 95951, 95953, and 95956. The technical component (TC) involved in long-term EEG is significant enough that separate codes are needed to report TC services. In addition, video recording is performed with EEG (VEEG) in greater frequency in current practice, and new codes are necessary to reflect this service. New long-term EEG codes (95700-95726) have been added to replace the outdated codes to accurately reflect current clinical practice.

Code 95700 is listed in a new subsection, "Long-term EEG Setup." This is a TC services code that is reported by an EEG technologist on the date set-up is performed. An EEG technologist is qualified by education, training, and licensure/certification/regulation (when applicable) in seizure recognition. Code 95700 is reported once per recording period, and describes EEG recording with or without video, set-up of supplies and equipment, patient education, and take-down when performed. Code 95700 requires the EEG technologist to perform the services in person. If the services are performed by someone who does not meet the definition of EEG technologist, including if they are remotely supervised by an EEG technologist, then unlisted code 95999 should be reported in lieu of code 95700. There may be instances when an EEG is performed on a patient using patient-placed electrode sets. In these instances, code 95999 should be reported in lieu of code 95700.

Codes 95705-95726 are listed in the new subsection, "Monitoring," which is divided into TC services (95705-95716) and professional component (PC) services (95717-95726). TC services (95705-95716) are performed by an EEG technologist. Codes 95705-95716 are time-based and include review of EEG/VEEG data and a technical description. A technical description is the EEG technologist's written record of the data. Codes 95706, 95707, 95709, 95710, 95712, 95713, 95715, and 95716 include maintenance of the long-term EEG equipment.

TC services codes 95705-95716 are structured by: (1) whether the EEG was performed with video (VEEG); (2) duration of recording; and (3) type of monitoring performed (ie, unmonitored, intermittent monitoring, continuous, real-time monitoring).

Table 1 illustrates the structure of TC services codes. (Note that Table 1 does not contain the full code descriptors.)

Table 1. Technical Component Services Codes

95705	**EEG without video, 2-12 hours;** unmonitored
95706	intermittent monitoring
95707	continuous, real-time monitoring
95708	**EEG, without video, each increment of 12-26 hours;** unmonitored
95709	intermittent monitoring
95710	continuous, real-time monitoring
95711	**EEG with video, 2-12 hours;** unmonitored
95712	intermittent monitoring
95713	continuous, real-time monitoring
95714	**EEG with video, each increment of 12-26 hours;** unmonitored
95715	intermittent monitoring
95716	continuous, real-time monitoring

Codes 95705-95707 and 95711-95713 describe 2-12 hours of EEG recording time, and may only be reported once per long-term EEG service to report either: (1) an EEG service that lasts only 2-12 hours; or (2) the final 2-12-hour increment of an EEG service that extends beyond 26 hours. For example, if 26 hours plus one minute of EEG services were performed, then one unit of code 95708 and one unit of code 95705 would be reported together. Codes 95708-95710 and 95714-95716 describe each increment of 12-26 hours of EEG services. For example, if a 52-hour EEG were performed (95708), then the EEG technologist would report code 95708 twice. A Long-Term EEG Monitoring Table is included in the new guidelines to assist users in code selection based on the duration of EEG/VEEG recording for both TC and PC services.

PC services codes 95717-95726 describe services performed by a physician or other qualified health care professional (QHP) and are time-based. Codes 95717-95726 include review of recorded EEG events, analysis of spike and seizure detection, and interpretation and report. For EEG recordings of greater than 12 hours' duration (95719-95720, 95721-95726), the report may be written after each 24-hour period or at the end of the complete study. Codes 95717-95726 are structured by: (1) duration of recording; (2) when the physician or other QHP report is generated; and (3) whether the EEG is performed with video (VEEG).

Codes 95717, 95718 describe 2-12 hours of EEG recording and may only be reported once per long-term EEG service, to report either: (1) an EEG service that lasts only 2-12 hours; or (2) the final 2-12-hour increment of an EEG service that extends beyond 24 hours. Codes 95719 and 95720 describe each increment of greater than 12 hours up to 26 hours of EEG recording. Codes 95721 and 95722 describe greater than 36 hours up to 60 hours of EEG recording. Codes 95723 and 95724 describe greater than 60 hours up to 84 hours of EEG recording. Codes 95725 and 95726 describe greater than 84 hours of EEG recording.

Table 2 illustrates the structure of the PC services codes. (Note that Table 2 does not contain the full code descriptors.)

Table 2. Professional Component Services Codes

95717	**EEG, interpretation and report, 2-12 hours;** without video
95718	with video
95719	**EEG, each increment of greater than 12 hours, up to 26 hours, interpretation and report after each 24-hour period;** without video
95720	with video
95721	**EEG, interpretation, summary report, complete study;** greater than 36 hours, up to 60 hours, without video
95722	greater than 36 hours, up to 60 hours, with video
95723	greater than 60 hours, up to 84 hours, without video
95724	greater than 60 hours, up to 84 hours, with video
95725	greater than 84 hours, without video
95726	greater than 84 hours, with video

In addition to the Long-Term EEG Monitoring Table, the new guidelines describe long-term EEG services and some of the clinical situations in which long-term EEG services may be performed. The guidelines also explain the long-term EEG coding structure and proper use of the codes; provide definitions of terms used in the technical component services codes (ie, EEG technologist, technical description, maintenance, unmonitored service, intermittent monitoring, continuous, real-time monitoring, set-up); and descriptions for TC and PC. The guidelines provide examples of EEG recording scenarios and how to apply the new codes. New parenthetical notes have been added throughout the Monitoring subsection to provide additional guidance on the proper use of the new codes. It is important to carefully review these extensive guidelines and parenthetical notes when reporting long-term EEG services.

Clinical Example (95700)

A 44-year-old male with a history of tonic-clonic seizures reports seizure freedom for the past year. A 72-hour electroencephalogram (EEG) with 20 channels is ordered to confirm seizure freedom and assist physician to determine if medications can be reduced or withdrawn entirely.

Description of Procedure (95700)

Prepare and sanitize equipment. Collect supplies to complete set-up (paste, gauze, solvent, electrodes, etc.), and test equipment.

Explain service and set-up process to patient or family. Obtain signed consent and answer patient or family questions regarding the procedure, logs, operation of equipment, and how to get technical assistance.

Set up room, supplies, and video equipment, tripod, laptop or computer, and Internet connections (when used). Check or test and/or reposition, reactivate, or reset video equipment (when used); laptop or computer; and Internet connections (when used).

Prepare patient and obtain patient's vital signs and BP. Clean patient's skin or scalp; measure and mark head for EEG electrodes; and apply and secure EEG electrodes with protective material for long-term use. Position patient and position EEG wires, EEG monitor, and belt. Check or test and/or reposition or reattach EEG monitor, wires, and belt, and check impedances of each EEG electrode.

After set up, review documented events with patient or family to gather additional context and/or note. Explain how the electrodes will be removed. Answer patient or family questions on use of EEG and video data. Explain what will happen next regarding physician review and interpretation.

Remove electrodes, collodion, and wires, and clean patient.

Clinical Example (95705)

An 8-year-old male with a history of absence seizures reports seizure freedom for the past year. A 24-hour unmonitored without video EEG is ordered to confirm seizure freedom and assist physician to determine if medications can be reduced or withdrawn. The patient removes the electrode wires after 10 hours.

Description of Procedure (95705)

N/A

Clinical Example (95706)

A 48-year-old male has daily intermittent mental status changes. An eight-hour intermittent monitored without video EEG is ordered to evaluate for subclinical seizures.

Description of Procedure (95706)

N/A

Clinical Example (95707)

A 36-year-old female with a known seizure disorder reports feeling dizzy and disoriented. A 10-hour continuous monitoring without video EEG is performed to evaluate effect of recent medication changes.

Description of Procedure (95707)

N/A

Clinical Example (95708)

A 25-year-old male, who was in a motorcycle accident two years ago, was placed on anticonvulsant medication prophylactically. A 24-hour unmonitored without video EEG was ordered to evaluate prior to medication ween.

Description of Procedure (95708)

N/A

Clinical Example (95709)

A 54-year-old male previously presented in nonconvulsive status epilepticus. A 48-hour intermittently monitored without video EEG is ordered to evaluate that nonconvulsive seizures have resolved.

Description of Procedure (95709)

N/A

Clinical Example (95710)

A 65-year-old female postcardiac arrest was placed in a medically induced coma. A 48-hour continuously monitored without video EEG was ordered to evaluate level of medication-induced coma.

Description of Procedure (95710)

N/A

Clinical Example (95711)

A 15-year-old female has frequent jerking movements in the morning. An eight-hour unmonitored video EEG is ordered to evaluate for juvenile myoclonic epilepsy.

Description of Procedure (95711)

N/A

Clinical Example (95712)

A 13-year-old autistic male has frequent episodes of eyelid flutter. An eight-hour with intermittent monitoring video EEG is ordered to evaluate for absence seizures.

Description of Procedure (95712)

N/A

Clinical Example (95713)

A newborn female has atypical movements. An eight-hour continuously monitored video EEG is ordered to evaluate for seizures.

Description of Procedure (95713)

N/A

Clinical Example (95714)

A 30-year-old male presents with known seizure disorder. A 24-hour unmonitored video EEG, is ordered to evaluate breakthrough seizures.

Description of Procedure (95714)

N/A

Clinical Example (95715)

A 15-year-old female is experiencing episodes described as collapsing with convulsions. Episodes have occurred during school where she reports feeling stressed. A 72-hour with intermittent monitoring video EEG is ordered to determine if the patient is having nonepileptic or epileptic seizures.

Description of Procedure (95715)

N/A

Clinical Example (95716)

A 5-year-old autistic male is having sudden head drops and is unresponsive for a few seconds after the event. The events occur several times per week. A 72-hour continuous monitoring with video EEG to capture the event(s) is ordered.

Description of Procedure (95716)

N/A

Clinical Example (95717)

An 8-year-old male with a history of absence seizures reports seizure freedom for the past year. A 24-hour continuous recording without video EEG is ordered to confirm seizure freedom and assist physician to determine if medications can be reduced or withdrawn. The patient removes the electrode wires after 10 hours.

Description of Procedure (95717)

The physician or other QHP reviews patient log of previous seizures and EEG technologist log that includes clinical history, medication history, brain imaging findings if applicable, patient alertness, orientation during awake state, and other EEG technologist notes or observations. In addition, review seizure detection software to identify time of possible seizures or events. Review the EEG recording for artifacts, background activity, normal variants, sleep stages, interictal epileptiform abnormalities, and/or ictal patterns suggestive of clinical or subclinical seizures. Analyze the field potential of each type of epileptiform activity to determine localization. For each seizure or event, review acquired EEG data and annotate the EEG recording before, during, and after the event, describing EEG findings for each recorded event. Review and interpret ECG. Annotate relevant sections of EEG to be archived by EEG technologists. Prepare a report that contains interpretation of EEG background activity, interictal or ictal abnormalities, localization of the seizures or events, and clinical correlation of findings.

Clinical Example (95718)

An 8-year-old male with a history of absence seizures reports seizure freedom for the past year. A 24-hour continuous recording with video EEG is ordered to confirm seizure freedom and assist physician to determine if medications can be reduced or withdrawn. The study is concluded after 10 hours after sufficient data have been recorded.

Description of Procedure (95718)

The physician or other QHP reviews patient log of previous seizures and EEG technologist log that includes clinical history, medication history, brain imaging findings if applicable, patient alertness and orientation during awake state, and other EEG technologist notes or observations. In addition, review seizure detection software to identify time of possible seizures or events. Review the EEG recording for artifacts, background activity, normal variants, sleep stages, interictal epileptiform abnormalities, and/or ictal patterns suggestive of clinical or subclinical seizures. Analyze the field potential of each type of epileptiform activity to determine localization. For each seizure or event, review acquired EEG and video data and the EEG recording and video before, during, and after the event is annotated, describing EEG/video findings for each recorded event. Review and interpret ECG. Annotate relevant sections of EEG along with video to be archived by EEG technologists. Prepare a report that contains interpretation of pertinent video findings along with EEG background activity, interictal or ictal abnormalities, localization of the seizures or events, and clinical correlation of findings.

Clinical Example (95719)

A critically ill 56-year-old female with intracerebral hemorrhage has fluctuating mental status, with periods of unresponsiveness several times per day. A 24-hour continuous recording without video EEG is ordered to determine if these episodes are epileptic seizures.

Description of Procedure (95719)

The physician or other QHP reviews EEG technologist log that includes clinical history, medication history including sedatives, brain imaging findings, patient alertness and orientation during awake state, and other EEG technologist notes or observations. In addition, review seizure detection software to identify time of possible seizures or events. Review the EEG recording for artifacts, background activity, normal variants, sleep stages, interictal epileptiform abnormalities and/or ictal patterns suggestive of clinical or subclinical seizures. Analyze the field potential of each type of epileptiform activity to determine localization. For each seizure or event, review acquired EEG and the EEG recording before, during, and after the event is annotated, describing EEG findings for each recorded event. Review and interpret ECG. Annotate relevant sections of EEG to be archived by EEG technologists. Each 24 hours prepare a report that contains interpretation of EEG background activity, interictal or ictal abnormalities, localization of the seizures or events, and clinical correlation of findings.

Clinical Example (95720)

A 40-year-old female with intractable epilepsy is admitted to the epilepsy monitoring unit for seizure characterization and presurgical evaluation. Anti-epileptic medications are withdrawn. Continuous recording with video EEG is ordered to localize site of seizure onset.

Description of Procedure (95720)

The physician or other QHP reviews patient log, EEG technologist log, EEG technologist technical description summary, nurse notes, and other medical team notes if appropriate. Review seizure detection software to identify possible seizures and/or spells. Review the EEG recording for artifacts, background activity, sleep stages, and interictal epileptiform abnormalities. Analyze the field potential of each type of epileptiform activity to determine localization. For each seizure or event, review the video and EEG data during the entire event to make correlations of changes in video and EEG to localize the site of seizure onset. Review nursing or EEG technologist interaction with the patient during the seizure (nursing ictal and postictal assessment) for language, motor, and memory assessment, including vital signs. Annotate the recording before, during, and after each event, describing clinical and EEG findings and their relative timing. Correlate clinical and EEG findings determine localization of each seizure. Compare seizure features to determine if seizures arise from multiple locations. Annotate relevant sections of EEG and video to be archived by EEG technologists. Communicate any electrode or recording issues, and any required modification to recording (eg, additional electrodes, or changes to seizure or spike detection parameters) to the EEG technologist when necessary. Each 24 hours the physician or other QHP prepares a written report that contains interpretation of EEG background activity, interictal abnormalities, detailed description of electrographic seizure onset, and evolution and offset in relation to detailed description of clinical manifestations based on video data interpretation. Based on these data, report localization of the seizures or events, and clinical correlation of findings.

Clinical Example (95721)

A 14-year-old male with a history of absence seizures experiences staring spells nearly daily. A 48-hour continuous recording without video EEG is ordered to determine if the patient's staring spells are seizures.

Description of Procedure (95721)

The physician or other QHP reviews patient log, EEG technologist log, and EEG technologist technical description summary, including medication history.

Review seizure detection software to identify possible seizures and/or spells. Review the EEG recording for artifacts, background activity, sleep stages, and interictal epileptiform abnormalities. Analyze the field potential of each type of epileptiform activity to determine localization. Review EEG data for each seizure or event during the entire event to make correlations of changes and EEG to localize the site of seizure onset. Annotate the recording before, during, and after each event, describing EEG findings. Correlate clinical and EEG findings to determine localization of each seizure. Compare seizure features to determine if seizures arise from multiple locations. Review and interpret ECG. Annotate relevant sections of EEG to be archived by EEG technologists. At the end of 48 hours of testing, prepare a written report that contains interpretation of EEG background activity, interictal abnormalities, detailed description of electrographic seizure onset, evolution, and offset, and clinical correlation of findings for each 24 hours of recording.

Clinical Example (95722)

A 35-year-old male with a history of focal epilepsy has episodes of amnesia nearly daily. A 48-hour continuous recording with video EEG is ordered to determine if the patient's amnestic episodes are seizures and to determine the clinical manifestations of the seizures.

Description of Procedure (95722)

The physician or other QHP reviews patient log, EEG technologist log, and EEG technologist technical description summary, including medication history. Review seizure detection software to identify possible seizures and/or spells. Review the EEG recording for artifacts, background activity, sleep stages, and interictal epileptiform abnormalities. Analyze the field potential of each type of epileptiform activity to determine localization. Review video and EEG data for each seizure or event during the entire event to make correlations of changes and EEG to localize the site of seizure onset. Annotate the recording before, during, and after each event, describing EEG findings. Correlate clinical and EEG findings to determine localization of each seizure. Compare seizure features to determine if seizures arise from multiple locations. Annotate relevant sections of EEG and video to be archived by EEG technologists. At the end of the 48 hours of testing, prepare a written report that contains interpretation of pertinent video findings along with EEG background activity, interictal abnormalities, detailed description of electrographic seizure onset, evolution and offset, and clinical correlation of findings for each 24 hours of recording.

Clinical Example (95723)

A 14-year-old male with a history of absence seizures experiences staring spells two to three times per week. A 72-hour continuous recording without video EEG is ordered to determine if the patient's staring spells are seizures.

Description of Procedure (95723)

The physician or other QHP reviews patient log, EEG technologist log, and EEG technologist technical description summary, including medication history. Review seizure detection software to identify possible seizures and/or spells. Review the EEG recording for artifacts, background activity, sleep stages, and interictal epileptiform abnormalities. Analyze the field potential of each type of epileptiform activity to determine localization. Review the EEG data for each seizure or event during the entire event to make correlations of changes and EEG to localize the site of seizure onset. Annotate the recording before, during, and after each event, describing EEG findings. Correlate clinical and EEG findings to determine localization of each seizure. Compare seizure features to determine if seizures arise from multiple locations. Review and interpret ECG. Annotate relevant sections of EEG to be archived by EEG technologists. At the end of 72 hours of testing, the physician or other QHP prepares a written report that contains interpretation of EEG background activity, interictal abnormalities, detailed description of electrographic seizure onset, evolution and offset, and clinical correlation of findings for each 24 hours of recording.

Clinical Example (95724)

A 35-year-old male with a history of focal epilepsy has episodes of amnesia two to three times per week. A 72-hour continuous recording with video EEG is ordered to determine if the patient's amnestic episodes are seizures and to determine the clinical manifestations of the seizures.

Description of Procedure (95724)

The physician or other QHP reviews patient log, EEG technologist log, and EEG technologist technical description summary, including medication history. Review seizure detection software to identify possible seizures and/or spells. Review the EEG recording for artifacts, background activity, sleep stages, and interictal epileptiform abnormalities. Analyze the field potential of each type of epileptiform activity to determine localization. Review video and EEG data for each seizure or event during the entire event to make correlations of changes and EEG to localize the site of seizure onset. Annotate the recording before, during, and after each event, describing EEG findings. Correlate clinical and EEG findings to determine localization of each seizure. Compare seizure features to determine if seizures arise from multiple locations. Annotate relevant sections of EEG and video to be archived by EEG technologists. At the end of the 72 hours of testing, the physician or other QHP prepares a written report that contains interpretation of pertinent video findings along with EEG background activity, interictal abnormalities, detailed description of electrographic seizure onset, evolution and offset, and clinical correlation of findings for each 24 hours of recording.

Clinical Example (95725)

A 14-year-old male with a history of absence seizures experiences staring spells approximately once a week. A 96-hour continuous recording without video EEG is ordered to determine if the patient's staring spells are seizures.

Description of Procedure (95725)

The physician or other QHP reviews patient log, EEG technologist log, and EEG technologist technical description summary, including medication history. Review seizure detection software to identify possible seizures and/or spells. Review the EEG recording for artifacts, background activity, sleep stages, and interictal epileptiform abnormalities. Analyze the field potential of each type of epileptiform activity to determine localization. Review the EEG data for each seizure or event during the entire event to make correlations of changes and EEG to localize the site of seizure onset. Annotate the recording before, during, and after each event, describing EEG findings. Correlate clinical and EEG findings to determine localization of each seizure. Compare seizure features to determine if seizures arise from multiple locations. Review and interpret ECG. Annotate relevant sections of EEG to be archived by EEG technologists. At the end of 96 hours of testing, the physician or other QHP prepares a written report that contains interpretation of EEG background activity, interictal abnormalities, detailed description of electrographic seizure onset, evolution and offset, and clinical correlation of findings for each 24 hours of recording.

Clinical Example (95726)

A 35-year-old male with a history of focal epilepsy has episodes of amnesia approximately once per week. A 96-hour continuous recording with video EEG is ordered to determine if the patient's amnestic episodes are seizures and to determine the clinical manifestations of the seizures.

Description of Procedure (95726)

The physician or other QHP reviews patient log, EEG technologist log, and EEG technologist technical description summary, including medication history. Review seizure detection software to identify possible seizures and/or spells. Review the EEG recording for artifacts, background activity, sleep stages, and interictal epileptiform abnormalities. Analyze the field potential of each type of epileptiform activity to determine localization. Review video and EEG data for each seizure or event during the entire event to make correlations of changes and EEG to localize the site of seizure onset. Annotate the recording before, during, and after each event, describing EEG findings. Correlate clinical and EEG findings to determine localization of each seizure. Compare seizure features to determine if seizures arise from multiple locations. Annotate relevant sections of EEG and video to be archived by EEG technologists. At the end of the 96-hour period of testing, the physician or other QHP prepares a written report that contains interpretation of pertinent video findings along with EEG background activity, interictal abnormalities, detailed description of electrographic seizure onset, evolution and offset, and clinical correlation of findings for each 24 hours of recording.

Neurostimulators, Analysis-Programming

(For insertion of neurostimulator pulse generator, see 61885, 61886, 63685, 64568, 64590)

(For revision or removal of neurostimulator pulse generator or receiver, see 61888, 63688, 64569, 64570, 64595)

(For implantation of neurostimulator electrodes, see 43647, 43881, 61850-61870, 63650, 63655, 64553-64581. For revision or removal of neurostimulator electrodes, see 43648, 43882, 61880, 63661, 63662, 63663, 63664, 64569, 64570, 64585)

▶(For analysis and programming of implanted integrated neurostimulation system, posterior tibial nerve, see 0589T, 0590T)◀

95970 Electronic analysis of implanted neurostimulator pulse generator/transmitter (eg, contact group[s], interleaving, amplitude, pulse width, frequency [Hz], on/off cycling, burst, magnet mode, dose lockout, patient selectable parameters, responsive neurostimulation, detection algorithms, closed loop parameters, and passive parameters) by physician or other qualified health care professional; with brain, cranial nerve, spinal cord, peripheral nerve, or sacral nerve, neurostimulator pulse generator/transmitter, without programming

(Do not report 95970 in conjunction with 43647, 43648, 43881, 43882, 61850, 61860, 61863, 61864, 61867, 61868, 61870, 61880, 61885, 61886, 61888, 63650, 63655, 63661, 63662, 63663, 63664, 63685, 63688, 64553, 64555, 64561, 64566, 64568, 64569, 64570, 64575, 64580, 64581, 64585, 64590, 64595, during the same operative session)

(Do not report 95970 in conjunction with 95971, 95972, 95976, 95977, 95983, 95984)

95971 with simple spinal cord or peripheral nerve (eg, sacral nerve) neurostimulator pulse generator/transmitter programming by physician or other qualified health care professional

(Do not report 95971 in conjunction with 95972)

95972 with complex spinal cord or peripheral nerve (eg, sacral nerve) neurostimulator pulse generator/transmitter programming by physician or other qualified health care professional

▶(For percutaneous implantation or replacement of integrated neurostimulation system, posterior tibial nerve, use 0587T)◀

(95974, 95975 have been deleted. To report, see 95976, 95977)

95976 with simple cranial nerve neurostimulator pulse generator/transmitter programming by physician or other qualified health care professional

(Do not report 95976 in conjunction with 95977)

95977 with complex cranial nerve neurostimulator pulse generator/transmitter programming by physician or other qualified health care professional

 # 95983 with brain neurostimulator pulse generator/transmitter programming, first 15 minutes face-to-face time with physician or other qualified health care professional

#+ 95984 with brain neurostimulator pulse generator/transmitter programming, each additional 15 minutes face-to-face time with physician or other qualified health care professional (List separately in addition to code for primary procedure)

(Use 95984 in conjunction with 95983)

▶(Do not report 95970, 95971, 95972, 95976, 95977, 95983, 95984 in conjunction with 0587T, 0588T, 0589T, 0590T)◀

▶(For percutaneous implantation or replacement of integrated neurostimulation system, posterior tibial nerve, use 0587T)◀

(95978, 95979 have been deleted. To report, see 95983, 95984)

Rationale

In accordance with the establishment of Category III codes 0587T, 0588T, 0589T, and 0590T, several parenthetical notes have been added to the Neurostimulators, Analysis-Programming subsection to reflect the new codes.

Refer to the codebook and the Rationale for codes 0587T, 0588T, 0589T, and 0590T for a full discussion of these changes.

Adaptive Behavior Services

Adaptive Behavior Assessments

 # 97152 **Behavior identification-supporting assessment,** administered by one technician under the direction of a physician or other qualified health care professional, face-to-face with the patient, each 15 minutes

(97151, 97152, 0362T may be repeated on the same or different days until the behavior identification assessment [97151] and, if necessary, supporting assessment[s] [97152, 0362T], is complete)

(For psychiatric diagnostic evaluation, see 90791, 90792)

(For speech evaluations, see 92521, 92522, 92523, 92524)

(For occupational therapy evaluation, see 97165, 97166, 97167, 97168)

(For medical team conference, see 99366, 99367, 99368)

▶(For health and behavior assessment/intervention, see 96156, 96158, 96159, 96164, 96165, 96167, 96168, 96170, 96171)◀

(For neurobehavioral status exam, see 96116, 96121)

(For neuropsychological testing, see 96132, 96133, 96136, 96137, 96138, 96139, 96146)

Rationale

In accordance with the deletion of codes 96150, 96151, 96152, 96153, 96154, and 96155 and the establishment of codes 96156, 96158, 96159, 96164, 96165, 96167, 96168, 96170, and 96171, the cross-reference parenthetical note following code 97152 has been revised to reflect these changes.

Refer to the codebook and the Rationale for codes 96156, 96158, 96159, 96164, 96165, 96167, 96168, 96170, and 96171 for a full discussion of these changes.

Medicine | CPT Changes 2020

Adaptive Behavior Treatment

 # 97153 **Adaptive behavior treatment by protocol,** administered by technician under the direction of a physician or other qualified health care professional, face-to-face with one patient, each 15 minutes

▶(Do not report 97153 in conjunction with 90785-90899, 92507, 96105-96171, 97129)◀

 # 97154 **Group adaptive behavior treatment by protocol,** administered by technician under the direction of a physician or other qualified health care professional, face-to-face with two or more patients, each 15 minutes

(Do not report 97154 if the group has more than 8 patients)

▶(Do not report 97154 in conjunction with 90785-90899, 92508, 96105-96171, 97150)◀

 # 97155 **Adaptive behavior treatment with protocol modification,** administered by physician or other qualified health care professional, which may include simultaneous direction of technician, face-to-face with one patient, each 15 minutes

▶(Do not report 97155 in conjunction with 90785-90899, 92507, 96105-96171, 97129)◀

Rationale

In accordance with the deletion of codes 96150, 96151, 96152, 96153, 96154, 96155, and 97127 and the establishment of codes 96156, 96158, 96159, 96164, 96165, 96167, 96168, 96170, 96171, and 97129, the exclusionary parenthetical notes following codes 97153, 97154, and 97155 have been revised to reflect these changes.

Refer to the codebook and the Rationale for codes 96156, 96158, 96159, 96164, 96165, 96167, 96168, 96170, 96171, and 97129 for a full discussion of these changes.

 # 97156 **Family adaptive behavior treatment guidance,** administered by physician or other qualified health care professional (with or without the patient present), face-to-face with guardian(s)/caregiver(s), each 15 minutes

▶(Do not report 97156 in conjunction with 90785-90899, 96105-96171)◀

 # 97157 **Multiple-family group adaptive behavior treatment guidance,** administered by physician or other qualified health care professional (without the patient present), face-to-face with multiple sets of guardians/caregivers, each 15 minutes

(Do not report 97157 if the group has more than 8 families)

▶(Do not report 97156, 97157 in conjunction with 90785-90899, 96105-96171)◀

 # 97158 **Group adaptive behavior treatment with protocol modification,** administered by physician or other qualified health care professional, face-to-face with multiple patients, each 15 minutes

(Do not report 97158 if the group has more than 8 patients)

▶(Do not report 97158 in conjunction with 90785-90899, 96105-96171, 92508, 97150)◀

Rationale

In accordance with the deletion of codes 96150, 96151, 96152, 96153, 96154, and 96155 and the establishment of codes 96156, 96158, 96159, 96164, 96165, 96167, 96168, 96170, and 96171, the exclusionary parenthetical notes following codes 97156, 97157, and 97158 have been revised to reflect these changes.

Refer to the codebook and the Rationale for codes 96156, 96158, 96159, 96164, 96165, 96167, 96168, 96170, and 96171 for a full discussion of these changes.

Central Nervous System Assessments/Tests (eg, Neuro-Cognitive, Mental Status, Speech Testing)

The following codes are used to report the services provided during testing of the central nervous system functions. The central nervous system assessments include, but are not limited to, memory, language, visual motor responses, and abstract reasoning/problem-solving abilities. It is accomplished by the combination of several types of testing procedures. Testing procedures include assessment of aphasia and cognitive performance testing, developmental screening and behavioral assessments and testing, and psychological/neuropsychological testing. The administration of these tests will generate material that will be formulated into a report or an automated result.

▶(For development of cognitive skills, see 97129, 97533)◀

(For dementia screens, [eg, Folstein Mini-Mental State Examination, by a physician or other qualified health care professional], see **Evaluation and Management** services codes)

(Do not report assessment of aphasia and cognitive performance testing services [96105, 96125], developmental/behavioral screening and testing services [96110, 96112, 96113, 96127], and psychological/neuropsychological testing services [96116, 96121, 96130, 96131, 96132, 96133, 96136, 96137, 96138, 96139, 96146] in conjunction with 97151, 97152, 97153, 97154, 97155, 97156, 97157, 97158, 0362T, 0373T)

Rationale

In support of the establishment of code 97129 and the deletion of code 97127, the cross-reference parenthetical note following the Central Nervous System Assessments/Tests (eg, Neuro-Cognitive, Mental Status, Speech Testing) guidelines has been revised to reflect these changes.

Refer to the codebook and the Rationale for codes 97127 and 97129 for a full discussion of these changes.

▶Health Behavior Assessment and Intervention◀

▶Health behavior assessment and intervention services are used to identify and address the psychological, behavioral, emotional, cognitive, and interpersonal factors important to the assessment, treatment, or management of physical health problems.

The patient's primary diagnosis is physical in nature and the focus of the assessment and intervention is on factors complicating medical conditions and treatments. These codes describe assessments and interventions to improve the patient's health and well-being utilizing psychological and/or psychosocial interventions designed to ameliorate specific disease-related problems.

Health behavior assessment: includes evaluation of the patient's responses to disease, illness or injury, outlook, coping strategies, motivation, and adherence to medical treatment. Assessment is conducted through health-focused clinical interviews, observation, and clinical decision making.

Health behavior intervention: includes promotion of functional improvement, minimizing psychological and/or psychosocial barriers to recovery, and management of and improved coping with medical conditions. These services emphasize active patient/family engagement and involvement. These interventions may be provided individually, to a group (two or more patients), and/or to the family, with or without the patient present.

Codes 96156, 96158, 96159, 96164, 96165, 96167, 96168, 96170, 96171 describe services offered to patients who present with primary physical illnesses, diagnoses, or symptoms and may benefit from assessments and interventions that focus on the psychological and/or psychosocial factors related to the patient's health status. These services do not represent preventive medicine counseling and risk factor reduction interventions.

For patients that require psychiatric services (90785-90899), adaptive behavior services (97151, 97152, 97153, 97154, 97155, 97156, 97157, 97158, 0362T, 0373T) as well as health behavior assessment and intervention (96156, 96158, 96159, 96164, 96165, 96167, 96168, 96170, 96171), report the predominant service performed. Do not report 96156, 96158, 96159, 96164, 96165, 96167, 96168, 96170, 96171 in conjunction with 90785-90899 on the same date.

Evaluation and management services codes (including counseling risk factor reduction and behavior change intervention [99401-99412]) should not be reported on the same day as health behavior assessment and intervention codes 96156, 96158, 96159, 96164, 96165, 96167, 96168, 96170, 96171 by the same provider.

Health behavior assessment and intervention services (96156, 96158, 96159, 96164, 96165, 96167, 96168, 96170, 96171) can occur and be reported on the same date of service as evaluation and management services (including counseling risk factor reduction and behavior change intervention [99401, 99402, 99403, 99404, 99406, 99407, 99408, 99409, 99411, 99412]), as long as the health behavior assessment and intervention service is reported by a physician or other qualified health care professional and the evaluation and management service is performed by a physician or other qualified health care professional who may report evaluation and management services.◀

▶Do not report 96158, 96164, 96167, 96170 for less than 16 minutes of service.◀

▶(For health behavior assessment and intervention services [96156, 96158, 96159, 96164, 96165, 96167, 96168, 96170, 96171] performed by a physician or other qualified health care professional who may report evaluation and management services, see **Evaluation and Management** or **Preventive Medicine Services** codes)◀

▶(Do not report 96156, 96158, 96159, 96164, 96165, 96167, 96168, 96170, 96171 in conjunction with 97151, 97152, 97153, 97154, 97155, 97156, 97157, 97158, 0362T, 0373T)◀

▶(96150, 96151, 96152 have been deleted. To report, see 96156, 96158, 96159)◀

Medicine

▶(96153 has been deleted. To report, see 96164, 96165)◀

▶(96154 has been deleted. To report, see 96167, 96168)◀

▶(96155 has been deleted. To report, see 96170, 96171)◀

●96156 Health behavior assessment, or re-assessment (ie, health-focused clinical interview, behavioral observations, clinical decision making)

●96158 Health behavior intervention, individual, face-to-face; initial 30 minutes

+●96159 each additional 15 minutes (List separately in addition to code for primary service)

▶(Use 96159 in conjunction with 96158)◀

#●96164 Health behavior intervention, group (2 or more patients), face-to-face; initial 30 minutes

#+●96165 each additional 15 minutes (List separately in addition to code for primary service)

▶(Use 96165 in conjunction with 96164)◀

#●96167 Health behavior intervention, family (with the patient present), face-to-face; initial 30 minutes

#+●96168 each additional 15 minutes (List separately in addition to code for primary service)

▶(Use 96168 in conjunction with 96167)◀

#●96170 Health behavior intervention, family (without the patient present), face-to-face; initial 30 minutes

#+●96171 each additional 15 minutes (List separately in addition to code for primary service)

▶(Use 96171 in conjunction with 96170)◀

96160 Administration of patient-focused health risk assessment instrument (eg, health hazard appraisal) with scoring and documentation, per standardized instrument

96161 Administration of caregiver-focused health risk assessment instrument (eg, depression inventory) for the benefit of the patient, with scoring and documentation, per standardized instrument

96164 Code is out of numerical sequence. See 96158-96161

96165 Code is out of numerical sequence. See 96158-96161

96167 Code is out of numerical sequence. See 96158-96161

96168 Code is out of numerical sequence. See 96158-96161

96170 Code is out of numerical sequence. See 96158-96161

96171 Code is out of numerical sequence. See 96158-96161

Rationale

Revisions made to the Health Behavior Assessment and Intervention subsection now enable the reporting of services provided to improve a patient's health and well-being utilizing psychological and/or psychosocial interventions. Specifically, codes 96150, 96151, 96152, 96153, 96154, and 96155 have been deleted and codes 96156, 96158, 96159, 96164, 96165, 96167, 96168, 96170, and 96171 have been established. The heading has been revised to more clearly describe the services in this subsection. Several parenthetical notes have been added and revised throughout this subsection to provide instruction on the proper reporting for these assessments and interventions.

Additional guidelines have been added to describe the difference between assessment and interventions, including definitions for health behavior assessment and health behavior intervention.

Clinical Example (96156)

A 65-year-old male with osteoarthritis, chronic back pain, and medication-related somnolence is referred for health behavior assessment to determine the psychological factors requiring intervention as part of the patient's overall treatment plan.

Description of Procedure (96156)

QHP meets with patient to assess adjustment to the medical illness or injury; psychological, motivational, and interpersonal factors affecting medical management; outlook; coping strategies; treatment compliance; and health risk behaviors.

Clinical Example (96158)

A 55-year-old female with heart disease, migraines, and hypertension is referred for health behavior services to improve patient treatment compliance and engagement in self-management.

Description of Procedure (96158)

QHP actively promotes the patient's compliance and full participation in medical treatment by engaging the patient in jointly reviewing treatment progress, outlook, understanding of the medical condition(s), and attitudes toward treatment goals and care team members. Employ psychological and behavioral treatment approaches to address health risk behaviors and factors impeding adjustment to, management of, and recovery from the patient's medical condition. QHP documentation includes description of patient's status in addition to services provided and progress toward and/or modification of treatment goals based on patient progress or other confounding factors that arise.

Clinical Example (96159)

A 55-year-old female with heart disease, migraines, and hypertension is referred for health behavior services to improve patient treatment compliance and engagement in self-management. Patient requires an additional 15 minutes of health behavior services beyond the first 30 minutes.

Description of Procedure (96159)

QHP actively promotes the patient's compliance and full participation in medical treatment by engaging the patient in jointly reviewing treatment progress, outlook, understanding of the medical condition(s), and attitudes toward treatment goals and care team members. Employ psychological and behavioral treatment approaches to address health risk behaviors and factors impeding adjustment to, management of, and recovery from the patient's medical condition.

Clinical Example (96164)

A 26-year-old obese female post-bariatric surgery with poor adherence to treatment regimens and multiple medical complications is referred for group health behavior intervention.

Description of Procedure (96164)

Initiate or continue health behavior interventions within the group setting, including providing educational information about the disease process or injury, training members in psychologically based self-management procedures, and improving social support. QHP documentation in the medical record for each patient includes description of patient's status in addition to services provided and progress toward and/or modification of treatment goals based on patient progress or other confounding factors that arise.

Clinical Example (96165)

A 26-year-old obese female post-bariatric surgery with poor adherence to treatment regimens and multiple medical complications is referred for group health behavior intervention. Patient requires an additional 15 minutes of health behavior services beyond the first 30 minutes.

Description of Procedure (96165)

Continue health behavior interventions within the group setting, including providing educational information about the disease process or injury, training members in psychologically based self-management procedures, and improving social support.

Clinical Example (96167)

A 36-year-old married female diagnosed with breast cancer, who is undergoing aggressive chemotherapy and radiation therapy with poor adherence to treatment regimens and multiple medical complications, is referred for family intervention.

Description of Procedure (96167)

Conduct face-to-face interaction with the patient and family members. Facilitate family communication and provide education about the patient's illness or injury. Engage and mobilize family support and problem-solving regarding treatment adherence and prognosis. Clarify family roles and caregiver responsibilities. QHP documents in the medical record includes description of the patient's status, family involvement, and progress toward and/or modification of treatment goals based on patient progress or other confounding factors that arise.

Clinical Example (96168)

A 36-year-old married female diagnosed with breast cancer, who is undergoing aggressive chemotherapy and radiation therapy with poor adherence to treatment regimens and multiple medical complications, is referred for family intervention. Patient and family require an additional 15 minutes of health behavior services beyond the first 30 minutes.

Description of Procedure (96168)

Conduct face-to-face interaction with the patient and family members. Facilitate family communication and provide education about the patient's illness or injury. Engage and mobilize family support and problem-solving regarding treatment adherence and prognosis. Clarify family roles and caregiver responsibilities.

Clinical Example (96170)

The family of a 9-year-old boy, who was diagnosed with type 1 diabetes two years ago, is referred for intervention because of the patient's continuing refusal to self-inject his insulin and to test his own glucose levels.

Description of Procedure (96170)

Conduct face-to-face interaction with family members without the patient present. Facilitate family communication and provide education about the patient's illness or injury and resistance to change. Engage and mobilize family support and problem-solving regarding treatment adherence. Clarify family roles and caregiver responsibilities. QHP documents in the medical record includes description of the patient's status, family involvement, and progress toward and/or modification of treatment goals based on patient progress or other confounding factors that arise.

Medicine | CPT Changes 2020

Clinical Example (96171)

The family of a 9-year-old boy, who was diagnosed with type 1 diabetes two years ago, is referred for intervention because of the patient's continuing refusal to self-inject his insulin and to test his own glucose levels. The family requires an additional 15 minutes of family health behavior services beyond the first 30 minutes.

Description of Procedure (96171)

Conduct face-to-face interaction with family members without the patient present. Facilitate family communication and provide education about the patient's illness or injury and resistance to change. Engage and mobilize family support and problem-solving regarding treatment adherence. Clarify family roles and caregiver responsibilities.

Physical Medicine and Rehabilitation

Codes 97010-97763 should be used to report each distinct procedure performed. Do not append modifier 51 to 97010-97763.

The work of the physician or other qualified health care professional consists of face-to-face time with the patient (and caregiver, if applicable) delivering skilled services. For the purpose of determining the total time of a service, incremental intervals of treatment at the same visit may be accumulated.

The meanings of terms in the Physical Medicine and Rehabilitation section are not the same as those in the Evaluation and Management Services section (99201-99350). Do not use the Definitions of Commonly Used Terms in the Evaluation and Management (E/M) Guidelines for Physical Medicine and Rehabilitation services.

►(For range of joint motion, see 95851, 95852)◄

(For biofeedback training by EMG, use 90901)

(For transcutaneous nerve stimulation [TENS], use 97014 for electrical stimulation requiring supervision only, or use 97032 for electrical stimulation requiring constant attendance)

Rationale

In accordance with the deletion of codes 95831-95834, the cross-reference parenthetical note following the Physical Medicine and Rehabilitation introductory guidelines has been revised to reflect these changes.

Refer to the codebook and the Rationale for codes 95831-95834 for a full discussion of these changes.

Therapeutic Procedures

►(97127 has been deleted. To report, use 97129)◄

● 97129 Therapeutic interventions that focus on cognitive function (eg, attention, memory, reasoning, executive function, problem solving, and/or pragmatic functioning) and compensatory strategies to manage the performance of an activity (eg, managing time or schedules, initiating, organizing, and sequencing tasks), direct (one-on-one) patient contact; initial 15 minutes

►(Report 97129 only once per day)◄

+● 97130 each additional 15 minutes (List separately in addition to code for primary procedure)

►(Use 97130 in conjunction with 97129)◄

►(Do not report 97129, 97130 in conjunction with 97153, 97155)◄

97139 Unlisted therapeutic procedure (specify)

Rationale

Code 97127 has been deleted and codes 97129 and 97130 established to report therapeutic interventions that focus on cognitive function for an initial 15 minutes (97129) and each additional 15 minutes (97130) of therapeutic interventions.

Code 97129 includes therapeutic interventions and lists examples of elements of cognitive function that may be addressed during therapy. It also includes the use of compensatory strategies. Code 97130 is an add-on code to code 97129, which can be reported for each additional 15 minutes of service. Parenthetical notes have been revised and added regarding the proper use of these codes.

Clinical Example (97129)

A 30-year-old male presents with traumatic brain injury sustained in a vehicular accident resulting in memory problems, distractibility, depression, inappropriate social interaction, inability to self-monitor, and impaired organizational skills for executive function. He is seen for cognitive function intervention.

Description of Procedure (97129)

The clinician implements therapeutic activities that may include attention tasks (eg, gradually increasing levels of distracting background noise); memory tasks (eg, visualization, mnemonics, environmental adaptations); problem-solving activities (eg, techniques to define a problem, set a goal, and organize an action); and pragmatic activities to improve social communication skills and increase self-awareness of limitations and disabilities (eg, use of internal dialogue). Tools (eg, technology-assisted activities, role-playing activities) and compensatory strategies (eg, memory log) may be used to accomplish functional outcomes.

Clinical Example (97130)

A 30-year-old male presents with traumatic brain injury sustained in a vehicular accident resulting in memory problems, distractibility, depression, inappropriate social interaction, inability to self-monitor, and impaired organizational skills for executive function. He is seen for cognitive function intervention and requires an additional 15 minutes of treatment beyond the initial 15 minutes.

Description of Procedure (97130)

The clinician implements therapeutic activities that may include attention tasks (eg, gradually increasing levels of distracting background noise); memory tasks (eg, visualization, mnemonics, environmental adaptations); problem solving activities (eg, techniques to define a problem, set a goal, and organize an action); and pragmatic activities to improve social communication skills and increase self-awareness of limitations and disabilities (eg, use of internal dialogue). Tools (eg, technology-assisted activities, role-playing activities) and compensatory strategies (eg, memory log) may be used to accomplish functional outcomes.

97140 Manual therapy techniques (eg, mobilization/manipulation, manual lymphatic drainage, manual traction), 1 or more regions, each 15 minutes

►(For needle insertion[s] without injection[s] [eg, dry needling, trigger-point acupuncture], see 20560, 20561)◄

Rationale

In accordance with the establishment of codes 20560 and 20561, a cross-reference parenthetical note has been added following code 97140 directing users to the new codes for needle insertion(s) without injections(s).

Refer to the codebook and the Rationale for codes 20560 and 20561 for a full discussion of these changes.

97530 Therapeutic activities, direct (one-on-one) patient contact (use of dynamic activities to improve functional performance), each 15 minutes

►(97532 has been deleted. To report, use 97129)◄

Rationale

In support of the deletion of code 97127 and the establishment of code 97129, the cross-reference parenthetical note following code 97530 has been revised to reflect these changes.

Refer to the codebook and the Rationale for codes 97127 and 97129 for a full discussion of these changes.

Tests and Measurements

Requires direct one-on-one patient contact.

►(For joint range of motion, see 95851, 95852; for electromyography, see 95860-95872, 95885, 95886, 95887; for nerve velocity determination, see 95905, 95907, 95908, 95909, 95910, 95911, 95912, 95913)◄

97750 Physical performance test or measurement (eg, musculoskeletal, functional capacity), with written report, each 15 minutes

Rationale

In accordance with the deletion of codes 95831-95834 (manual muscle testing), the cross-reference parenthetical note listed in the Physical Medicine and Rehabilitation Test and Measurements subsection has been revised to remove references to muscle testing.

Refer to the codebook and the Rationale for codes 95831-95834 for a full discussion of these changes.

Acupuncture

Acupuncture is reported based on 15-minute increments of personal (face-to-face) contact with the patient, not the duration of acupuncture needle(s) placement.

If no electrical stimulation is used during a 15-minute increment, use 97810, 97811. If electrical stimulation of any needle is used during a 15-minute increment, use 97813, 97814.

Only one code may be reported for each 15-minute increment. Use either 97810 or 97813 for the initial 15-minute increment. Only one initial code is reported per day.

Evaluation and management services may be reported in addition to acupuncture procedures when performed by physicians or other health care professionals, who may report evaluation and management services, including new or established patient office or other outpatient services (99201-99215), hospital observation care (99217-99220, 99224-99226), hospital care (99221-99223, 99231-99233), office or other outpatient consultations (99241-99245), inpatient consultations (99251-99255), critical care services (99291, 99292), inpatient neonatal intensive care services and pediatric and neonatal critical care services (99466-99480), emergency department services (99281-99285), nursing facility services (99304-99318), domiciliary, rest home, or custodial care services (99324-99337), and home services (99341-99350) may be reported separately using modifier 25 if the patient's condition requires a significant, separately identifiable E/M service above and beyond the usual preservice and postservice work associated with the acupuncture services. The time of the E/M service is not included in the time of the acupuncture service.

▶For needle insertion(s) without injection(s) (eg, dry needling, trigger point acupuncture), see 20560, 20561.◀

Rationale

In accordance with the addition of codes 20560 and 20561, a sentence has been added to the Acupuncture subsection guidelines directing users to the correct codes to report needle insertion(s) without injection(s).

Refer to the codebook and the Rationale for codes 20560 and 20561 for a full discussion of these changes.

97810 Acupuncture, 1 or more needles; without electrical stimulation, initial 15 minutes of personal one-on-one contact with the patient

(Do not report 97810 in conjunction with 97813)

+ 97811 without electrical stimulation, each additional 15 minutes of personal one-on-one contact with the patient, with re-insertion of needle(s) (List separately in addition to code for primary procedure)

(Use 97811 in conjunction with 97810, 97813)

97813 with electrical stimulation, initial 15 minutes of personal one-on-one contact with the patient

(Do not report 97813 in conjunction with 97810)

+ 97814 with electrical stimulation, each additional 15 minutes of personal one-on-one contact with the patient, with re-insertion of needle(s) (List separately in addition to code for primary procedure)

(Use 97814 in conjunction with 97810, 97813)

▶(Do not report 97810, 97811, 97813, 97814 in conjunction with 20560, 20561. When both time-based acupuncture services and needle insertion[s] without injection[s] are performed, report only the time-based acupuncture codes)◀

Rationale

In accordance with the establishment of codes 20560 and 20561, an exclusionary parenthetical note has been added following code 97814 to restrict reporting of acupuncture services (97810, 97811, 97813, 97814) in conjunction with the new needle insertion(s) without injection(s) services codes 20560 and 20561. In addition, the parenthetical note provides instructions regarding how to report when both time-based acupuncture and needle insertions without injection(s) are performed.

Refer to the codebook and the Rationale for codes 20560 and 20561 for a full discussion of these changes.

Education and Training for Patient Self-Management

(For counseling and education provided by a physician to a group, use 99078)

(For counseling and/or risk factor reduction intervention provided by a physician to patient[s] without symptoms or established disease, see 99401-99412)

(For medical nutrition therapy, see 97802-97804)

▶(For health behavior assessment and intervention that is not part of a standardized curriculum, see 96156, 96158, 96159, 96164, 96165, 96167, 96168, 96170, 96171)◀

(For education provided as genetic counseling services, use 96040. For education to a group regarding genetic risks, see 98961, 98962)

98960 Education and training for patient self-management by a qualified, nonphysician health care professional using a standardized curriculum, face-to-face with the patient (could include caregiver/family) each 30 minutes; individual patient

98961 2-4 patients

98962 5-8 patients

Rationale

In accordance with the deletion of codes 96150, 96151, 96152, 96153, 96154, and 96155 and the establishment of codes 96156, 96158, 96159, 96164, 96165, 96167, 96168, 96170, and 96171, the cross-reference parenthetical note preceding code 98960 has been revised to reflect these changes.

Refer to the codebook and the Rationale for codes 96156, 96158, 96159, 96164, 96165, 96167, 96168, 96170, and 96171 for a full discussion of these changes.

Non-Face-to-Face Nonphysician Services

Telephone Services

▶Telephone services are non-face-to-face assessment and management services provided by a qualified health care professional to a patient using the telephone. These codes are used to report episodes of care by the qualified health care professional initiated by an established patient or guardian of an established patient. If the telephone service ends with a decision to see the patient within 24 hours or the next available urgent visit appointment, the code is not reported; rather the encounter is considered part of the preservice work of the subsequent assessment and management service, procedure, and visit. Likewise, if the telephone call refers to a service performed and reported by the qualified health care professional within the previous seven days (either qualified health care professional requested or unsolicited patient follow-up) or within the postoperative period of the previously completed procedure, then the service(s) are considered part of that previous service or procedure. (Do not report 98966-98968 if reporting 98966-98968 performed in the previous seven days.)◀

(For telephone services provided by a physician, see 99441-99443)

Rationale

In accordance with the deletion of code 98969, the Telephone Services guidelines have been revised to reflect this change.

Refer to the codebook and the Rationale for codes 98969, 99421, 99422, and 99423 for a full discussion of these changes.

▶Qualified Nonphysician Health Care Professional Online Digital Evaluation and Management Service◀

▶Qualified nonphysician health care professional online digital evaluation and management (E/M) services are patient-initiated digital services with qualified nonphysician health care professionals that require qualified nonphysician health care professional patient evaluation and decision making to generate an assessment and subsequent management of the patient. These services are not for the nonevaluative electronic communication of test results, scheduling of appointments, or other communication that does not include E/M. While the patient's problem may be new to the qualified nonphysician health care professional, the patient is an established patient. Patients initiate these services through Health Insurance Portability and Accountability Act (HIPAA)-compliant, secure platforms, such as through the electronic health record (EHR) portal, email, or other digital applications, which allow digital communication with the qualified nonphysician health care professional.

Qualified nonphysician health care professional online digital E/M services are reported once for the qualified nonphysician health care professional's cumulative time devoted to the service during a seven-day period. The seven-day period begins with the qualified nonphysician health care professional's initial, personal review of the patient-generated inquiry. Qualified nonphysician health care professional cumulative service time includes review of the initial inquiry, review of patient records or data pertinent to assessment of the patient's problem, personal qualified nonphysician health care professional interaction with clinical staff focused on the patient's problem, development of management plans, including qualified nonphysician health care professional generation of prescriptions or ordering of tests, and subsequent communication with the patient through online, telephone, email, or other digitally supported communication. All qualified nonphysician health care professionals in the same group practice who are involved in the online digital E/M service contribute to

Medicine

the cumulative service time devoted to the patient's online digital E/M service. Qualified nonphysician health care professional online digital E/M services require visit documentation and permanent storage (electronic or hard copy) of the encounter.

If the patient generates the initial online digital inquiry within seven days of a previous treatment or E/M service and both services relate to the same problem, or the online digital inquiry occurs within the postoperative period of a previously completed procedure, then the qualified nonphysician health care professional's online digital E/M service may not be reported separately. If the patient generates an initial online digital inquiry for a new problem within seven days of a previous service that addressed a different problem, then the qualified nonphysician health care professional online digital E/M service is reported separately. If a separately reported evaluation service occurs within seven days of the qualified nonphysician health care professional's initial review of the online digital E/M service, 98970, 98971, 98972 are not reported. If the patient presents a new, unrelated problem during the seven-day period of an online digital E/M service, then the qualified nonphysician health care professional's time spent on the evaluation and management of the additional problem is added to the cumulative service time of the online digital E/M service for that seven-day period.◄

▶(For an online digital E/M service provided by a physician or other qualified health care professional, see 99421, 99422, 99423)◄

▶(98969 has been deleted. To report, see 98970, 98971, 98972)◄

● **98970** Qualified nonphysician health care professional online digital evaluation and management service, for an established patient, for up to 7 days, cumulative time during the 7 days; 5-10 minutes

● **98971** 11-20 minutes

● **98972** 21 or more minutes

▶(Report 98970, 98971, 98972 once per 7-day period)◄

▶(Do not report online digital E/M services for cumulative visit time less than 5 minutes)◄

▶(Do not count 98970, 98971, 98972 time otherwise reported with other services)◄

▶(Do not report 98970, 98971, 98972 for home and outpatient INR monitoring when reporting 93792, 93793)◄

▶(Do not report 98970, 98971, 98972 when using 99091, 99339, 99340, 99374, 99375, 99377, 99378, 99379, 99380, 99487, 99489, 99495, 99496, for the same communication[s])◄

Rationale

A new subsection, Qualified Nonphysician Health Care Professional Online Digital Evaluation and Management Service, with new guidelines, and three new codes (98970, 98971, 98972) have been added. Code 98969 has been deleted.

Codes 98970, 98971, and 98972 describe patient-initiated digital communications performed by a qualified nonphysician health care professional that require a clinical decision that otherwise would have been typically provided in the office.

Codes 98970, 98971, and 98972 are reported for established patients and time-based. Code 98970 is for the first 5-10 minutes, 98971 for 11-20 minutes, and 98972 for 21 or more minutes of service. Guidelines have been added to outline the components of these codes and correct reporting.

An instructional parenthetical note has been added to remind users that codes 98970, 98971, and 98972 may only be reported once per 7-day period. Exclusionary parenthetical notes have been added to: (1) indicate if the online digital evaluation cumulative visit time is less than 5 minutes, reporting of these codes is not appropriate; (2) preclude the use of codes 98970, 98971, and 98972 when using codes 99091, 99339, 99340, 99374, 99375, 99377, 99378, 99379, 99380, 99487, 99489, 99495, and 99496, for the same communication(s); and (3) preclude the use of codes 98970, 98971, and 98972 when reporting codes 93792 and 93793 for home and outpatient INR monitoring.

In addition, an exclusionary parenthetical note has been added indicating do not count codes 98970, 98971, and 98972 time otherwise reported with other services.

Clinical Example (98970)

A 70-year-old male, who has insulin-dependent diabetes, submits an online query through his registered dietitian nutritionist's (RDN's) electronic health record (EHR) portal reporting nausea and vomiting due to the flu and seeking guidance on diabetes self-management.

Description of Procedure (98970)

Review the initial patient inquiry, review the medical history, review documents sent by the patient, and check online data registries or information exchanges. Assess medical or nutrition condition described in the patient query. Review current medications and laboratory test results. Formulate and send the registered dietitian response (eg, a nutrition diagnosis and intervention plan and/or requests for additional information) to the patient. Implement, initiate, or modify orders for therapeutic diets, pharmacotherapy management, or nutrition-related services (eg, medical foods, nutrition or dietary supplements, enteral and parenteral nutrition, laboratory test, or medications) using approved clinical privileges, delegated orders, protocols, or other organization-approved processes. Conduct follow-up communication with the patient. Communicate with patient's physician to coordinate care. Complete necessary referrals to programs and/or providers as indicated. Complete medical record documentation of all communications.

Clinical Example (98971)

A 65-year-old male with congestive heart failure submits an online query through HIPAA-compliant encrypted email to his RDN regarding a recent 7-lb weight gain.

Description of Procedure (98971)

Review the initial patient inquiry, review the medical history, review documents sent by the patient, and check online data registries or information exchanges. Assess medical or nutrition condition described in the patient query. Review current medications and laboratory test results. Formulate and send the registered dietitian response (eg, a nutrition diagnosis and intervention plan and/or requests for additional information) to the patient. Implement, initiate, or modify orders for therapeutic diets, pharmacotherapy management, or nutrition-related services (eg, medical foods, nutrition or dietary supplements, enteral and parenteral nutrition, laboratory test, or medications) using approved clinical privileges, delegated orders, protocols, or other organization-approved processes. Conduct follow-up communication with the patient. Communicate with patient's physician to coordinate care. Complete necessary referrals to programs and/or providers as indicated. Complete medical record documentation of all communications.

Clinical Example (98972)

A 40-year-old female, who is newly diagnosed with type 2 diabetes, submits an online query through her RDN's EHR portal after noticing her morning fasting blood glucose levels were gradually increasing.

Description of Procedure (98972)

Review the initial patient inquiry, review the medical history, review documents sent by the patient, and check online data registries or information exchanges. Assess medical or nutrition condition described in the patient query. Review current medications and laboratory test results. Formulate and send the registered dietitian response (eg, a nutrition diagnosis and intervention plan and/or requests for additional information) to the patient. Implement, initiate, or modify orders for therapeutic diets, pharmacotherapy management, or nutrition-related services (eg, medical foods, nutrition or dietary supplements, enteral and parenteral nutrition, laboratory test, or medications) using approved clinical privileges, delegated orders, protocols, or other organization-approved processes. Conduct follow-up communication with the patient. Communicate with patient's physician to coordinate care. Complete necessary referrals to programs and/or providers as indicated. Complete medical record documentation of all communications.

Notes

Category II Codes

Summary of Additions, Deletions, and Revisions

The summary of changes shows the actual changes that have been made to the code descriptors.

New codes appear with a bullet (●) and are indicated as "Code added." Revised codes are preceded with a triangle (▲). Within revised codes, or if a code symbol has been deleted, the deleted language and code symbol appear with a ~~strikethrough~~ (⊖), while new text appears underlined.

The ⁄ symbol is used to identify codes for vaccines that are pending FDA approval. The # symbol is used to identify codes that have been resequenced. CPT add-on codes are annotated by the + symbol. The ⊘ symbol is used to identify codes that are exempt from the use of modifier 51. The ★ symbol is used to identify codes that may be used for reporting telemedicine services. The ⋈ is used to identify proprietary laboratory analyses (PLA) test that has an identical descriptor as another PLA test. A PLA code that satisfies Category I code criteria and has been accepted by the CPT Editorial Panel is annotated with the ↑↓ symbol.

Code	Description
▲2022F	Dilated retinal eye exam with interpretation by an ophthalmologist or optometrist documented and reviewed; with evidence of retinopathy (DM)[2,4]
●2023F	Code added
▲2024F	7 standard field stereoscopic retinal photos with interpretation by an ophthalmologist or optometrist documented and reviewed; with evidence of retinopathy (DM)[2,4]
●2025F	Code added
▲2026F	Eye imaging validated to match diagnosis from 7 standard field stereoscopic retinal photos results documented and reviewed; with evidence of retinopathy (DM)[2,4]
#●2033F	Code added
3045F	~~Most recent hemoglobin A1c (HbA1c) level 7.0-9.0% (DM)[2,4]~~
#●3051F	Code added
#●3052F	Code added

▲ = Revised code   ● = New code   ▶◀ = Contains new or revised text   ⋈ = Duplicate PLA test   ↑↓ = Category I PLA

Category II Codes

Physical Examination

Physical examination codes describe aspects of physical examination or clinical assessment.

	2021F	Dilated macular or fundus exam performed, including documentation of the presence or absence of macular edema **and** level of severity of retinopathy (EC)[2]
▲	2022F	Dilated retinal eye exam with interpretation by an ophthalmologist or optometrist documented and reviewed; with evidence of retinopathy (DM)[2]
●	2023F	without evidence of retinopathy (DM)[2]
▲	2024F	7 standard field stereoscopic retinal photos with interpretation by an ophthalmologist or optometrist documented and reviewed; with evidence of retinopathy (DM)[2]
●	2025F	without evidence of retinopathy (DM)[2]
▲	2026F	Eye imaging validated to match diagnosis from 7 standard field stereoscopic retinal photos results documented and reviewed; with evidence of retinopathy (DM)[2]
#●	2033F	without evidence of retinopathy (DM)[2]
	2033F	Code is out of numerical sequence. See 2025F-2028F

Rationale

Codes 2022F, 2024F, and 2026F have been revised and codes 2023F, 2025F, and 2033F have been added to allow more specific reporting for the Appropriate Eye Exam for People with Diabetes measure. This includes the revision of the Alphabetical Clinical Topics Listing (Alpha Listing) included on the AMA website. The changes that have been made for reporting compliance for this measure were made to simplify reporting by the physician or other qualified health care professional (ie, ophthalmologist or optometrist) responsible for the patient for this aspect of care (ie, to ensure eye examination for diabetic retinal disease for patients who have diabetes). This simplification is intended to assist with reporting when the examination by the eye care professional actually occurs. This has been accomplished by revising the existing codes to include language that indicates "with evidence of retinopathy" (2022F, 2024F, 2026F) and adding new codes that allow for reporting "without evidence of retinopathy (2023F, 2025F, 2033F). The changes allow for reporting with more specificity in identifying whether the dilated retinal eye examination, 7 standard field stereoscopic retinal photos, or eye imaging validated to match diagnosis from 7 standard field stereoscopic retinal photos (all performed by the ophthalmologist/optometrist) noted evidence with or without retinopathy. This specificity allows more specific information to be captured regarding compliance with the National Commission for Quality Assurance (NCQA) measure. Changes have also been made to the Alpha Listing on the AMA website (https://www.ama-assn.org/practice-management/cpt/category-ii-codes). This includes changes to the NCQA Appropriate Eye Exam for People with Diabetes measure snapshot listings. The changes made to the Alpha Listing reflect the revisions made to the NCQA measure, as well as the code changes described in the previous explanation. The changes to the NCQA measure listing include: (1) revisions to the reporting instructions that direct users to report one of the codes listed to note measure compliance, as well as the addition of language that specifies that the date of service for report of the codes should match the service date of the service with the eye care professional; (2) revision of the percentage statement to reflect "retinal" instead of "dilated"; and (3) revisions to the numerator statement removing the term "at least once." (**Note:** Code 3072F should be reported with a date of service for the current year to appropriately reflect the prior year experience.) For additional instructions regarding compliance with the measure specifications, what the specifications are, and other intended use of the NCQA's healthcare effectiveness data and information set (HEDIS) measures for this condition, please refer to the NCQA website (NCQA, Health Employer Data Information Set [HEDIS®] www.ncqa.org).

Diagnostic/Screening Processes or Results

	3044F	Most recent hemoglobin A1c (HbA1c) level less than 7.0% (DM)[2,4]
		▶(3045F has been deleted. To report control of HbA1c, see 3051F, 3052F)◀
#●	3051F	Most recent hemoglobin A1c (HbA1c) level greater than or equal to 7.0% and less than 8.0% (DM)[2]
#●	3052F	Most recent hemoglobin A1c (HbA1c) level greater than or equal to 8.0% and less than or equal to 9.0% (DM)[2]
	3046F	Most recent hemoglobin A1c level greater than 9.0% (DM)[4]
		▶(To report most recent hemoglobin A1c level less than or equal to 9.0%, see 3044F, 3051F, 3052F)◀

3051F	Code is out of numerical sequence. See 3042F-3048F
3052F	Code is out of numerical sequence. See 3042F-3048F
3066F	Documentation of treatment for nephropathy (eg, patient receiving dialysis, patient being treated for ESRD, CRF, ARF, or renal insufficiency, any visit to a nephrologist) (DM)[2]
3072F	Low risk for retinopathy (no evidence of retinopathy in the prior year) (DM)[2]

Rationale

Code 3045F has been deleted and replaced with two new codes (3051F and 3052F) to allow more specific reporting for most recent hemoglobin A1c levels. This includes the revision of the Alphabetical Clinical Topics Listing (Alpha Listing) included on the AMA website. In addition, a number of parenthetical notes have been added or revised to accommodate the change. Code 3045F was originally used to identify "Most recent hemoglobin A1c (HbA1c) level 7.0-9.0%" as part of the NCQA and National Diabetes Quality Improvement Alliance (NDQIA) diabetes mellitus (DM) measure set. However, in the wake of the disbandment of the NDQIA, the NCQA as the sole proprietor of the measure has revised the measure to more specifically identify appropriate control of HbA1c with a lower threshold— ie, less than 8.0% (previously appropriate control was identified at 9.0%). Specifically, the measure has been updated to note that any HbA1c level that is not less than 8.0% is not compliant with the new measure specifications. The codes previously included in the Category II section that identify HbA1c levels of less than 7.0% (3044F), and greater than 9.0% (3046F) remain. In order to allow for reporting between 7.0% and 8.0%, code 3045F (A1c [HbA1c] level 7.0%-9.0%) has been deleted and code 3051F has been added to identify control of HbA1c at 7.0% to less than 8.0%. In addition, code 3052F has been added to identify a level of HbA1c of 8.0%-9.0%. A deletion cross-reference has been added in place of code 3045F to direct users to the appropriate code to report identification of HbA1c levels in the 7.0%-9.0% range. In addition, a cross-reference following code 3046F has also been revised to reflect the addition of the new codes. Changes have also been made to the Alpha Listing on the AMA website (https://www.ama-assn.org/practice-management/cpt/category-ii-codes). This includes changes to both the measure for the NCQA A1c Management measure snapshot and the NDQIA A1c Management measure snapshot listings (**Note:** The changes made to the NDQIA snapshot have been made to update the listing with the changes to the codes as no changes were made to the measure snapshot listing.) The changes made to the Alpha Listing reflect the revisions made to the NCQA measure as well as the code changes described in the previous explanation. The changes to the NCQA measure listing include: (1) revisions to the reporting instructions; (2) revision of the exclusion language included for the measure "snapshot" to provide an example of an acceptable medical exclusion; and (3) revisions to the measure and numerator statements to better reflect the levels that now identify appropriate HbA1c control according to the NCQA measure set. Instructions have also been provided to direct users to the NCQA's HEDIS measure set for instructions regarding intended use and reporting for their measure.

Notes

Category III Codes

Summary of Additions, Deletions, and Revisions

The summary of changes shows the actual changes that have been made to the code descriptors.

New codes appear with a bullet (●) and are indicated as "Code added." Revised codes are preceded with a triangle (▲). Within revised codes, or if a code symbol has been deleted, the deleted language and code symbol appear with a ~~strikethrough~~ (⊖), while new text appears underlined.

The ∕ symbol is used to identify codes for vaccines that are pending FDA approval. The # symbol is used to identify codes that have been resequenced. CPT add-on codes are annotated by the + symbol. The ⊘ symbol is used to identify codes that are exempt from the use of modifier 51. The ★ symbol is used to identify codes that may be used for reporting telemedicine services. The ⋈ is used to identify proprietary laboratory analyses (PLA) test that has an identical descriptor as another PLA test. A PLA code that satisfies Category I code criteria and has been accepted by the CPT Editorial Panel is annotated with the ↿⇂ symbol.

Code	Description
0205T	~~Intravascular catheter-based coronary vessel or graft spectroscopy (eg, infrared) during diagnostic evaluation and/or therapeutic intervention including imaging supervision, interpretation, and report, each vessel (List separately in addition to code for primary procedure)~~
0206T	~~Computerized database analysis of multiple cycles of digitized cardiac electrical data from two or more ECG leads, including transmission to a remote center, application of multiple nonlinear mathematical transformations, with coronary artery obstruction severity assessment~~
0249T	~~Ligation, hemorrhoidal vascular bundle(s), including ultrasound guidance~~
0254T	~~Endovascular repair of iliac artery bifurcation (eg, aneurysm, pseudoaneurysm, arteriovenous malformation, trauma, dissection) using bifurcated endograft from the common iliac artery into both the external and internal iliac artery, including all selective and/or nonselective catheterization(s) required for device placement and all associated radiological supervision and interpretation, unilateral~~
0341T	~~Quantitative pupillometry with interpretation and report, unilateral or bilateral~~
0357T	~~immature oocyte(s)~~
0375T	~~Total disc arthroplasty (artificial disc), anterior approach, including discectomy with end plate preparation (includes osteophytectomy for nerve root or spinal cord decompression and microdissection), cervical, three or more levels~~
0377T	~~Anoscopy with directed submucosal injection of bulking agent for fecal incontinence~~
0380T	~~Computer-aided animation and analysis of time series retinal images for the monitoring of disease progression, unilateral or bilateral, with interpretation and report~~
0399T	~~Myocardial strain imaging (quantitative assessment of myocardial mechanics using image-based analysis of local myocardial dynamics) (List separately in addition to code for primary procedure)~~
▲0402T	Collagen cross-linking of cornea ~~(~~, including removal of the corneal epithelium and intraoperative pachymetry~~)~~, when performed <u>(Report medication separately)</u>
0482T	~~Absolute quantitation of myocardial blood flow, positron emission tomography (PET), rest and stress (List separately in addition to code for primary procedure)~~
●0543T	Code added

▲ = Revised code ● = New code ▶◀ = Contains new or revised text ⋈ = Duplicate PLA test ↿⇂ = Category I PLA

Category III Codes

Code	Description
●0544T	Code added
●0545T	Code added
●0546T	Code added
●0547T	Code added
●0548T	Code added
●0549T	Code added
●0550T	Code added
●0551T	Code added
●0552T	Code added
●0553T	Code added
●0554T	Code added
●0555T	Code added
●0556T	Code added
●0557T	Code added
●0558T	Code added
●0559T	Code added
+●0560T	Code added
●0561T	Code added
+●0562T	Code added
#●0563T	Code added
●0564T	Code added
●0565T	Code added
●0566T	Code added
●0567T	Code added
●0568T	Code added
●0569T	Code added
+●0570T	Code added
●0571T	Code added
●0572T	Code added
●0573T	Code added
●0574T	Code added
●0575T	Code added
●0576T	Code added

Category III Codes

Code	Description
●0577T	Code added
●0578T	Code added
●0579T	Code added
●0580T	Code added
●0581T	Code added
●0582T	Code added
●0583T	Code added
●0584T	Code added
●0585T	Code added
●0586T	Code added
●0587T	Code added
●0588T	Code added
●0589T	Code added
●0590T	Code added
●0591T	Code added
●0592T	Code added
●0593T	Code added

Category III Codes

0058T Cryopreservation; reproductive tissue, ovarian

▶(For cryopreservation of mature oocyte(s), use 89337)◀

▶(0357T has been deleted)◀

▶(For cryopreservation of immature oocyte[s], use 89398)◀

(For cryopreservation of embryo(s), sperm and testicular reproductive tissue, see 89258, 89259, 89335)

Rationale

In accordance with CPT guidelines for archiving Category III codes, code 0357T and related cross-references have been deleted. Report code 89398, *Unlisted reproductive medicine laboratory procedure*, if cryopreservation of immature oocyte(s) is performed. To reflect the change, all related parenthetical notes have also been revised.

0202T Posterior vertebral joint(s) arthroplasty (eg, facet joint[s] replacement), including facetectomy, laminectomy, foraminotomy, and vertebral column fixation, injection of bone cement, when performed, including fluoroscopy, single level, lumbar spine

(Do not report 0202T in conjunction with 22511, 22514, 22840, 22853, 22854, 22857, 22859, 63005, 63012, 63017, 63030, 63042, 63047, 63056 at the same level)

▶(0205T has been deleted)◀

▶(For intravascular catheter-based coronary vessel or graft spectroscopy [eg, infrared] during diagnostic evaluation and/or therapeutic intervention including imaging supervision, interpretation, and report, each vessel, use 93799)◀

Rationale

In accordance with CPT guidelines for archiving Category III codes, code 0205T (intravascular catheter-based coronary vessel or graft spectroscopy) and all related cross-references have been deleted. Report code 93799, *Unlisted cardiovascular service or procedure*, if intravascular catheter-based coronary vessel or graft spectroscopy [eg, infrared] during diagnostic evaluation and/or therapeutic intervention, including imaging supervision, interpretation, and report of each vessel is performed. To reflect the change, all related parenthetical notes have also been revised.

▶(0206T has been deleted)◀

▶(For computerized database analysis of multiple cycles of digitized cardiac electrical data from 2 or more ECG leads, including transmission to a remote center, application of multiple nonlinear mathematical transformations, with coronary artery obstruction severity assessment, use 93799)◀

Rationale

In accordance with CPT guidelines for archiving Category III codes, code 0206T and related cross-references have been deleted. Report code 93799, *Unlisted cardiovascular service or procedure*, if computerized database analysis of multiple cycles of digitized cardiac electrical data from two or more ECG leads, including transmission to a remote center, application of multiple nonlinear mathematical transformations, with coronary artery obstruction severity assessment is performed. To reflect the change, all related parenthetical notes have also been revised.

0207T Evacuation of meibomian glands, automated, using heat and intermittent pressure, unilateral

▶(For evacuation of meibomian glands using heat-delivered through wearable, open-eye eyelid treatment devices and manual gland expression, use 0563T. For evacuation of meibomian gland using manual gland expression only, use the appropriate evaluation and management code)◀

#● **0563T** Evacuation of meibomian glands, using heat delivered through wearable, open-eye eyelid treatment devices and manual gland expression, bilateral

▶(For evacuation of meibomian gland using manual gland expression only, use the appropriate evaluation and management code)◀

Rationale

Code 0563T has been established to report evacuation of meibomian glands using heat delivered through a wearable open-eye device treating the eyelids and manual gland expression. Additional parenthetical notes have been added following the new code and in other sections of the code set to accommodate the addition of the new code.

The procedure described by code 0207T differs from the procedure described in code 0563T because the new procedure is not performed using automated means. Instead, as noted in the descriptor, after the meibum is heated, it is manually expressed from the gland. The procedure is typically done for both eyes due to the needs of dry eye disease and meibomian gland dysfunction. As a result the code descriptor includes language that identifies bilateral provision of the service.

Parenthetical notes listed with the codes and within the code set in other appropriate locations provide additional instructions regarding reporting this service. This includes instruction following code 0563T to report the appropriate evaluation and management (E/M) services code for manual expression of the gland without the use of heat, instruction following code 0207T regarding appropriate reporting for heat-delivered manual gland expression vs automated meibomian gland expression, and a cross-reference within the Surgery section following code 68040 that directs users to the new code for this procedure.

Clinical Example (0563T)

A 47-year-old female presents to the ophthalmologist or optometrist complaining of chronic dryness and redness and irritation of both eyes that has not been relieved with artificial tears. After appropriate diagnostic testing, it is determined that the patient suffers from dry eye disease secondary to meibomian gland disease.

Description of Procedure (0563T)

Ophthalmologist or optometrist performs entire procedure. Thoroughly clean and dry all four eyelids to remove any oil and make-up. Carefully affix four adhesive, single use, disposable devices to the outside (skin side) of the tarsal plates of each of the four eyelids. Then affix temple pads to each temple and wire behind the ears. Plug the adhesive, disposable devices that are affixed to the eyelids into the control unit. Activate the control unit to begin the software-controlled heat treatment. The system initiates treatment at 41°C to a maximum temperature of 45°C and is maintained for 15 minutes to effectively melt all meibomian gland obstructions. Advise patient to blink throughout treatment to begin the natural clearance of melted meibum. At the conclusion of the 15-minute thermal cycle, gently remove the single use, disposable adhesive devices from all four eyelids and discard. Instill topical anesthetic in both eyes. Using a disposable meibomian gland clearance instrument on each of the four eyelids, manually express the meibum from each meibomian gland in each of the four eyelids. Section each eyelid into three zones and progress nasally (Zone 1) to medially (Zone 2) to temporally (Zone 3). Begin clearing the glands at the base of the tarsal plate, then middle, and then the lid margin. Complete clearing of the meibomian glands after two thorough passes on the upper and lower eyelid of each eye. Discard the single use, disposable meibomian gland clearance instrument.

0213T Injection(s), diagnostic or therapeutic agent, paravertebral facet (zygapophyseal) joint (or nerves innervating that joint) with ultrasound guidance, cervical or thoracic; single level

(To report bilateral procedure, use 0213T with modifier 50)

+ 0214T second level (List separately in addition to code for primary procedure)

(Use 0214T in conjunction with 0213T)

▶(For bilateral procedure, report 0214T twice. Do not report modifier 50 in conjunction with 0214T)◀

+ 0215T third and any additional level(s) (List separately in addition to code for primary procedure)

(Do not report 0215T more than once per day)

(Use 0215T in conjunction with 0213T, 0214T)

▶(For bilateral procedure, report 0215T twice. Do not report modifier 50 in conjunction with 0215T)◀

0216T Injection(s), diagnostic or therapeutic agent, paravertebral facet (zygapophyseal) joint (or nerves innervating that joint) with ultrasound guidance, lumbar or sacral; single level

(To report bilateral procedure, use 0216T with modifier 50)

+ 0217T second level (List separately in addition to code for primary procedure)

(Use 0217T in conjunction with 0216T)

▶(For bilateral procedure, report 0217T twice. Do not report modifier 50 in conjunction with 0217T)◀

+ 0218T third and any additional level(s) (List separately in addition to code for primary procedure)

(Do not report 0218T more than once per day)

(Use 0218T in conjunction with 0216T, 0217T)

(If injection(s) are performed using fluoroscopy or CT, see 64490-64495)

▶(For bilateral procedure, report 0218T twice. Do not report modifier 50 in conjunction with 0218T)◀

Rationale

In support of the revision to instructions for reporting add-on procedures, the instructional parenthetical notes for add-on codes 0214T, 0215T, 0217T, and 0218T have been revised to instruct that these codes should be reported twice when the procedure is performed bilaterally.

Refer to the codebook and the Rationale for modifier 50, *Bilateral Procedure*, for a full discussion of these changes.

Category III Codes

0232T Injection(s), platelet rich plasma, any site, including image guidance, harvesting and preparation when performed

▶(Do not report 0232T in conjunction with 15769, 15771, 15772, 15773, 15774, 20550, 20551, 20600, 20604, 20605, 20606, 20610, 20611, 36415, 36592, 76942, 77002, 77012, 77021, 86965, 0481T)◀

(Do not report 38220-38230 for bone marrow aspiration for platelet rich stem cell injection. For bone marrow aspiration for platelet rich stem cell injection, use 0232T)

Rationale

In accordance with the deletion of code 20926 and the addition of codes 15769, 15771, 15772, 15773, 15774, the parenthetical note following code 0232T has been revised to remove the deleted code from its listing and add the new tissue and fat grafting codes.

Refer to the codebook and the Rationale for code 20926 and codes 15769, 15771, 15772, 15773, 15774 for a full discussion of these changes.

▶(0249T has been deleted. To report, use 46948)◀

Rationale

Code 0249T has been deleted and converted to Category I code 46948. A deletion parenthetical note has been added in its place. In addition, the exclusionary parenthetical note associated with this code has been deleted.

Refer to the codebook and the Rationale for code 46948 for a full discussion of these changes.

0253T Code is out of numerical sequence. See 0184T-0200T

▶(0254T has been deleted. To report, see 34717, 34718)◀

▶(0255T has been deleted. To report, see 34717, 34718)◀

Rationale

In accordance with the conversion of Category III code 0254T to Category I codes 34717 and 34718, code 0254T has been deleted. A cross-reference parenthetical note has been added directing users to codes 34717 and 34718. In addition, the existing parenthetical note for code 0255T has been revised to remove code 0254T and replace it with codes 34717 and 34718.

Refer to the codebook and the Rationale for codes 34717, 34718 for a full discussion of these changes.

▶(0341T has been deleted)◀

▶(For quantitative pupillometry with interpretation and report, unilateral or bilateral, use 92499)◀

Rationale

In accordance with CPT guidelines for archiving Category III codes, code 0341T has been deleted. Report code 92499, *Unlisted ophthalmological service or procedure,* if quantitative pupillometry with interpretation and report, unilateral or bilateral, is performed.

0342T Therapeutic apheresis with selective HDL delipidation and plasma reinfusion

Fluoroscopy (76000) and radiologic supervision and interpretation are inherent to the transcatheter mitral valve repair (TMVR) procedure and are not separately reportable. Diagnostic cardiac catheterization (93451, 93452, 93453, 93454, 93455, 93456, 93457, 93458, 93459, 93460, 93461, 93530, 93531, 93532, 93533) should **not** be reported with transcatheter mitral valve repair (0345T) for:

- Contrast injections, angiography, roadmapping, and/or fluoroscopic guidance for the transcatheter mitral valve repair (TMVR),
- Left ventricular angiography to assess mitral regurgitation, for guidance of TMVR, or
- Right and left heart catheterization for hemodynamic measurements before, during, and after TMVR for guidance of TMVR.

Diagnostic right and left heart catheterization (93451, 93452, 93453, 93456, 93457, 93458, 93459, 93460, 93461, 93530, 93531, 93532, 93533), and diagnostic coronary angiography (93454, 93455, 93456, 93457, 93458, 93459, 93460, 93461, 93563, 93564) not inherent to the TMVR, may be reported with 0345T, appended with modifier 59 if:

1. No prior study is available and a full diagnostic study is performed, or
2. A prior study is available, but as documented in the medical record:
   a. There is inadequate visualization of the anatomy and/or pathology, or
   b. The patient's condition with respect to the clinical indication has changed since the prior study, or
   c. There is a clinical change during the procedure that requires new evaluation.

Percutaneous coronary interventional procedures may be reported separately, when performed.

Other cardiac catheterization services may be reported separately, when performed for diagnostic purposes not intrinsic to the TMVR.

When transcatheter ventricular support is required, the appropriate code may be reported with the appropriate ventricular assist device (VAD) procedure (33990, 33991, 33992, 33993) or balloon pump insertion (33967, 33970, 33973).

0345T Transcatheter mitral valve repair percutaneous approach via the coronary sinus

(For transcatheter mitral valve repair percutaneous approach including transseptal puncture when performed, see 33418, 33419)

(Do not report 0345T in conjunction with 93451, 93452, 93453, 93456, 93457, 93458, 93459, 93460, 93461 for diagnostic left and right heart catheterization procedures intrinsic to the valve repair procedure)

(Do not report 0345T in conjunction with 93453, 93454, 93563, 93564 for coronary angiography intrinsic to the valve repair procedure)

(For transcatheter mitral valve implantation/replacement [TMVI], see 0483T, 0484T)

►(For transcatheter mitral valve annulus reconstruction, use 0544T)◄

Rationale

A cross-reference parenthetical note has been included following code 0345T to direct users to the appropriate code to report transcatheter mitral valve annulus reconstruction.

Refer to the codebook and the Rationale for codes 0544T and 0545T for a full discussion of these changes.

Adaptive Behavior Assessments and Treatment

0362T **Behavior identification supporting assessment,** each 15 minutes of technicians' time face-to-face with a patient, requiring the following components:

- administration by the physician or other qualified health care professional who is on site;

- with the assistance of two or more technicians;

- for a patient who exhibits destructive behavior;

- completion in an environment that is customized to the patient's behavior.

(0362T is reported based on a single technician's face-to-face time with the patient and not the combined time of multiple technicians [eg, one hour with three technicians equals one hour of service])

(0362T may be repeated on different days until the behavior identification assessment [97151] and, if necessary, supporting assessment[s] [97152, 0362T], is complete)

(For psychiatric diagnostic evaluation, see 90791, 90792)

(For speech evaluations, see 92521, 92522, 92523, 92524)

(For occupational therapy evaluation, see 97165, 97166, 97167, 97168)

(For medical team conference, see 99366, 99367, 99368)

►(For health behavior assessment and intervention, see 96156, 96158, 96159, 96164, 96165, 96167, 96168, 96170, 96171)◄

(For neurobehavioral status examination, see 96116, 96121)

(For neuropsychological testing, see 96132, 96133, 96136, 96137, 96138, 96139, 96146)

Rationale

In accordance with the deletion of codes 96150, 96151, 96152, 96153, 96154, and 96155 and the establishment of codes 96156, 96158, 96159, 96164, 96165, 96167, 96168, 96170, and 96171, the cross-reference parenthetical note following code 0362T has been revised to reflect these changes.

Refer to the codebook and the Rationale for codes 96156, 96158, 96159, 96164, 96165, 96167, 96168, 96170, and 96171 for a full discussion of these changes.

(0363T, 0364T, 0365T, 0366T, 0367T, 0368T, 0369T, 0370T, 0371T, 0372T have been deleted. To report, see 97153, 97154, 97155, 97156, 97157, 97158, 0373T)

0373T **Adaptive behavior treatment with protocol modification,** each 15 minutes of technicians' time face-to-face with a patient, requiring the following components:

- administration by the physician or other qualified health care professional who is on site;

- with the assistance of two or more technicians;

- for a patient who exhibits destructive behavior;

- completion in an environment that is customized to the patient's behavior.

Category III Codes

(0373T is reported based on a single technician's face-to-face time with the patient and not the combined time of multiple technicians)

▶(Do not report 0373T in conjunction with 90785-90899, 96105, 96110, 96116, 96121, 96156, 96158, 96159, 96164, 96165, 96167, 96168, 96170, 96171)◀

Rationale

In accordance with the deletion of codes 96150, 96151, 96152, 96153, 96154, and 96155 and the establishment of codes 96156, 96158, 96159, 96164, 96165, 96167, 96168, 96170, and 96171, the cross-reference parenthetical note following code 0373T has been revised to reflect these changes.

Refer to the codebook and the Rationale for codes 96156, 96158, 96159, 96164, 96165, 96167, 96168, 96170, and 96171 for a full discussion of these changes.

(0374T has been deleted. To report, use 0373T)

▶(0375T has been deleted)◀

▶(For total disc arthroplasty [artificial disc], anterior approach, including discectomy with end-plate preparation [includes osteophytectomy for nerve root or spinal cord decompression and microdissection], cervical, 3 or more levels, use 22899)◀

Rationale

In accordance with CPT guidelines for archiving Category III codes, code 0375T and all related cross-reference parenthetical notes have been deleted. Report code 22899, *Unlisted procedure, spine,* if total disc arthroplasty (artificial disc), anterior approach, including discectomy with end plate preparation (includes osteophytectomy for nerve root or spinal cord decompression and microdissection), cervical, three or more levels is performed. To reflect the change, all related parenthetical notes have also been revised.

0376T Code is out of numerical sequence. See 0184T-0200T

▶(0377T has been deleted)◀

▶(For anoscopy with directed submucosal injection of bulking agent for fecal incontinence, use 46999)◀

Rationale

In accordance with CPT guidelines for archiving Category III codes, code 0377T has been deleted. Report code 46999, *Unlisted procedure, anus,* if anoscopy with directed submucosal injection of bulking agent for fecal incontinence is performed. To reflect the change, all related parenthetical notes have been revised as well.

0378T Visual field assessment, with concurrent real time data analysis and accessible data storage with patient initiated data transmitted to a remote surveillance center for up to 30 days; review and interpretation with report by a physician or other qualified health care professional

0379T technical support and patient instructions, surveillance, analysis, and transmission of daily and emergent data reports as prescribed by a physician or other qualified health care professional

▶(0380T has been deleted)◀

▶(For computer-aided animation and analysis of time series retinal images for the monitoring of disease progression, unilateral or bilateral, with interpretation and report, use 92499)◀

Rationale

In accordance with CPT guidelines for archiving Category III codes, code 0380T has been deleted. Report code 92499, *Unlisted ophthalmological service or procedure,* if computer-aided animation and analysis of time series retinal images for the monitoring of disease progression, unilateral or bilateral, with interpretation and report are performed.

0398T Magnetic resonance image guided high intensity focused ultrasound (MRgFUS), stereotactic ablation lesion, intracranial for movement disorder including stereotactic navigation and frame placement when performed

(Do not report 0398T in conjunction with 61781, 61800)

▶(0399T has been deleted. To report, use 93356)◀

Rationale

Code 0399T has been deleted and converted to Category I code 93356 to report myocardial strain imaging using speckle tracking-derived assessment of myocardial mechanics, when performed. In addition, a deletion parenthetical note has been added in its place and all related parenthetical notes have also been revised.

CPT Changes 2020 — Category III Codes

Refer to the codebook and the Rationale for code 93356 for a full discussion of these changes.

0400T Multi-spectral digital skin lesion analysis of clinically atypical cutaneous pigmented lesions for detection of melanomas and high risk melanocytic atypia; one to five lesions

0401T six or more lesions

(Do not report 0401T in conjunction with 0400T)

▲ **0402T** Collagen cross-linking of cornea, including removal of the corneal epithelium and intraoperative pachymetry, when performed (Report medication separately)

(Do not report 0402T in conjunction with 65435, 69990, 76514)

Rationale

Code 0402T has been revised to state that medication should be reported separately. This revision provides additional language to indicate that the FDA-approved drug utilized as part of this procedure should be reported separately. This revision reflects current practice and clarifies that the drug is not included in this procedure, and is, therefore, not bundled into the CPT code.

0481T Injection(s), autologous white blood cell concentrate (autologous protein solution), any site, including image guidance, harvesting and preparation, when performed

▶(Do not report 0481T in conjunction with 15769, 15771, 15772, 15773, 15774, 20550, 20551, 20600, 20604, 20605, 20606, 20610, 20611, 36415, 36592, 76942, 77002, 77012, 77021, 86965, 0232T)◀

(Do not report 38220, 38221, 38222, 38230 for bone marrow aspiration for autologous white blood cell concentrate [autologous protein solution] injection. For bone marrow aspiration for autologous white blood cell concentrate [autologous protein solution] injection, use 0481T)

Rationale

In accordance with the deletion of code 20926 and the addition of codes 15769, 15771, 15772, 15773, and 15774, the parenthetical note following code 0481T has been revised to remove the deleted code from its listing and to add the new tissue and fat grafting codes.

Refer to the codebook and the Rationale for code 20926 and codes 15769, 15771, 15772, 15773, and 15774 for a full discussion of these changes.

▶(0482T has been deleted)◀

▶(For absolute quantitation of myocardial blood flow [AQMBF] for cardiac PET, use 78434)◀

Rationale

Code 0482T has been deleted and a new Category I code 78434 has been added to report absolute quantitation of myocardial blood flow positron emission tomography (PET) at rest and stress. In addition, a parenthetical note to instruct the use of code 78434 has been added.

Refer to the codebook and the Rationale for code 78434 for a full discussion of these changes.

Codes 0483T, 0484T include vascular access, catheterization, balloon valvuloplasty, deploying the valve, repositioning the valve as needed, temporary pacemaker insertion for rapid pacing, and access site closure, when performed.

Angiography, radiological supervision and interpretation, intraprocedural roadmapping (eg, contrast injections, fluoroscopy) to guide the TMVI, left ventriculography (eg, to assess mitral regurgitation for guidance of TMVI), and completion angiography are included in codes 0483T, 0484T.

Diagnostic right and left heart catheterization codes (93451, 93452, 93453, 93456, 93457, 93458, 93459, 93460, 93461, 93530, 93531, 93532, 93533) should **not** be used with 0483T, 0484T to report:

1. contrast injections, angiography, roadmapping, and/or fluoroscopic guidance for the transcatheter mitral valve implantation (TMVI),
2. left ventricular angiography to assess or confirm valve positioning and function,
3. right and left heart catheterization for hemodynamic measurements before, during, and after TMVI for guidance of TMVI.

Diagnostic right and left heart catheterization codes (93451, 93452, 93453, 93456, 93457, 93458, 93459, 93460, 93461, 93530, 93531, 93532, 93533) and diagnostic coronary angiography codes (93454, 93455, 93456, 93457, 93458, 93459, 93460, 93461, 93563, 93564) performed at the time of TMVI may be separately reportable, if:

1. no prior study is available and a full diagnostic study is performed, or
2. a prior study is available, but as documented in the medical record:

Category III Codes

a. there is inadequate visualization of the anatomy and/or pathology, or

b. the patient's condition with respect to the clinical indication has changed since the prior study, or

c. there is a clinical change during the procedure that requires new evaluation.

For same session/same day diagnostic cardiac catheterization services, report the appropriate diagnostic cardiac catheterization code(s) appended with modifier 59, indicating separate and distinct procedural service from TMVI.

When cardiopulmonary bypass is performed in conjunction with TMVI, 0483T, 0484T may be reported with the appropriate add-on code for percutaneous peripheral bypass (33367), open peripheral bypass (33368), or central bypass (33369).

▶For percutaneous transcatheter tricuspid valve annulus reconstruction, with implantation of adjustable annulus reconstruction device, use 0545T.◀

0483T Transcatheter mitral valve implantation/replacement (TMVI) with prosthetic valve; percutaneous approach, including transseptal puncture, when performed

▶(For transcatheter mitral valve annulus reconstruction, use 0544T)◀

▶(For transcatheter mitral valve repair percutaneous approach including transseptal puncture when performed, see 33418, 33419)◀

▶(For transcatheter mitral valve repair percutaneous approach via the coronary sinus, use 0345T)◀

0484T transthoracic exposure (eg, thoracotomy, transapical)

Rationale

Guidelines and multiple cross-reference parenthetical notes have been placed before and after code 0483T to direct users to the appropriate codes for reporting percutaneous transcatheter tricuspid valve annulus reconstruction with implantation of an adjustable annulus reconstruction device (0545T), mitral valve annulus reconstruction (0544T), percutaneous transcatheter mitral valve repair completed with transseptal puncture (33418, 33419), and percutaneous transcatheter mitral valve repair done via coronary sinus approach (0345T).

Refer to the codebook and the Rationale for codes 0544T and 0545T for a full discussion of these changes.

0487T Biomechanical mapping, transvaginal, with report

0488T Code is out of numerical sequence. See 0402T-0405T

0489T Autologous adipose-derived regenerative cell therapy for scleroderma in the hands; adipose tissue harvesting, isolation and preparation of harvested cells including incubation with cell dissociation enzymes, removal of non-viable cells and debris, determination of concentration and dilution of regenerative cells

▶(Do not report 0489T in conjunction with 15769, 15771, 15772, 15773, 15774, 15876, 15877, 15878, 15879, 20600, 20604)◀

0490T multiple injections in one or both hands

▶(Do not report 0490T in conjunction with 15769, 15771, 15772, 15773, 15774, 15876, 15877, 15878, 15879, 20600, 20604)◀

(Do not report 0490T for a single injection)

(For complete procedure, use 0490T in conjunction with 0489T)

Rationale

In accordance with the deletion of code 20926 and the addition of codes 15769, 15771, 15772, 15773, and 15774, the parenthetical notes following codes 0489T and 0490T have been revised to remove the deleted code from the listing and to add the new tissue and fat grafting codes.

Refer to the codebook and the Rationale for code 20926 and codes 15769, 15771, 15772, 15773, and 15774 for a full discussion of these changes.

0541T Myocardial imaging by magnetocardiography (MCG) for detection of cardiac ischemia, by signal acquisition using minimum 36 channel grid, generation of magnetic-field time-series images, quantitative analysis of magnetic dipoles, machine learning–derived clinical scoring, and automated report generation, single study;

0542T interpretation and report

●**0543T** Transapical mitral valve repair, including transthoracic echocardiography, when performed, with placement of artificial chordae tendineae

▶(For transesophageal echocardiography image guidance, use 93355)◀

Rationale

Code 0543T has been established to report transapical mitral valve repair, including transthoracic echocardiography when performed, with placement of artificial chordae tendineae. In addition, a parenthetical note has been added to direct users to report the appropriate code.

Existing codes for mitral valve repair refer to the approach for the procedure using traditional "open" or "transcatheter" approaches. However, there was no code that specifically described the transapical approach mitral valve repair without use of cardiopulmonary bypass. The absence of provision of cardiopulmonary bypass and the transapical approach for accomplishing the mitral valve repair inherently change the work being performed. As a result, code 0543T has been established to allow reporting for this procedure. A cross-reference parenthetical note has been added following code 0543T to direct users to the appropriate code (93355) to report transesophageal echocardiography (TEE) image guidance. The cross-reference parenthetical note (in combination with the code descriptor) provides additional instruction regarding imaging guidance that is inherently included (transthoracic echocardiography [TTE]) vs imaging that is separately reportable (TEE).

Clinical Example (0543T)

A 58-year-old male diagnosed with severe degenerative mitral valve regurgitation (insufficiency) due to mitral valve prolapse involving the posterior leaflet secondary to elongated or ruptured native mitral chords (chordae tendineae) presents for transapical mitral valve repair with placement of artificial chordae tendineae.

Description of Procedure (0543T)

Under general anesthesia, expose the heart via thoracotomy, open the pericardium, and insert a soft tissue retractor to maximize access to the heart. Transthoracic echocardiography (TTE) (typically performed by the primary surgeon) is used to guide proper location of the thoracotomy. Pass a transesophageal echocardiography (TEE) probe and use it throughout the procedure (report separately by a different provider, eg cardiac anesthesiologist or cardiologist). On the beating heart, place concentric pledgeted sutures around the identified target entry location in the left ventricle. Insert a custom introducer into the ventricle using standard techniques. Insert the shaft of the hemostatic delivery system via a Seldinger technique and navigate under TEE guidance to the targeted location on the underside of the prolapsed mitral valve leaflet. The delivery system houses an artificial cord (eg, ePTFE, expanded polytetrafluoroethylene) wrapped around a needle in a preformed knot. Once the tip of the device is properly positioned on the edge of the prolapsing mitral leaflet, attach the artificial cord to the prolapsing leaflet and deploy a preformed knot. Slowly withdraw the delivery system from the heart and discard. Repeat the procedure sequence until the appropriate number (typically 3 to 5) of artificial cords have been implanted into the prolapsing leaflet. Once complete, remove the introducer, tighten the concentric sutures, and secure hemostasis. Under TEE guidance adjust the length of each artificial cord to minimize mitral regurgitation. Once properly adjusted, tie each of the artificial cords over a pledget. Place chest tube(s). Close the incision in layers and place dressings.

►Codes 0544T and 0545T include vascular access, catheterization, deploying and adjusting the reconstruction device(s), temporary pacemaker insertion for rapid pacing if required, and access site closure, when performed.

Angiography, radiological supervision and interpretation, intraprocedural roadmapping (eg, contrast injections, fluoroscopy) to guide the device implantation, ventriculography (eg, to assess target valve regurgitation for guidance of device implantation and adjustment), and completion angiography are included in 0544T and 0545T.

Diagnostic right and left heart catheterization codes (93451, 93452, 93453, 93454, 93455, 93456, 93457, 93458, 93459, 93460, 93461, 93530, 93531, 93532, 93533, 93565, 93566) may not be used in conjunction with 0544T, 0545T to report:

1. contrast injections, angiography, road-mapping, and/or fluoroscopic guidance for the implantation and adjustment of the transcatheter mitral or tricuspid valve annulus reconstruction device, or

2. right or left ventricular angiography to assess or confirm transcatheter mitral or tricuspid valve annulus reconstruction device positioning and function, or

3. right and left heart catheterization for hemodynamic measurements before, during, and after transcatheter mitral or tricuspid valve annulus reconstruction for guidance.

Diagnostic right and left heart catheterization codes (93451, 93452, 93453, 93456, 93457, 93458, 93459, 93460, 93461, 93530, 93531, 93532, 93533) and diagnostic coronary angiography codes (93454, 93455, 93456, 93457, 93458, 93459, 93460, 93461, 93563, 93564) performed at the time of transcatheter mitral or tricuspid valve annulus reconstruction may be separately reportable if:

1. no prior study is available and a full diagnostic study is performed, or

2. a prior study is available, but as documented in the medical record:

   a. there is inadequate visualization of the anatomy and/or pathology, or

b. the patient's condition with respect to the clinical indication has changed since the prior study, or

c. there is a clinical change during the procedure that requires new evaluation.

Other cardiac catheterization services may be reported separately, when performed for diagnostic purposes not intrinsic to the transcatheter mitral valve annulus reconstruction.

For same session/same day diagnostic cardiac catheterization services, report the appropriate diagnostic cardiac catheterization code(s) appended with modifier 59 indicating separate and distinct procedural service from transcatheter mitral or tricuspid valve annulus reconstruction.

Percutaneous coronary interventional procedures may be reported separately, when performed.

When cardiopulmonary bypass is performed in conjunction with transcatheter mitral valve or tricuspid valve annulusreconstruction, 0544T, 0545T should bereported with the appropriate add-on code for percutaneous peripheral bypass (33367), open peripheral bypass (33368), or central bypass (33369).

When transcatheter ventricular support is required, the appropriate code may be reported with the appropriate ventricular assist device (VAD) procedure (33990, 33991, 33992, 33993) or balloon pump insertion (33967, 33970, 33973).

For percutaneous transcatheter mitral valve repair, use 0345T. For percutaneous transcatheter mitral valve implantation/replacement (TMVI) with prosthetic valve, use 0483T.◄

● **0544T** Transcatheter mitral valve annulus reconstruction, with implantation of adjustable annulus reconstruction device, percutaneous approach including transseptal puncture

▶(For transcatheter mitral valve repair percutaneous approach including transseptal puncture when performed, see 33418, 33419)◄

▶(For transcatheter mitral valve repair percutaneous approach via the coronary sinus, use 0345T)◄

▶(For transcatheter mitral valve implantation/replacement [TMVI] with prosthetic valve percutaneous approach, use 0483T)◄

● **0545T** Transcatheter tricuspid valve annulus reconstruction with implantation of adjustable annulus reconstruction device, percutaneous approach

▶(Do not report 0544T, 0545T in conjunction with 76000)◄

▶(Do not report 0544T, 0545T in conjunction with 93451, 93452, 93453, 93456, 93457, 93458, 93459, 93460, 93461, 93530, 93531, 93532, 93533, 93565, 93566 for diagnostic left and right heart catheterization procedures intrinsic to the annular repair procedure)◄

▶(Do not report 0544T, 0545T in conjunction with 93454, 93455, 93456, 93457, 93458, 93459, 93460, 93461, 93563, 93564 for coronary angiography procedures intrinsic to the annular repair procedure)◄

Rationale

New Category III codes (0544T, 0545T), new guidelines and instructions, and new cross-references and exclusionary parenthetical notes have been added to the Category III section to identify percutaneous transcatheter mitral and tricuspid valve annulus reconstruction procedures with implantation of an adjustable annulus reconstruction device. Changes have also been made throughout the Surgery and Medicine sections to accommodate the addition of the new codes for these services.

Codes 0544T and 0545T were developed to identify percutaneous valve annuloplasty reconstruction procedures performed for the mitral and tricuspid valves. These services are differentiated from other existing mitral and tricuspid valve procedures in that they are percutaneous versus open and are for mitral or tricuspid valve annulus reconstruction versus repair. As a result, cross-reference parenthetical notes have been placed in key areas to direct users to the appropriate codes to use depending on the procedure being performed.

However, these codes also inherently include component services that are included with other mitral and tricuspid valve procedures. This includes catheterizations necessary to access the anatomy for the procedure, deploy the device, and temporary pacemaker insertion done for rapid pacing when needed, as well as site closure when performed; the use of radiological supervision and interpretation; intraprocedural road-mapping to guide the device implantation; ventriculography for assessing target valve regurgitation, for guidance of device implantation, and adjustment of the device; completion of angiography; diagnostic cardiac catheterization codes to report contrast injections, angiography, road-mapping, and/or fluoroscopy for implantation and adjustment of the device; angiography to assess/confirm device positioning and function; and catheterization done for hemodynamic measurement before, during, and after reconstruction for guidance. When these procedures are done to accomplish mitral/tricuspid valve reconstruction, no additional codes should be reported.

Other similarities to other existing mitral and tricuspid valve procedures are instructions that provide guidance regarding when separate left/right heart cauterization services are appropriate for separate reporting, such as when no prior study is available and a full diagnostic study is performed, or when an available prior study does not serve the purpose needed, such as to adequately visualize the anatomy and pathology within the heart, when the patient's condition has changed since the last documented catheterization, and/or when a new evaluation is necessary because of a change in the clinical circumstances during the procedure.

As a result, the code language, guidelines, and parenthetical notes have all been developed to instruct users of services that are inherently included as part of the reconstruction/implantation procedure and not separately reported. These instructions have been included throughout the code set, both in the Category III section and in other sections of the book where related code instructions are needed to eliminate confusion regarding appropriate reporting for these services. This includes placement of cross-reference and exclusionary parenthetical notes to direct users to appropriate codes for these or other services that better identify the procedure being performed and to restrict reporting of services that are inherently included and should not be reported in conjunction with one another. Instructions have also been provided to direct reporting when other reportable service codes may be used in place of or in conjunction with these services. This includes direction regarding modifier use to further validate or otherwise provide information regarding reporting and listings of the specific codes that may be reported for various additionally reportable procedures.

Clinical Example (0544T)

A 67-year-old female presents with progressive shortness of breath and established symptomatic heart failure despite guideline-directed medical therapy. Echocardiography demonstrates chronic functional or secondary mitral regurgitation (≥+3). She is considered high risk for mitral valve surgery due to multiple comorbidities.

Description of Procedure (0544T)

Following percutaneous puncture of the femoral vein, the left atrium (LA) is accessed using standard transvenous, transseptal equipment and an extra stiff guidewire is placed in the LA. Echocardiography or fluoroscopy is used for guidance and observation. A dilator of 18 French (18Fr) or wider is used to pre-dilate femoral access. Standard heart catheterization procedures are used to insert the transseptal steerable sheath (TSS). The tip of the TSS is steered into the LA under transesophageal echocardiography (TEE) or fluoroscopy guidance, and the guidewire is left in the LA to confirm the tip of the TSS is across the septum using TEE. Prior to implantation of the first anchor, verification is obtained that TEE imaging adequately supports the implantation. The implant catheter (IC) tip is navigated to the anterior lateral commissure using 3-dimensional (3D) TEE. The size adjustment tool (SAT) leading wire is gently pulled back from the guide catheter (GC) handle in order to place the adjustment mechanism as proximal as possible from the implant tip. The tip of the IC is positioned in the first deployment site, anterior to the commissure. Echocardiography under 2-dimensional plane view is used to verify tissue contact and the angle between the IC and the annulus plane. The first anchor is deployed by rotating the torque limiter clockwise under imaging guidance until the anchor is fully out from the implant. The system is navigated along the annulus to the next anchoring location by using left anterior oblique (LAO) fluoroscopy and 3D echocardiography. Anchor deployment steps are repeated until all necessary anchors have been implanted. After deployment of the last anchor, the implant is disengaged and released from the catheter and the catheter is carefully removed using fluoroscopic guidance. Implant adjustment is optimized by assessing mitral regurgitation, measuring after each degree of reduction, and allowing four minutes waiting time between one reduction degree to another. The TSS is steered to a straight position and retracted into the right atrium (RA), then carefully removed from the body.

Clinical Example (0545T)

A 75-year-old female presents with progressive shortness of breath and established symptomatic heart failure despite guideline-directed medical therapy. Echocardiography demonstrates chronic functional or secondary tricuspid regurgitation (2+-4+) with annular diameter ≥40 mm with systolic pulmonary pressure ≤60 mmHg and left ventricular ejection fraction (LVEF) ≥30%. She is considered high risk for tricuspid valve surgery due to multiple comorbidities.

Description of Procedure (0545T)

Select implant size based on preoperative measurement of the tricuspid annulus size using cardiac computed tomography (CT) scan. Following percutaneous puncture of the femoral vein, access the RA using standard transvenous, transfemoral equipment. Use TEE or fluoroscopy for guidance and observation. Use a dilator of 18Fr or wider to pre-dilate femoral access. Use standard heart catheterization procedures to insert the TSS with the dilator through the femoral vein and over a high support guidewire that was previously deployed up to the RA. Prior to implantation of the first anchor, verify that TEE imaging adequately supports the implantation. Navigate the IC tip to the anterior leaflet, anterior to the aortic root segment, using fluoroscopic projections (LAO). Gently pull back the SAT leading wire from the guide catheter (GC) handle in order to place the adjustment mechanism as proximal as possible from the implant tip. Position the tip of the IC in the first deployment site, on the annulus of the anterior leaflet segment, anterior to the aortic root. Use

Category III Codes

echocardiography under 2D plane view and fluoroscopy under perpendicular (RAO) view to verify tissue contact and the angle between the IC and the annulus plane. Deploy the first anchor by rotating the torque limiter clockwise under imaging guidance until the anchor is fully out from the implant. Navigate the system along the annulus to the next anchoring location by using LAO fluoroscopy and 3D echo. Repeat anchor deployment steps until all necessary anchors have been implanted. After deployment of the last anchor, disengage the implant and release from the catheter. Optimize implant adjustment by assessing tricuspid regurgitation, measuring after each degree of reduction, and allowing four minutes waiting time between one reduction degree to the next. Release the SAT and implant guidewire from the implant. Retract the SAT into the TSS and remove. Retract the TSS into the RA, unlock from the stand, and carefully remove from the body.

●0546T   Radiofrequency spectroscopy, real time, intraoperative margin assessment, at the time of partial mastectomy, with report

▶(Use 0546T only once for each partial mastectomy site)◀

▶(Do not report 0546T for re-excision)◀

Rationale

Category III code 0546T has been established for reporting real-time radiofrequency (RF) spectroscopy for intraoperative margin assessment at the time of a partial mastectomy. This procedure is performed at the time of partial mastectomy (eg, lumpectomy) as described by Category I codes 19301, 19302 to identify any remaining cancerous tissue at the margins of the partial mastectomy site. It is important to note that RF spectroscopy as described by code 0546T is intended to be performed once per partial mastectomy site. It is not intended to be performed on additional margins or re-excision of the same partial mastectomy site. Parenthetical notes have been added following code 0546T to clarify this.

Clinical Example (0546T)

A 65-year-old female, who is undergoing breast conserving surgery to remove the cancerous lesion in her breast, during partial mastectomy (eg, lumpectomy) requires an additional procedure in which her ex-vivo lumpectomy specimen is evaluated using radiofrequency spectroscopy to assess the surgical margins for microscopic disease during surgery.

Description of Procedure (0546T)

In the operating room following partial mastectomy, after the cancerous tumor specimen is removed, physician assesses the specimen margins for microscopic residual disease using radiofrequency spectroscopy. Confirm probe-to-console attachment and console calibration. Using the sterile, disposable, radiofrequency spectroscopy probe, position the probe face perpendicular to each of the six-specimen tissue faces (lateral, medial, anterior, superior, inferior, and posterior) of the main tumor or partial mastectomy specimen. Identify probe-to-tissue contact by the system, allowing a measurement only when the probe ensures adequate tissue contact with the sensor. Continue measurements until the entire specimen's surface has been fully assessed. Review the binary data provided on the console screen once all specimen measurements have been completed. Device-positive findings displayed on the radiofrequency spectroscopy console screen inform an immediate surgical decision to take a directed cavity excision (or shaving) from the partial mastectomy cavity. Dictate report of radiofrequency spectroscopy assessment findings, including all device-identified positive margins, and surgeon response (eg, anterior device positive margin was excised) for the medical record.

●0547T   Bone-material quality testing by microindentation(s) of the tibia(s), with results reported as a score

Rationale

Code 0547T has been established to report bone material quality testing by microindentation of the tibia. This emerging technology is typically performed in an office setting and involves work by the physician that includes an overall assessment of a patient's bone health. The procedure described in code 0547T reflects current practice not previously described in the CPT code set.

Clinical Example (0547T)

A 65-year-old female with a five-year history of type 2 diabetes (T2D) has sustained a peripheral fracture. The physician suspects that her bone quality may be poor and performs a touch biopsy to assess her bone material quality.

Description of Procedure (0547T)

Disinfect the midshaft of the left or right tibia. Apply a local anesthetic. Load a single-use sterile tip to the device and insert the tip through the skin to the tibial surface. Perform multiple measurements in a 1- to 2-cm area. After 10 valid measurements are obtained, remove the tip from the skin and, optionally, place a small adhesive bandage over the measurement site. Then measure a reference material to complete the calculation of the patient's bone quality measure. Results are displayed immediately to the physician. Review the result and based on training, incorporate it into decision making.

● **0548T** Transperineal periurethral balloon continence device; bilateral placement, including cystoscopy and fluoroscopy

● **0549T** unilateral placement, including cystoscopy and fluoroscopy

● **0550T** removal, each balloon

● **0551T** adjustment of balloon(s) fluid volume

▶(Do not report 0551T in conjunction with 0548T, 0549T, 0550T)◀

Rationale

In the Category III code section, four new Category III codes (0548T, 0549T, 0550T, 0551T) have been added to report transperineal periurethral balloon continence device procedures. In addition, a parenthetical note has also been added following code 0551T to restrict reporting of this service with the other new codes.

Currently codes exist in the CPT code set to describe the insertion, removal, replacement, and repair of an artificial urinary sphincter. In addition, more codes exist in the CPT code set to further describe the placement, removal, and revision of a male mesh sling. However, no codes exist to describe transperineal periurethral balloon continence device procedures. Code 0548T is used to report bilateral placement of this device and includes cystoscopy and fluoroscopy. The additional codes (0549T, 0550T, 0551T) are used to report specific procedures that may be performed for this device. For example, if balloon removal is performed, code 0550T should be reported for each balloon removal. An exclusionary parenthetical note has been added following code 0551T to restrict reporting codes for transperineal periurethral balloon continence device bilateral placement (0548T), unilateral placement (0549T), and balloon removal (0550T) in conjunction with adjustment of balloon(s) fluid volume (0551T).

Clinical Example (0548T)

A 70-year-old male underwent radical prostatectomy four years ago. His prostate-specific antigen is undetectable; however, he has intractable stress incontinence secondary to intrinsic sphincter deficiency and has failed all conservative measures. After appropriate counseling it was decided that he would not be a good candidate for an artificial urinary sphincter or male sling; therefore, it was elected to perform transperineal implantation of two permanent adjustable balloon continence devices.

Description of Procedure (0548T)

After induction of general anesthesia, sterilely prepare and drape the patient's perineum. Perform cystoscopy to evaluate the urethra and bladder neck. Remove the cystoscopy lens with the cystoscope sheath in place and fill the bladder with contrast and saline. Prime the adjustable continence device with isotonic solution, emptied and submerged in antibiotic solution. Make two 0.5-cm incisions on either side of the midline of the perineum. Direct the sharp trocar with a mated U-channel sheath toward the bladder neck under fluoroscopy, using the cystoscopy sheath as a urethral landmark for balloon placement at the bladder neck. Remove the sharp trocar and replace it with the blunt trocar to dilate the last 0.5 cm to minimize the risk of bladder or urethral perforation. Remove the balloon device from the antibiotic solution and push the push wire to the tip of the balloon. Lubricate the device and slide into the U-channel sheath trough up to the bladder neck. Once the balloon is in the correct position and confirmed by fluoroscopic imaging, pull back the U-channel sheath 2 cm, keeping the balloon at the bladder neck. Inflate the device with 1.0 mL of isotonic contrast solution by inserting the provided needle into the device port. Re-check device positioning using fluoroscopy. Remove the U-channel sheath. Re-confirm the balloon's position to be correct by fluoroscopy. Then repeat the procedure on the contralateral side. Remove the push wires from both balloon devices. Use forceps to create a subcutaneous pocket from the perineal skin incision to the posterolateral wall of the scrotum. Place the ports in this pocket and close the perineal wound with two layers of absorbable sutures. Perform a second cystoscopy to access any possible urethral or bladder injury and then remove it.

Clinical Example (0549T)

A 70-year-old male with post-prostatectomy urinary stress incontinence underwent implantation of two permanent adjustable balloon devices one year ago, followed by removal of the left balloon ten months later due to balloon migration and recurrence of his incontinence. After sufficient healing, he has elected to undergo reimplantation of a single permanent adjustable balloon continence device on the left side.

Description of Procedure (0549T)

After induction of general anesthesia, sterilely prepare and drape the patient's perineum. Perform cystoscopy to evaluate the urethra and bladder neck. Remove the cystoscopy lens with the cystoscope sheath in place and fill the bladder with contrast and saline. Prime the adjustable continence device with isotonic solution, emptied and submerged in antibiotic solution. Make a perineal 0.5-cm incision on one side. Direct the sharp trocar with a mated U-channel sheath toward the bladder neck under fluoroscopy, using the cystoscopy sheath as a urethral landmark for balloon placement at the bladder neck. Remove the sharp trocar and replace with the blunt trocar to dilate the last 0.5 cm to minimize the risk of bladder or urethral perforation. Remove the balloon device from the antibiotic solution and push the push wire to the tip of the balloon. Lubricate the device and slide into the U-channel sheath trough up to the bladder neck. Once the balloon is in the correct position, confirmed by fluoroscopic imaging, pull back the U-channel sheath 2 cm, keeping the balloon at the bladder neck. Inflate the device with 1.0 ml of isotonic contrast solution by inserting the provided needle into the device port. Re-check the device positioning using fluoroscopy. Remove the U-channel sheath. Re-confirm the balloon's position to be correct by fluoroscopy and remove the push wire. Use forceps to create a subcutaneous pocket from the perineal skin incision to the posterolateral wall of the scrotum. Place the port in this pocket and close the perineal wound with two layers of absorbable sutures. Perform a second cystoscopy to access any possible urethral or bladder injury and then remove it.

Clinical Example (0550T)

A 65-year-old male with post-prostatectomy urinary stress incontinence underwent implantation of two permanent adjustable balloon continence devices two years ago with excellent initial results. Approximately six months ago, he noted sudden recurrence of his incontinence. An abdominal X ray shows absence of the left balloon consistent with slow leak because the patient denies any trauma. He undergoes removal of the left balloon.

Description of Procedure (0550T)

Place the patient in the dorsal decubitus position and sterilely prepare and drape his perineum. Palpate the titanium port of the left-sided balloon through the skin for localization. Use lidocaine 1% for local anesthesia. Make a small skin incision over the port and through the subcutaneous tissue until the port is easily found. Using a 10-cc syringe and a 23-gauge (g) needle, remove any residual fluid from the left balloon. Once all liquid is removed from the balloon, place gentle traction on the port and tubing and explant the balloon. Close the skin and subcutaneous tissue with absorbable sutures.

Clinical Example (0551T)

A 66-year-old male with post-prostatectomy urinary stress incontinence underwent implantation of two permanent adjustable balloon continence devices six weeks ago. Postoperatively his continence is improved; however, he still has bothersome leakage. In the office, he will undergo addition of fluid to both balloons to increase urethral resistance and decrease urinary leakage.

Description of Procedure (0551T)

Place the patient in the dorsal decubitus position and sterilely prepare and drape his perineum. Palpate the titanium port through the skin for localization. Use lidocaine 1% for local anesthesia. Fill a 10-cc syringe with isotonic fluid and use a 23-g needle to puncture the septum contained in the titanium port. Once the needle is deep enough within the septum, add 0.5 to 1.0 cc to the balloon. Then repeat this on the contralateral balloon as well. Permit the patient to leave the office once he is able to void without significant leakage.

● **0552T** Low-level laser therapy, dynamic photonic and dynamic thermokinetic energies, provided by a physician or other qualified health care professional

Rationale

Code 0552T has been established to report low-level laser therapy provided by a physician or other qualified health care professional. The procedure described in code 0552T includes two forms of energy, dynamic photonic and dynamic thermokinetic.

Clinical Example (0552T)

A 60-year-old female presents herself to a clinic with bilateral knee pain exacerbated by exercise as well as decreased mobility. The patient has been taking nonsteroidal anti-inflammatory drugs (NSAIDs) for five years to control her pain symptoms; however, she requests consideration of alternate therapy because of complications of long-term NSAID use. Her primary care provider examines her knees, asks a series of questions, orders diagnostic X rays, then arrives at the diagnosis of osteoarthritis (OA). Low-level laser therapy is administered.

Description of Procedure (0552T)

Identify the area to be treated. Evaluate the performance and the subjective symptoms of the joint. Explain the device and procedure to the patient. Position the patient appropriately for application of low-level laser therapy. Apply low-level laser therapy to the appropriate area, turn the unit on, and select the proper mode of treatment for the condition. At the conclusion of the 25-minute treatment, remove the laser therapy device. Re-assess the patient's joint for symptoms and performance. If the treatment outcome is favorable, suggest either returning to the clinic for continued treatment, and/or if the patient so desires, arrange for the patient to obtain a unit for home use.

- **0553T** Percutaneous transcatheter placement of iliac arteriovenous anastomosis implant, inclusive of all radiological supervision and interpretation, intraprocedural roadmapping, and imaging guidance necessary to complete the intervention

    ▶(Do not report 0553T in conjunction with 36005, 36011, 36012, 36140, 36245, 36246, 37220, 37221, 37224, 37226, 37238, 37248, 75710, 75820)◀

Rationale

Code 0553T has been added to report percutaneous transcatheter placement of iliac arteriovenous (AV) anastomosis implant. In addition, a parenthetical note has also been added following code 0553T to guide users in the appropriate reporting of these services in conjunction with other services in the CPT code set. Code 0553T is described as transcatheter creation of an iliac AV anastomosis via implant. This code differs from other AV anastomosis procedures since this procedure creates an anastomosis in the iliac vein and artery using an implanted device. Similar to other vascular procedures, this procedure includes: (1) accessing and selectively catheterizing the vessels; (2) supervision and interpretation; (3) closure using any method of the arteriotomy and venotomy; and (4) documenting any imaging being performed for insertion of the implant. An exclusionary parenthetical note has been added to restrict reporting of certain procedures that are inherently included as part of the service.

Clinical Example (0553T)

A 65-year-old male presenting with uncontrolled primary hypertension is on a stable regimen of three antihypertensive drugs, including a calcium channel blocker, an angiotensin-converting-enzyme (ACE) inhibitor, and a diuretic. He elects to have the procedure of a transcatheter placement of iliac arteriovenous anastomosis implant to help reduce his blood pressure.

Description of Procedure (0553T)

Place patient in the supine position and administer anesthesia. Place introducer sheaths in both the right femoral vein and right femoral artery. Under fluoroscopy, mark target implant location in the central iliac artery and vein and insert crossing wire. Advance the implant delivery system from vein to artery and confirm the implant position using fluoroscopy. Deploy the arterial and venous arms of the implant. Dilate the anastomosis using a noncompliant balloon catheter. Conduct angiography to document implant placement. Apply manual compression, closure device, or surgical closure to achieve hemostasis. Dictate a procedure report for the medical record.

- **0554T** Bone strength and fracture risk using finite element analysis of functional data and bone-mineral density utilizing data from a computed tomography scan; retrieval and transmission of the scan data, assessment of bone strength and fracture risk and bone-mineral density, interpretation and report

    ▶(Do not report 0554T in conjunction with 0555T, 0556T, 0557T)◀

- **0555T** retrieval and transmission of the scan data
- **0556T** assessment of bone strength and fracture risk and bone-mineral density
- **0557T** interpretation and report
- **0558T** Computed tomography scan taken for the purpose of biomechanical computed tomography analysis

    ▶(Do not report 0558T in conjunction with 71250, 71260, 71270, 71275, 72125, 72126, 72127, 72128, 72129, 72130, 72131, 72132, 72133, 72191, 72192, 72193, 72194, 74150, 74160, 74170, 74174, 74175, 74176, 74177, 74178, 74261, 74262, 74263, 75571, 75572, 75573, 75574, 75635, 78816)◀

Rationale

Five codes (0554T, 0555T, 0556T, 0557T, 0558T) have been established to report bone strength and fracture risk using finite element analysis.

This code structure provides a comprehensive mechanism to obtain bone mass measurements for diagnosis and management. There are different aspects to reporting biomechanical computed tomography (BCT) and a combination of the services. The aspects are as follows:

- retrieval and transmission of the CT data
- assessment of bone strength and fracture risk and bone mineral density
- interpretation and report or
- a combination of the services

Code 0554T is intended for all aspects of BCT; it includes retrieval and transmission of the data, assessment of bone strength and fracture risk and bone mineral density, interpretation and report. Because code 0554T includes all aspects of BCT, an exclusionary parenthetical has been added to preclude the use of this code with codes 0555T, 0556T, 0557T.

Code 0555T is reported for retrieval and transmission of the scan data. Retrieval and transmission of CT data is unique, it uses previously taken CT scans, which will often have been acquired from a different medical facility than that of the ordering physician and usually weeks or months before the BCT procedure is ordered.

Code 0556T is reported for assessment of bone strength and fracture risk and bone mineral density, and code 0557T includes bone strength and fracture risk using finite element analysis with interpretation and report.

Code 0558T describes a CT scan that is taken for the purpose of the biomechanical study.

Clinical Example (0554T)

A 68-year-old female, based on her age and sex, is at risk of having osteoporosis. She recently had an abdominal CT scan to investigate stomach pain. To obtain a bone mass measurement, her physician orders a biomechanical CT procedure utilizing the separately acquired scan.

Description of Procedure (0554T)

The referring physician places an order with the testing laboratory to perform the biomechanical analysis of the CT scan. The laboratory arranges with the appropriate radiology facility to have the patient's scan retrieved and transmitted to the laboratory for analysis. Technical staff at the laboratory perform the biomechanical CT analysis of the CT scan using specialized analysis software and advanced engineering computation. First, calibrate the scan with a phantomless method utilizing the patient's internal tissues, and then create a biomechanical, finite element structural model of the patient's bone. Using finite element analysis, virtually load the model to failure to provide a measurement of the breaking strength of the patient's bone. Also measure bone mineral density (BMD). The analysis can be performed for the proximal femur, a vertebral body, or both. For the proximal femur, the virtual loading simulates a sideways fall. For the vertebral body, the virtual loading simulates a compressive overload. Compare the measurements of bone strength and BMD against validated clinical thresholds to identify the presence of fragile bone strength and osteoporosis, respectively, and to calculate an overall fracture-risk classification. Collate these data and images in a structured file and send to the qualified health care professional (QHP) for review and interpretation. Considering also any relevant patient factors, any prior bone density or bone strength reports if available, and practice guidelines, the QHP interprets this collective information, explains any discordance between bone density and bone strength results, may use fracture-risk calculators to combine clinical risk factors with the hip BMD T-score to calculate a fracture-risk value, and dictates a medical report.

Clinical Example (0555T)

A 68-year-old female, based on her age and sex, is at risk of having osteoporosis. She recently had an abdominal CT scan to investigate stomach pain. To obtain a bone mass measurement, her physician orders a biomechanical CT procedure utilizing the separately acquired scan.

Description of Procedure (0555T)

Upon receiving an order, the laboratory arranges with the appropriate radiology facility to have the patient's scan retrieved and transmitted to the laboratory for analysis.

Clinical Example (0556T)

A 68-year-old female, based on her age and sex, is at risk of having osteoporosis. She recently had an abdominal CT scan to investigate stomach pain. To obtain a bone mass measurement, her physician orders a biomechanical CT procedure utilizing the separately acquired scan.

Description of Procedure (0556T)

After receiving a patient's scan, technical staff at the laboratory perform the biomechanical CT analysis of the CT scan using specialized analysis software and advanced engineering computation. First, calibrate the scan with a phantomless method utilizing the patient's internal tissues, and then create a biomechanical, finite element structural model of the patient's bone. Using finite element analysis, virtually load the model to failure to provide a measurement of the breaking strength of the patient's bone. Also measure a BMD. The analysis can be performed for the proximal femur, a vertebral body, or both. For the proximal femur, the virtual loading simulates a sideways fall. For the vertebral body, the virtual loading simulates a compressive overload. Compare the measurements of bone strength and BMD against validated clinical thresholds to identify the presence of fragile bone strength and osteoporosis, respectively, and to calculate an overall fracture-risk classification. Collate these data and images in a structured file and send to the QHP for review and interpretation.

Clinical Example (0557T)

A 68-year-old female, based on her age and sex, is at risk of having osteoporosis. She recently had an abdominal CT scan to investigate stomach pain. To obtain a bone mass measurement, her physician orders a biomechanical CT procedure utilizing the separately acquired scan.

Description of Procedure (0557T)

After receiving the results from the biomechanical CT analysis, and considering also any relevant patient factors, any prior bone density or bone strength reports if available, and practice guidelines, interpret this collective information, explain any discordance between bone density and bone strength results, perhaps use fracture-risk calculators to combine clinical risk factors with the hip BMD T-score to calculate a fracture-risk value, and dictate a medical report.

Clinical Example (0558T)

A 68-year-old female has not had a bone mass measurement in the previous five years. Her primary care physician orders a CT scan of the pelvis without contrast solely for the purpose of biomechanical modeling of bone strength, measurement of bone density, and fracture-risk assessment.

Description of Procedure (0558T)

Determine the appropriate CT protocol for the examination and communicate it to the CT technologists. Acquisition settings for a typical abdominal or spine CT examination can be used, with a large field of view and 1-mm axial slice spacing in the reconstruction. An external calibration phantom is not necessary. Review scout radiographs. Review the initial and subsequent series of CT image data to confirm the adequacy of anatomic coverage and assess the need for repeat sections. Review the scans for abnormalities and prepare a diagnostic report.

►Codes 0559T, 0560T represent production of 3D-printed models of individually prepared and processed components of structures of anatomy. These individual components of structures of anatomy include, but are not limited to, bones, arteries, veins, nerves, ureters, muscles, tendons and ligaments, joints, visceral organs, and brain. Each 3D-printed anatomic model of a structure can be made up of one or more separate components. The 3D anatomic printings can be 3D printed in unique colors and/or materials.

Codes 0561T, 0562T represent the production of 3D-printed cutting or drilling guides using individualized imaging data. 3D-printed guides are cutting or drilling tools used during surgery and are 3D printed so that they precisely fit an individual patient's anatomy to guide the surgery. A cutting guide does not have multiple parts, but instead is a unique single tool. It may be necessary to make a 3D-printed model and a 3D-printed cutting or drilling guide on the same patient to assist with surgery.◄

● 0559T Anatomic model 3D-printed from image data set(s); first individually prepared and processed component of an anatomic structure

+● 0560T each additional individually prepared and processed component of an anatomic structure (List separately in addition to code for primary procedure)

►(Use 0560T in conjunction with 0559T)◄

►(Do not report 0559T, 0560T in conjunction with 76376, 76377)◄

● 0561T Anatomic guide 3D-printed and designed from image data set(s); first anatomic guide

+● 0562T each additional anatomic guide (List separately in addition to code for primary procedure)

►(Use 0562T in conjunction with 0561T)◄

►(Do not report 0561T, 0562T in conjunction with 76376, 76377)◄

Rationale

Four new codes (0559T, 0560T, 0561T, 0562T) have been added with accompanying guidelines and parenthetical notes to identify anatomic model 3D printing. This includes addition of the new codes to existing parenthetical language in the Diagnostic Radiology subsection to accommodate the addition of the new codes.

Two different sets of codes have been developed to represent the procedures for 3D printing: anatomic models and anatomic guides. Three-dimensional printed models allow surgeons and/or interventionalists to anticipate and plan for intraprocedural needs and requirements for safe outcomes. Three-dimensional printed models offer a framework of the patient's complex anatomy and help the surgeon appreciate depth, angles, and contours to aid in presurgical decision making. The effort of making 3D models is separate for each individual component of structure of anatomy. Therefore, each component represents separate work to create.

Model development is intended to increase safety, decrease surgical risk, potentially decrease time in surgery, and improve outcomes. These anatomic models are used as a reference during surgery. For example, a model of the kidney with a tumor, parenchyma, collecting system, and vessels would be represented as individually prepared and processed components of the patient's anatomic structure as these are frequently performed from different data sets, ie, arterial phase of enhancement for arteries, venous phase for parenchyma and veins, and delayed phase imaging for collecting system. Making a 3D-printed model of the renal parenchyma alone, or a kidney and renal pelvis/ureter, is substantially less work than making a kidney with a tumor in the parenchyma and demonstrating the relationship of the tumor to the collecting system and vessels. As a result, each component (ie, building block of the final printed product to help an intervention) is separately reportable for data collection so that the typical number of components for a structure may be determined, for example, for a patient with kidney cancer. Therefore, to adequately represent the efforts and analysis conducted to develop each component, reporting has been developed to identify these individual components using code 0559T for the first individually prepared and processed component and code 0560T for each additional component.

This is different from the development of 3D guides. Although also made using individualized imaging data, guides do not reflect patient anatomy and thus are not anatomic parts. Instead, they are cutting tools used during surgery and are 3D-printed so that they precisely fit an individual patient's anatomy to guide the surgery. As a result, these components are separately developed from 3D-printed models and are separately represented using code 0561T for the first component and code 0562T for each additional component.

The guidelines included for these services help users to understand the differences between "anatomic models" and "anatomic guides." In addition, the parenthetical notes following codes 0560T and 0562T provide instruction to users regarding use of the add-on codes and exclusion from reporting these codes in conjunction with 3D imaging codes. This instruction has also been included following the 3D-rendering section codes 76376 and 76377.

Clinical Example (0559T)

A 7-year-old male presents with long segment scoliosis secondary to multiple congenital vertebral anomalies. Complex pedicle screw and posterior rod placement is necessary to improve the spinal curvature and prevent progression. A life-size physical anatomic model is created to plan the surgical approach and guide pedicle screw placement. The model is used to obtain consent from the parents and as reference during surgery.

Description of Procedure (0559T)

Conduct an initial consultation with the requesting physician or other QHP to discuss the requested model. This discussion includes the clinical scenario, surgical needs, and critical anatomy needed in the model. Review imaging data to determine if it is adequate to use to create an accurate model. Then export the image data to dedicated segmentation software, where a physician or QHP separates the boney spine from adjacent anatomy. Export the final segmented data of the anatomic part of the spine into a computer-aided design (CAD) file format, where it undergoes further processing to meet technical requirements for 3D printing. Digitally imprint a unique patient identifier on the model. Send the file to the 3D printer, where materials and color are assigned before printing. After printing, clean the model and post process as needed.

Perform a final consultation with the radiologist to review the anatomic relationships demonstrated in the model along with limitations encountered in model design. Photograph the model and place the image in the patient's electronic medical record.

Clinical Example (0560T)

A 12-month-old female with stridor and difficulty feeding is diagnosed with a double aortic arch and complete cartilaginous rings. In addition to the printed 3D physical anatomic model of the aorta and great vessels (separately reported with code 0559T), physical anatomic models of the airways are printed as a necessary additional part for demonstration of the patient-specific vascular and trachea relationship.

Description of Procedure (0560T)

Conduct an initial consultation between the requesting physician or other QHP and the consulting physician or other QHP to discuss the requested model. This discussion includes the patient's clinical scenario, surgical needs, and critical anatomy needed in the model. Besides the initial anatomic part of the aorta (separately reported with 0559T), an additional anatomic part of the tracheal bronchial tree is requested. The additional anatomic part of the trachea and proximal central bronchi requires separate processing. The work steps include segmentation of the image data, conversion of that data to a 3D printing compatible file type, and digital processing of the anatomic part file using CAD software by a physician or other QHP. Assemble the individually created tracheal anatomic part together with the aorta on the 3D printer–build tray. Color code each anatomic part and then print together as a single, larger multicontent physical model, with the combined model requiring more material, printing time, cleaning, and post-processing steps than a single anatomic part of the aorta. Conduct a final consultation with the ordering physician to review the anatomic parts of the model and limitations in model design. Photograph the model and place the image in the patient's electronic medical record. There may be separately reported services in the same setting when additional anatomic parts are created to include in the model.

Clinical Example (0561T)

A 45-year-old female, status post-radiation therapy for oral cancer, presents with progressive jaw pain and difficulty eating. CT revealed advanced osteonecrosis of the left mandibular ramus. The CT data is used to create a digital representation of the anatomy and surgical plan, from which an anatomic guide for mandibular osteotomy is designed. Subsequently, the digital design file is used to create the printed physical 3D anatomic guide.

Description of Procedure (0561T)

Consult initially with the requesting physician or other QHP to discuss the requested anatomic guide for mandibular osteotomy. The consultation with the physician or other QHP includes discussion of the patient's clinical scenario, surgical needs, and critical anatomy needed for the mandibular osteotomy guide. Assess imaging data to determine its adequacy for accurate anatomic guide creation. Export the image data to dedicated segmentation software, where a physician or other QHP separates the osseous mandible from adjacent anatomy. Convert the segmented mandible into a digital representation for virtual surgical planning. Digitally place the planned osteotomy cutting planes in the desired location of the mandible for optimal resection. Export the cutting planes and mandibular modeling files to CAD software, where the osteotomy cutting guide is designed to match the contour of the patient's mandible, including openings to match the desired osteotomy planes, which were created during the virtual surgical planning. Digitally overlay the finished design file on the segmented anatomy to ensure design accuracy. Imprint a unique patient identifying number on the anatomic guide. Convert this design file into a compatible format and export to a 3D printer. Three-dimensionally print the anatomic guide in biocompatible and sterilizable material. After printing, clean and process it according to guidelines for surgical material. Consult with the ordering physician to review the final anatomic guide and any specific considerations in guide design. Photograph the guide and place the image in the patient's electronic medical record.

Clinical Example (0562T)

A 45-year-old female, status post-radiation therapy for oral cancer undergoing mandibular resection, additionally requires a fibular free-flap graft to replace her resected mandible. CT data from the patient's lower extremity CT is used to create a digital representation of her fibula. This digital representation is used for surgical planning and design of a fibular osteotomy anatomic guide. The resulting design is used to create a separate physical 3D-printed fibular osteotomy anatomic guide in addition to the previously created mandibular osteotomy anatomic guide.

Description of Procedure (0562T)

In addition to the initial anatomic part of the maxillary cutting guide (separately reported with 0561T), a separate anatomic cutting guide for fibular osteotomy is needed. Consult with the physician or other QHP to discuss the patient's clinical scenario, surgical needs, and critical anatomy needed for the fibular osteotomy guide. Assess imaging data to determine its adequacy for accurate anatomic guide creation. Export fibular imaging data to dedicated segmentation software, where a physician or other QHP separates the osseous fibula from adjacent anatomy. Convert the segmented fibula into a digital representation for virtual surgical planning. Digitally place the planned osteotomy cutting lines on the desired location of the fibula for graft creation. Export the cutting planes and fibular modeling data to CAD software, where the osteotomy guide is designed to match the contour of the patient's fibula, including openings to match the desired osteotomy planes, which were created during the virtual surgical planning. Digitally overlay the finished design file on the segmented anatomy to ensure design accuracy. Imprint a unique patient identifying number on the anatomic guide. Convert this design file into a compatible format and export to a 3D printer. Three-dimensionally print the anatomic guide in biocompatible and sterilizable material. After printing, clean and process it according to guidelines for surgical material. Consult with the ordering physician to review the final anatomic guide and any specific considerations in guide design. Photograph the guide and place the image in the patient's electronic medical record.

0563T   Code is out of numerical sequence. See 0202T-0209T

● 0564T   Oncology, chemotherapeutic drug cytotoxicity assay of cancer stem cells (CSCs), from cultured CSCs and primary tumor cells, categorical drug response reported based on percent of cytotoxicity observed, a minimum of 14 drugs or drug combinations

Rationale

Category III code 0564T has been established to report chemotherapeutic drug cytotoxicity assay using cultured cancer stem cells (CSCs) and primary tumor cells, and reporting categorical drug response based on the percent of observed cytotoxicity for a minimum of 14 drugs or drug combinations.

Cytotoxicity is the presence of cell death observed among tumor cells and CSCs following chemotherapy and is indicative of cancerous cell response to chemotherapeutic drugs. This assay can assist in determining the patient's responsiveness to chemotherapy treatment.

Category III Codes

Clinical Example (0564T)

A 55-year-old female with headache, disorientation, and double vision complaints is seen by a neurosurgeon. Magnetic resonance imaging (MRI) scan showed a 2-cm irregular ring-enhancing lesion in the left posterior temporal lobe and two 3-cm lesions in the left mid-temporal lobe. A biopsy shows glioblastoma. A sample of tissue is submitted for chemotherapeutic drug cytotoxicity testing to aid in selecting optimal therapy.

Description of Procedure (0564T)

An unfixed, 5-mm^3 sample of tumor tissue is submitted for drug response testing. Disassociate the tissue, culture the tumor cells, and enrich the cancer stem cells (CSCs). Plate the cultured tumor cells and CSCs separately into 96-well plates and treat with chemotherapy agents, singly or in combination. Assess cytotoxicity by monitoring cell metabolic activity 48 hours following treatments by a colorimetric assay relative to untreated control cells. Measure mitochondrial activity in quadruplicates and normalize relative to their control cells. Report results as a percentage of cells killed by the treatment: Responsive (60%-100% cytotoxicity); intermediate (30%-60% cytotoxicity); nonresponsive (<10%-30% cytotoxicity).

● **0565T** Autologous cellular implant derived from adipose tissue for the treatment of osteoarthritis of the knees; tissue harvesting and cellular implant creation

▶(Do not report 0565T in conjunction with 15769, 15771, 15772, 15773, 15774)◀

● **0566T** injection of cellular implant into knee joint including ultrasound guidance, unilateral

▶(Do not report 0566T in conjunction with 20610, 20611, 76942, 77002)◀

▶(For bilateral procedure, report 0566T with modifier 50)◀

Rationale

Two new Category III codes (0565T, 0566T) have been established to report autologous cellular implant derived from adipose tissue for the treatment of osteoarthritis of the knees; tissue harvesting and cellular implant creation. These new codes have been established to allow reporting for autologous cellular implant for the treatment of osteoarthritis of the knees. Code 0565T differs from other codes in the code set, as it has various steps that must be followed for processing cellular implant into the joints. These include tissue harvest and incision closure; tissue washing; tissue enzymatic dissociation; cellar implant concentration from dissociated tissue; cellular implant resuspension and extraction; viability and yield assay for cellular implant; dose construction; endotoxin assay; microbial assay; and cellular implant release for injection. In addition, code 0566T has been added to allow reporting for injection procedures for this service when performed. An exclusionary parenthetical note following code 0565T has been added to restrict reporting grafting autologous codes. In addition, an exclusionary parenthetical note has been added to restrict users reporting code 0566T in conjunction with codes 20610, 20611 (arthrocentesis, aspiration); 76942 (ultrasonic guidance procedures); and 77002 (fluoroscopic guidance). In addition, an instructional parenthetical note has been added to describe reporting code 0566T with modifier 50 for bilateral procedures.

Refer to the codebook and the Rationale for codes 15769, 15771, 15772, 15773, and 15774 for a full discussion of these changes.

Clinical Example (0565T)

A 65-year-old female complains of persistent, chronic knee pain and decrease in her ability to perform activities of daily living. She has taken prescribed and over-the-counter anti-inflammatories and pain medication, but the pain persists to an impeding level. Radiographs show decreasing joint space and evidence of osteoarthritis. Without further intervention, joint degeneration will likely progress to a point in which total knee replacement is indicated.

Description of Procedure (0565T)

A physician or other QHP creates an autologous cellular implant from adipose tissue. Prepare patient and administer local anesthetic. Harvest tissue and close incision. Wash tissue and perform enzymatic dissociation of tissue, cellular implant concentration from dissociated tissue, cellular implant resuspension and extraction, viability and yield assay for cellular implant, dose construction, endotoxin assay, microbial assay, and cellular implant release for injection.

Clinical Example (0566T)

A 65-year-old female complains of persistent chronic knee pain and decrease in her ability to perform activities of daily living. She has taken prescribed and over-the-counter anti-inflammatories and pain medication, but the pain persists to an impeding level. Radiographs show decreasing joint space and evidence of osteoarthritis. Without further intervention, joint degeneration will likely progress to a point in which total knee replacement is indicated.

Description of Procedure (0566T)

Physician or other QHP injects cellular implant to the knee joint with image guidance. Injection is performed on same day and in same setting as adipose tissue harvest.

- **0567T** Permanent fallopian tube occlusion with degradable biopolymer implant, transcervical approach, including transvaginal ultrasound

    ▶(Do not report 0567T in conjunction with 58340, 58565, 74740, 74742, 76830, 76856, 76857)◀

- **0568T** Introduction of mixture of saline and air for sonosalpingography to confirm occlusion of fallopian tubes, transcervical approach, including transvaginal ultrasound and pelvic ultrasound

    ▶(Do not report 0568T in conjunction with 58340, 74740, 74742, 76830, 76831, 76856, 76857)◀

Rationale

Codes 0567T and 0568T have been established to report permanent fallopian tube occlusion using a degradable biopolymer implant via transcervical approach and the follow-up procedure of introducing a mixture of saline and air to confirm occlusion of the fallopian tubes. In addition, parenthetical notes have been added following the codes to restrict use of these code in conjunction with related, included services.

Code 0567T identifies a procedure that is intended to occlude the fallopian tubes via use of a biopolymer implant that is introduced via a transcervical approach. Transvaginal ultrasound is used for guidance during the procedure. The polymer is temporary and eventually degrades over time leaving the tubes occluded because of the procedure. Code 0568T identifies the procedure used to confirm that the tubes were successfully occluded and involves the introduction of a saline/air mixture for conformation of the occlusion. This confirmation is commonly performed months after the treatment to occlude the tubes is performed.

Since ultrasound is inherently included as a necessary component of both services, exclusionary parenthetical notes accompany both codes to provide instruction to users that certain diagnostic imaging (ie, hystosalpingographic [74740], radiological supervision and interpretation for transcervical catheterization [74742]) and ultrasound procedures (ie, transvaginal ultrasound [76830]), saline infusion sonohysterographic ultrasound [76831], pelvic ultrasound complete or limited [76856, 76857]) are inherently included as part of the procedure and not separately reported.

Clinical Example (0567T)

A 35-year-old multiparous female desires permanent sterilization. She has been counseled regarding the various options available to her and her partner. Permanent options include vasectomy, laparoscopic and hysteroscopic techniques, and the transcervical nonsurgical technique. She has opted for the transcervical nonsurgical approach.

Description of Procedure (0567T)

A sonographer or the physician perform a transvaginal ultrasound evaluation to determine uterine cavity direction and uterine measurements. The physician then performs the remainder of the procedure including a bimanual pelvic examination, insertion of a speculum into the vagina, and cleansing of the cervix. Place a tenaculum on the anterior or posterior lip of the cervix. Administer cervical anesthesia if deemed necessary. Insert a uterine sound to measure the depth of the uterine cavity and confirm cavity direction. Set the flange on the insertion tube of the delivery system to the measurement determined by the uterine sound or, if ultrasound assistance is needed, a sonographer may assist the physician in confirming the uterine sound measurement. Serially dilate the cervix as necessary to accommodate the delivery system. Insert the insertion tube through the cervix until the flange is at the external cervical os. Place the tip of the insertion tube at the fundus and secure the tenaculum to the device handle. Achieve access to both cornua with the advancement of two balloon catheters. Inflate both balloons and deliver biopolymer through the catheters to the cornua directed towards the fallopian tubes. Remove the delivery system from the patient after the balloons are deflated and the tenaculum is detached from the handle. Remove the tenaculum and speculum and control bleeding from the site of the cervical tenaculum, if necessary. Counsel the patient to rely on her choice of birth control for the next three months or until the confirmation procedure is performed. Counsel the patient to return for the confirmation procedure in three months.

Clinical Example (0568T)

A 35-year-old female, who had a transcervical nonsurgical fallopian tube occlusion procedure three months previously.

Description of Procedure (0568T)

Following a transvaginal ultrasound evaluation performed by a sonographer or the physician, perform a bimanual pelvic examination, insert a speculum into the vagina, and cleanse the cervix. Place a tenaculum on the anterior or posterior lip of the cervix if necessary to facilitate intrauterine catheter insertion. Administer cervical anesthesia if deemed necessary. Introduce an intrauterine balloon catheter through the cervix. Inflate the balloon and place above the internal cervical os. Remove the speculum. The transvaginal probe is inserted by the physician or sonographer. Attach the confirmation device to the catheter and deliver saline and air contrast. Confirm uterine distension visually with ultrasound and bubbles viewed moving in the pressure indicator window of the confirmation device, indicating 200 mm Hg of intrauterine pressure has been reached. The sonographer or physician orients the transvaginal probe to obtain views of the cornua, right and left cornu, right and left tubal course, right and left adnexa or ovary, and cul-de-sac, while observing bubbles flowing in the pressure indicator window to confirm uterine distension has been maintained throughout the evaluation. Confirm tubal occlusion with the absence of bubbles flowing into each tube, through the tubal course, near the adnexa or ovary, and in the cul-de-sac. The sonographer or physician removes the transvaginal probe. Remove the catheter from the patient. Inform the patient whether her tubal evaluation demonstrated bilateral occlusion and whether she can rely on tubal occlusion for birth control.

▶Tricuspid Valve Repair◀

▶Codes 0569T, 0570T include the work of percutaneous vascular access, placing the access sheath, cardiac catheterization, advancing the repair device system into position, repositioning the prosthesis as needed, deploying the prosthesis, and vascular closure. Code 0569T may only be reported once per session. Add-on code 0570T is reported in conjunction with 0569T for each additional prosthesis placed.

For open tricuspid valve procedures, see 33460, 33463, 33464, 33465, 33468.

Angiography, radiological supervision and interpretation performed to guide transcatheter tricuspid valve repair (TTVr) (eg, guiding device placement and documenting completion of the intervention) are included in these codes.

Intracardiac echocardiography (93662), when performed, is included in 0569T, 0570T. Transesophageal echocardiography (93355) performed by a separate operator for guidance of the procedure may be separately reported.

Fluoroscopy (76000) and diagnostic right and left heart catheterization codes (93451, 93452, 93453, 93456, 93457, 93458, 93459, 93460, 93461, 93530, 93531, 93532, 93533, 93566) may not be used with 0569T, 0570T to report the following techniques for guidance of TTVr:

1. Contrast injections, angiography, roadmapping, and/or fluoroscopic guidance for the TTVr,

2. Right ventricular angiography to assess tricuspid regurgitation for guidance of TTVr, or

3. Right and left heart catheterization for hemodynamic measurements before, during, and after TTVr for guidance of TTVr.

Diagnostic right and left heart catheterization codes (93451, 93452, 93453, 93456, 93457, 93458, 93459, 93460, 93461, 93530, 93531, 93532, 93533, 93566) and diagnostic coronary angiography codes (93454, 93455, 93456, 93457, 93458, 93459, 93460, 93461, 93563, 93564) may be reported with 0569T, 0570T, representing separate and distinct services from TTVr, if:

1. No prior study is available, and a full diagnostic study is performed, or

2. A prior study is available, but as documented in the medical record:

   a. There is inadequate evaluation of the anatomy and/or pathology, or

   b. The patient's condition with respect to the clinical indication has changed since the prior study, or

   c. There is a clinical change during the procedure that requires new diagnostic evaluation.

Other cardiac catheterization services may be reported separately when performed for diagnostic purposes not intrinsic to TTVr.

For same session/same day diagnostic cardiac catheterization services, report the appropriate diagnostic cardiac catheterization code(s) with modifier 59 indicating separate and distinct procedural service from TTVr.

Diagnostic coronary angiography performed at a separate session from an interventional procedure may be separately reportable.

Percutaneous coronary interventional procedures may be reported separately, when performed.

When transcatheter ventricular support is required in conjunction with TTVr, the procedure may be reported with the appropriate ventricular assist device (VAD) procedure code (33990, 33991, 33992, 33993) or balloon pump insertion code (33967, 33970, 33973).

When cardiopulmonary bypass is performed in conjunction with TTVr, 0569T, 0570T may be reported with the appropriate add-on code for percutaneous peripheral bypass (33367), open peripheral bypass (33368), or central bypass (33369).◀

- **0569T** Transcatheter tricuspid valve repair, percutaneous approach; initial prosthesis

+● **0570T** each additional prosthesis during same session (List separately in addition to code for primary procedure)

▶(Use 0570T in conjunction with 0569T)◀

▶(Do not report 0569T, 0570T in conjunction with 93451, 93452, 93453, 93456, 93457, 93458, 93459, 93460, 93461, 93566 for diagnostic left and right heart catheterization procedures intrinsic to the valve repair procedure)◀

▶(Do not report 0569T, 0570T in conjunction with 93454, 93563, 93564 for coronary angiography intrinsic to the valve repair procedure)◀

Rationale

A new Category III subsection and two new Category III codes (0569T, 0570T) have been established for reporting percutaneous transcatheter tricuspid valve repair. New guidelines and parenthetical notes have also been added to provide instruction on the appropriate use of the new codes.

Prior to 2020, only codes for open tricuspid valve repair procedures were available (33460, 33463, 33464, 33465, 33468). There were no specific codes for reporting percutaneous tricuspid valve repair procedures, therefore, unlisted code 33999 was reported.

Percutaneous transcatheter tricuspid valve repair, as described by these codes, involves the use of a prosthesis(es). Code 0569T is reported for repair using one or the initial prosthesis. Code 0570T is reported for each additional prosthesis placed. Codes 0569T and 0570T include percutaneous vascular access, access sheath placement, cardiac catheterization, positioning the repair device system, repositioning and deploying the prosthesis, closure, angiographic guidance of the procedure, and intracardiac echocardiography when performed. The new guidelines include instruction on the reporting of diagnostic left and right heart catheterization procedures and coronary angiography procedures with the new codes.

Clinical Example (0569T)

An 82-year-old male presents with exertional dyspnea and fatigue that has progressed over the past three years. Echocardiography shows severe tricuspid regurgitation (TR) with no other concomitant valvular heart disease to explain his symptoms. He has significant comorbidities. The patient has received guideline-directed medical therapy for heart failure (HF) but has persistent severe symptoms.

Description of Procedure (0569T)

Prepare the patient by sterilizing the vein access site, administer general anesthesia, and intubate the patient. Insert a Foley catheter. A separate health care professional inserts a TEE probe. Obtain pre-procedure images of the tricuspid valve and individual leaflets, with focus on identifying the regurgitant jet(s). Confirm such key measurements as the coaptation gap, leaflet length, and origin of the valve defect. Obtain right femoral vein access and verify location. Prepare the transcatheter tricuspid valve repair (TTVr) system with all components kept sterile. Inspect and flush the steerable guide catheter (SGC). Verify the competency of the hemostatic valve. Flush the dilator. Inspect and flush the clip delivery system (CDS) as well. Test the clip itself for opening and closing, then gently bring it back into the CDS shaft per the instructions for use. Predilate the femoral vein access site with step-up dilators and sheaths. Adjust the SGC deflection and torque to position the tip away from adjacent tissues, such as the walls of the right atrium and superior vena cava (SVC). Place a silicone rubber pad and stabilizer on the sterile drape over the lift. Once secure, retract the dilator approximately 5 cm into the guide, leaving the guidewire in the SVC. Then retract the guidewire into the dilator tip and remove both instruments while gently aspirating them with a 60-cc syringe. Cover the SGC hemostasis valve with a finger upon dilator removal. While flushing heparinized saline on the hemostatic valve, place the tip of the clip introducer (CI) against the valve of the SGC and advance it. Rotate the CI in small clockwise and counterclockwise motions until the clip is distal to the valve. Match the blue longitudinal alignment marker on the sleeve shaft with the blue alignment marker on the SGC hemostatic valve. Use alignment markers on the device, fluoroscopy, and echocardiography to guide the CDS through the SGC into the right atrium. Obtain positioning and continue until the clip is axially aligned over the desired line of coaptation of the tricuspid valve. Once the clip position and trajectory is established, open the arms to 180°. Translate the delivery catheter (DC) shaft multiple times to release stored torque and fully retract the DC handle. Using the transgastric view on echocardiography, verify the clip arms as perpendicular to the desired line of coaptation and the clip as not biased toward any of leaflets that are being captured. Advance the DC distally to position the clip below the tricuspid valve in the right ventricle. To grasp the leaflets, close the clip arms to 120° and retract the DC handle. Lower the grippers once leaflets are resting on the clip arms. Close the clip arms to 60° and secure the DC handle with the fastener. To confirm satisfactory leaflet insertion, check three features: (1) leaflet immobilization with creation of a single or multi-orifice valve; (2) limited leaflet mobility relative to the tips of both clip arms; and (3) decrease in TR. Exclude iatrogenic tricuspid stenosis on TEE imaging. The clip can still be repositioned by releasing the leaflets if needed. When ready to deploy the clip, re-establish the final arm angle to ensure clip remains closed when testing the locking mechanism. Confirm leaflet coaptation and insertion by allowing several minutes between shaft detachment and final deployment step, monitoring the TR reduction and patient hemodynamics, and using echocardiographic imaging. Perform the final step, removal of the gripper line, by gently pulling on one end of the gripper line, coaxially out of the gripper lever and completely over the CDS. Confirm clip position to be stable. Remove the CDS from the SGC, while ensuring the guide hemostasis valve is covered with a finger to ensure no air enters the guide lumen. Constantly monitor the patient's arterial pressure, electrocardiogram (ECG) waveforms, and oxygen saturation throughout the procedure. Review images to ensure no additional views are required before leaving the procedure suite. Close the groin site per physician and institutional practices. Transfer the patient to the recovery suite for additional monitoring.

Clinical Example (0570T)

An 83-year-old male who has just received the initial prosthesis for tricuspid repair during TTVr also requires the insertion of an additional prosthesis. Following deployment of the initial clip, evaluation indicates there was reduction in TR, but there is still a significant regurgitant jet present even with one clip now securely in place on the leaflets. The interventionalist and echosonographer agree that placing an additional clip is needed in order to decrease the TR further. [**Note:** This is an add-on service. Only consider the additional work related to TTVr, percutaneous approach, each additional prosthesis during same session.]

Description of Procedure (0570T)

Following deployment of the initial clip, prepare the second CDS on the back table to verify clip opening and closing, and to flush the device with heparinized saline. Unlike with the first clip, advance the second clip into the right ventricle with arms at greater than 60°, as to not disrupt or interact with the already implanted first clip. Confirm reduction in TR by echocardiography. The two clips should appear parallel to each other on fluoroscopy. In the transgastric echocardiographic view, the second clip arms appear perpendicular to the line of coaptation and the clip is not biased to either leaflet. Once it is established that the second clip will not interfere with the first clip, deploy the second clip in the same manner as the first clip. Perform the final step, removal of the gripper line, and confirm second clip

position to be stable. Reduction of TR is determined to be sufficient; therefore, no further intervention is needed.

▶Implantable Cardioverter-Defibrillator with Substernal Electrode◀

▶An implantable cardioverter-defibrillator system with substernal electrode (substernal implantable cardioverter-defibrillator) consists of a pulse generator and at least one substernal electrode. The generator is placed in a subcutaneous pocket over the lateral rib cage. The electrode is tunneled subcutaneously and placed into the substernal anterior mediastinum, without entering the pericardial cavity. The electrode performs defibrillation and pacing as needed. The system requires programming and interrogation of the device.

All imaging guidance (eg, fluoroscopy) required to complete the substernal implantable defibrillator procedure is included in 0571T, 0572T, 0573T, 0574T. The work of implantation, removal, repositioning, interrogation, or programming of substernal implantable cardioverter-defibrillator systems, generators, or leads may not be reported using 33202-33275, 93260-93298, 93640, 93641, 93642, 93644.◀

● 0571T   Insertion or replacement of implantable cardioverter-defibrillator system with substernal electrode(s), including all imaging guidance and electrophysiological evaluation (includes defibrillation threshold evaluation, induction of arrhythmia, evaluation of sensing for arrhythmia termination, and programming or reprogramming of sensing or therapeutic parameters), when performed

    ▶(Use 0571T in conjunction with 0573T, 0580T for removal and replacement of an implantable defibrillator pulse generator and substernal electrode)◀

    ▶(Do not report 0571T in conjunction with 93260, 93261, 93644, 0572T, 0575T, 0576T, 0577T)◀

    ▶(For insertion or replacement of permanent subcutaneous implantable defibrillator system with subcutaneous electrode, use 33270)◀

● 0572T   Insertion of substernal implantable defibrillator electrode

    ▶(Do not report 0572T in conjunction with 93260, 93261, 93644, 0571T, 0575T, 0576T, 0577T)◀

    ▶(For insertion of subcutaneous implantable defibrillator electrode, use 33271)◀

● 0573T   Removal of substernal implantable defibrillator electrode

▶(Do not report 0573T in conjunction with 93260, 93261, 93644, 0575T, 0576T, 0577T)◀

▶(For removal of subcutaneous implantable defibrillator electrode, use 33272)◀

● **0574T** Repositioning of previously implanted substernal implantable defibrillator-pacing electrode

▶(Do not report 0574T in conjunction with 93260, 93261, 93644, 0575T, 0576T, 0577T)◀

▶(For repositioning of previously implanted subcutaneous implantable defibrillator electrode, use 33273)◀

● **0575T** Programming device evaluation (in person) of implantable cardioverter-defibrillator system with substernal electrode, with iterative adjustment of the implantable device to test the function of the device and select optimal permanent programmed values with analysis, review and report by a physician or other qualified health care professional

▶(Do not report 0575T in conjunction with pulse generator or lead insertion or repositioning codes 0571T, 0572T, 0573T, 0574T, 0580T)◀

▶(Do not report 0575T in conjunction with 93260, 93282, 93287, 0576T)◀

● **0576T** Interrogation device evaluation (in person) of implantable cardioverter-defibrillator system with substernal electrode, with analysis, review and report by a physician or other qualified health care professional, includes connection, recording and disconnection per patient encounter

▶(Do not report 0576T in conjunction with pulse generator or lead insertion or repositioning codes 0571T, 0572T, 0573T, 0574T)◀

▶(Do not report 0576T in conjunction with 93261, 93289, 0575T)◀

● **0577T** Electrophysiological evaluation of implantable cardioverter-defibrillator system with substernal electrode (includes defibrillation threshold evaluation, induction of arrhythmia, evaluation of sensing for arrhythmia termination, and programming or reprogramming of sensing or therapeutic parameters)

▶(Do not report 0577T in conjunction with 93640, 93641, 93642, 93644, 0571T at the time of insertion or replacement of implantable defibrillator system with substernal lead)◀

▶(Do not report 0577T in conjunction with 0580T)◀

▶(For electrophysiological evaluation of subcutaneous implantable defibrillator system with subcutaneous electrode, use 93644)◀

● **0578T** Interrogation device evaluation(s) (remote), up to 90 days, substernal lead implantable cardioverter-defibrillator system with interim analysis, review(s) and report(s) by a physician or other qualified health care professional

▶(Do not report 0578T in conjunction with 93294, 93295, 93297, 93298, 0576T)◀

▶(Report 0578T only once per 90 days)◀

● **0579T** Interrogation device evaluation(s) (remote), up to 90 days, substernal lead implantable cardioverter-defibrillator system, remote data acquisition(s), receipt of transmissions and technician review, technical support and distribution of results

▶(Do not report 0579T in conjunction with 93296, 0576T)◀

▶(Report 0579T only once per 90 days)◀

● **0580T** Removal of substernal implantable defibrillator pulse generator only

▶(Use 0580T in conjunction with 0571T, 0573T for removal and replacement of an implantable cardioverter-defibrillator and substernal electrode[s])◀

▶(Do not report 0580T in conjunction with 0575T, 0576T, 0577T)◀

Rationale

In the Category III code section, 10 new Category III codes (0571T, 0572T, 0573T, 0574T, 0575T, 0576T, 0577T, 0578T, 0579T, 0580T) have been added to report implantable cardioverter-defibrillator system with substernal electrode (substernal implantable cardioverter-defibrillator) procedures. A new heading "Implantable Cardioverter-Defibrillator with Substernal Electrode" has also been added, along with new introductory guidelines to address the intended use for these implantable cardioverter-defibrillators procedures and accurate reporting. In addition, numerous parenthetical notes have been added following these new Category III codes to guide users in the appropriate reporting of these services in conjunction with other services in the CPT code set.

To accommodate these new Category III procedures, changes also have been made in the Surgery, Cardiovascular System, Heart and Pericardium, Pacemaker or Implantable Defibrillator subsection. These include revisions to the introductory guidelines section and addition of five parenthetical notes to provide additional coding guidance. The introductory guidelines section revisions explain the differences among the three general categories of implantable defibrillators that now exist in the CPT code set, including: (1) transvenous implantable pacing cardioverter-defibrillator (ICD); (2) subcutaneous implantable defibrillator (S-ICD); and (3) substernal implantable cardioverter-defibrillator. Further, parenthetical notes have been added to the Medicine, Cardiovascular, Implantable, Insertable, and Wearable Cardiac Device Evaluations subsection and the Intracardiac Electrophysiological Procedures/Studies subsection to enable the appropriate reporting of

Category III Codes

implantable cardioverter-defibrillator system with substernal electrode (substernal implantable cardioverter-defibrillator) procedures.

Currently codes exist in the CPT code set to describe transvenous implantable pacing cardioverter-defibrillator and subcutaneous implantable defibrillator. However, no codes existed to describe implantable cardioverter-defibrillator system with substernal electrode (substernal implantable cardioverter-defibrillator) procedures. It is for this reason a new subsection and ten Category III codes were added to the code set.

The new Category III codes are intended, as stated before, to describe a new type of defibrillator system with the lead subcutaneously tunneled and placed in the substernal anterior mediastinum, without entering the pericardial cavity. Substernal defibrillators differ from both subcutaneous (eg, 33270) and transvenous (eg, 33216) implantable pacing cardioverter-defibrillators in that they provide antitachycardia pacing, but not chronic pacing.

Although these new Category III codes describe substernal implantable cardioverter-defibrillator procedures, these codes are similar in structure/reporting for other cardioverter-defibrillator services. The new Category III services include codes for insertion or replacement (0571T), insertion (0572T), removal (0573T), repositioning (0574T), programming device evaluation (in person) (0575T), interrogation device evaluation (in person) (0576T), electrophysiological evaluation (0577T), interrogation device evaluation (remote) by a physician or other qualified health care provider (0578T), interrogation device evaluation (remote) technician review, technical support, and distribution of results (0579T), and generator removal (0580T).

It is important to note that the new Category III guidelines also describe the implantable cardioverter-defibrillator system. The guidelines also specify that all imaging guidance required to complete the substernal implantable defibrillator procedure is included in codes 0571T, 0572T, 0573T, and 0574T. The work of implantation, removal, repositioning, interrogation, programming of these systems is included in the new codes and should not be reported with existing codes 33202-33275, 93260-93298, 93640, 93641, 93642, and 93644.

Instructional, exclusionary, and cross-reference parenthetical notes have been added following each new Category III code to guide and instruct the user on appropriate reporting of these new services in conjunction with related or similar services. Notable instructions include: Insertion or replacement of implantable cardioverter defibrillator system (0571T) should be reported with codes 0573T and 0580T when performing removal and replacement of an implantable defibrillator pulse generator and substernal electrode. Code 0571T should not be reported with codes 93260, 93261, 93644, 0572T, 0575T, 0576T, and 0577T. Code 33270 should be reported for insertion or replacement of a permanent subcutaneous implantable defibrillator system, with a subcutaneous electrode. The two parenthetical notes following insertion of substernal implantable defibrillator electrode code (0572T) specify that this service should not be reported with codes 93260, 93261, 93644, 0571T, 0575T, 0576T, and 0577T. Code 33271 should be reported when performing the insertion of a subcutaneous implantable defibrillator electrode.

The two parenthetical notes following removal code 0573T specify that this service should not be reported with codes 93260, 93261, 93644, 0575T, 0576T, and 0577T. Code 33272 should be reported when performing the removal of a subcutaneous implantable defibrillator electrode.

The two exclusionary parenthetical notes following repositioning code 0574T specify that this service should not be reported with codes 93260, 93261, 93644, 0575T, 0576T, and 0577T. Code 33273 should be reported when performing repositioning of a previously implanted subcutaneous implantable defibrillator electrode.

The two exclusionary parenthetical notes following programming device evaluation (in person) of implantable cardioverter-defibrillator system (0575T) specify that this service should not be reported with pulse generator or lead insertion or repositioning codes 0571T, 0572T, 0573T, 0574T, and 0580T. Further, code 0575T should not be reported with codes 93260, 93282, 93287, and 0576T.

Interrogation device evaluation code 0576T should not be reported with pulse generator or lead insertion or repositioning codes 0571T, 0572T, 0573T, and 0574T. Further, code 0576T should not be reported with codes 93261 and 93289, and programming device evaluation (0575T).

The parenthetical notes following electrophysiological evaluation of implantable cardioverter-defibrillator system (0577T) specify that at the time of insertion or replacement of implantable defibrillator system with substernal lead, codes 93640, 93641, 93642, 93644, and 0571T should not be reported.

In addition, code 0577T should not be reported in conjunction with code 0580T. However, code 93644 should be reported when an electrophysiological evaluation of the subcutaneous implantable defibrillator system, with subcutaneous electrode, is performed.

Interrogation device evaluation(s) (remote) code 0578T should be reported only once per 90 days, and should not be reported in conjunction with codes 93294, 93295, 93297, 93298, and 0576T.

Interrogation device evaluation(s) (remote) code 0579T should only be reported once per 90 days, and should not be reported in conjunction with code 93296 or interrogation device evaluation service (0576T).

Removal of substernal implantable defibrillator pulse generator only (0580T) should be reported in conjunction with codes 0571T and 0573T when performing removal and replacement of an implantable cardioverter defibrillator and substernal electrode(s). However, code 0580T should not be reported with codes 0575T, 0576T, and 0577T.

Clinical Example (0571T)

A 57-year-old asymptomatic male presents with a history of prior myocardial infarction seven months ago and has since had documented runs of nonsustained ventricular tachycardia captured via Holter recordings. Echocardiography revealed a 32% left ventricular ejection fraction. The patient was referred for a substernal implantable cardioverter defibrillator.

Description of Procedure (0571T)

Prepare the sternum to the left chest and administer general anesthesia. Create a subxiphoid incision. Under fluoroscopic guidance, insert the prepared sternal tunneling rod, with introducer sheath anterior to the mediastinum while maintaining close contact with the underside of the sternum. Tunnel to the top of cardiac silhouette, just left of the sternal midline. Hold the introducer sheath in place while removing the sternal tunneling rod. Insert the lead into the sheath, then withdraw the sheath to expose the lead in its extravascular position, confirming that the defibrillation coil is directed towards the patient's right chest over the right ventricle. Fixate the lead. Confirm under fluoroscopy that the lead is in the substernal position without entering the mediastinum. Make a device pocket incision just below the left inframammary crease. Insert the transverse tunneling rod at the subxiphoid incision and tunnel above the coastal rib margin toward the device pocket. At the pocket, connect the lead to the pulse generator and place the system in the pocket. After closing the first tissue layer of the pocket, perform initial sensing, pacing, and lead impendence measurements. Program the device to detect and differentiate ventricular arrythmias and to deliver antitachycardia pacing and ventricular fibrillation therapy (included). Perform defibrillation threshold testing by inducing ventricular fibrillation through the device (included). Complete closure of the pocket, close subxiphoid incisions, and dress the wound. Dictate report of procedure for the medical record.

Clinical Example (0572T)

A 62-year-old male developed a mild infection of the substernal electrode of a substernal implantable cardioverter-defibrillator. The electrode was removed previously and followed by treatment with antibiotics. The patient presents for insertion of a new substernal electrode with connection to an existing functional pulse generator.

Description of Procedure (0572T)

Prepare the sternum to the left chest and administer general anesthesia. Create a subxiphoid incision. Under fluoroscopic guidance, insert the prepared sternal tunneling rod, with introducer sheath anterior to the mediastinum while maintaining close contact with the underside of the sternum. Tunnel to the top of cardiac silhouette, just left of the sternal midline. Hold the introducer sheath in place while removing the sternal tunneling rod. Insert the lead into the sheath, then withdraw the sheath to expose the lead in its extravascular position, confirming that the defibrillation coil is directed towards the patient's right chest over the right ventricle. Fixate the lead. Confirm under fluoroscopy that the lead is in the substernal position without entering the mediastinum. Make an incision in the existing generator pocket of the substernal implantable cardioverter-defibrillator generator, which is just below the left inframammary crease. Insert the transverse tunneling rod at the subxiphoid incision and tunnel above the coastal rib margin toward the device pocket. At the pocket, connect the lead to the existing pulse generator. After closing the first tissue layer of the pocket, perform initial sensing, pacing, and lead impendence measurements. Program the device to detect and differentiate ventricular arrythmias and to deliver antitachycardia pacing and ventricular fibrillation therapy (included). Perform defibrillation threshold testing by inducing ventricular fibrillation through the device (included). Complete closure of the pocket, close subxiphoid incisions, and dress the wound. Dictate report of procedure for the medical record.

Clinical Example (0573T)

A 62-year-old male with substernal cardioverter-defibrillator system implanted four months ago develops a mild infection at the substernal incision site. The electrode is removed followed by antibiotic treatment. Once the infection is resolved a new extravascular electrode will be placed.

Description of Procedure (0573T)

Prepare the sternum to the left chest and administer general anesthesia. Make an incision over the 5th and 6th ribs just below the left inframammary crease.

Perform subcutaneous dissection of the pulse generator and disconnect the lead from the generator. Open the subxiphoid incision to expose the lead and suture sleeve. Free the lead from the fascia and gently pull the lead from the pocket to the subxiphoid incision. If this is unable to be achieved, due to adhesions, cut the lead body at the subxiphoid incision and prepare the lead for extraction. Under fluoroscopy, gentle traction is used on the lead body to determine if an extraction sheath will be required or if the lead moves freely in the anterior mediastinum. Once the lead is withdrawn from the subxiphoid incision, close the pocket and subxiphoid incisions and dress the wounds. Dictate report of procedure for the medical record.

Clinical Example (0574T)

A 57-year-old male had a substernal cardioverter-defibrillator system implanted yesterday. Based on interrogation of the device and evaluation of anteroposterior and lateral chest X rays, there is indication the electrode has migrated and requires repositioning.

Description of Procedure (0574T)

Prepare the sternum to the left chest and administer general anesthesia. Using the incisions made from the prior implant procedure, perform subcutaneous dissection of the pulse generator and disconnect the lead from the generator. Next, open the subxiphoid incision and remove the sutures to free the lead. Reposition the lead, using fluoroscopy to confirm placement, and evaluate sensing performance. Reconnect the lead to the pulse generator. Perform defibrillation testing by induction of ventricular fibrillation through the device. Programming is completed. Close the pocket and subxiphoid incisions and dress the wounds. Dictate report of procedure for the medical record.

Clinical Example (0575T)

A 65-year-old male with ischemic cardiomyopathy and left ventricular ejection fraction of 30% had a substernal cardioverter-defibrillator implanted. The patient tells his physician that he "fainted" without palpitations, warning, or feeling a shock. The physician requests a programming device evaluation to assess device, battery, and lead function and subsequently performs programming adjustments to the device's rate cutoff and diagnostic parameters based upon the patient's interrogated data.

Description of Procedure (0575T)

Obtain verbal consent from the patient. Connect the patient to a single or multilead electrocardiographic recording system. Establish a communication link between the device and the programmer. Perform a full interrogation of the stored device parameters with assessment and recording of the current rhythm. Retrieve the stored pacing and tachyarrhythmia episode data and perform detailed physician analysis of these data. Review the stored summary and recorded rhythm data. Measure the lead impedance. Use this information to identify integrity issues with the existing lead and determine appropriate settings. Obtain the sensing threshold data by recording the signal from the ventricular chamber and utilizing iterative (step-wise) adjustment and identification of the appropriate implantable cardioverter defibrillator sensing level. After detailed analysis of the data, evaluate the appropriateness of the initial programmed anti-tachycardia pacing parameters and therapies relative to the patient's clinical status. If indicated, alter the device's programming at this time.

Clinical Example (0576T)

A 68-year-old male with history of nonsustained ventricular tachycardia treated with a substernal implantable cardioverter defibrillator system is followed with interrogation device evaluations (in person). The patient presents to the clinic for follow-up to assess device function.

Description of Procedure (0576T)

Interrogate the information from the device by telemetric communication, and either print for review or review on the programmer or computer monitor. Critically review the interrogated data with assessment of the appropriateness of the function of device and safety of the current programmed parameters, to assess whether the device function is normal. Also review the following data: presenting electrogram for appropriateness or presence of arrhythmia and appropriate sensing; stored episodes of data for appropriate sensing, appropriate magnet reversion, and noise reversions; alerts generated from the device; battery voltage and impedance, lead impedance, and sensed electrogram voltage amplitude for each lead; counters of events; and stored episodes of sensed events, including arrhythmias, ectopic beats, and nonsustained and sustained arrhythmias. Note the frequency, rate, and duration.

Clinical Example (0577T)

A 59-year-old male with a substernal implantable cardioverter defibrillator system has multiple appropriate shocks for ventricular tachycardia and is now placed on an antiarrhythmic medication. He is referred for defibrillator threshold testing, as there is concern for an increased threshold with the antiarrhythmic medication.

Description of Procedure (0577T)

Induce deep sedation prior to induction of ventricular fibrillation through the device. Using the two sensing electrodes, or either of the sensing electrodes or the pulse generator, detect cardiac rhythm. The substernal implantable cardioverter defibrillator system automatically selects an appropriate vector for rhythm detection. Use the feature analysis and rate detection to sort rhythm type and determine the need for therapy, once the signals have been validated as free of noise and double detection. A conditional discrimination zone that incorporates a feature extraction technique can be programmed between the rates of 170 and 240 beats per minute to distinguish supraventricular tachycardia from ventricular tachycardia, and to avoid inappropriate treatment of the former. Following capacitor charging, reconfirm ventricular tachyarrhythmia to avoid the delivery of shocks for nonsustained ventricular tachyarrhythmias.

Clinical Example (0578T)

A 63-year-old male with a history of sustained ventricular tachycardia treated with a substernal implantable cardioverter-defibrillator (ICD) is followed with interrogation device evaluations (remote) of the ICD from the patient's home. The patient has dyspnea on exertion and intermittent palpitations with light-headedness.

Description of Procedure (0578T)

Interrogate the information from the ICD by telemetric communication and either print for review or review on the programmer or computer monitor. Critically assess the interrogated data, with assessment of the appropriateness of the function of ICD, safety of the current programmed pacing, and anti-tachycardia parameters and assessment of device function. The data reviewed include the presenting electrograms for appropriateness of pacing and sensing; stored episodes of data; alerts generated from the device; battery voltage and impedance; pacing and shocking lead impedance; and sensed electrogram voltage amplitude for each lead. Note histogram and/or counters of paced and sensed events from each chamber and stored episodes of sensed arrhythmia events, including the type, frequency, rate, and duration. Evaluate adequacy of heart rate response.

Clinical Example (0579T)

A 63-year-old male with a history of sustained ventricular tachycardia treated with a substernal implantable cardioverter-defibrillator (ICD) is followed with interrogation device evaluations (remote) of the ICD from the patient's home. The patient has dyspnea on exertion and intermittent palpitations with light-headedness.

Description of Procedure (0579T)

Remote ICD device evaluation includes monitoring of all programmed parameters, leads, battery, capture and sensing function, presence or absence of therapy for ventricular tachyarrhythmias and underlying heart rhythm. Based on the physician's order, a patient with an ICD is registered for remote interrogation at a monitoring facility. The monitoring facility delivers the equipment to the patient with instructions for connection to the telephone system. Physician provides additional telephone support to help the patient complete the connections. Physician establishes a schedule for device interrogations based on the physician's order. An electrodiagnostic technician assembles the interrogated data and sends it to the physician. A nurse reviews it for device alerts and compares it to the physician-directed parameters for communication to the patient's physician. The interrogated data are both scheduled and triggered by the patient and/or device alarm-initiated episodes. The technician receives data through the device information system and inputs that data into the physician's database. The technician then reviews all of the data generated from the system. The data is then incorporated into the physician's system. The technician reviews and analyzes the parameters and, if present, documents patient symptoms. The technician reports to the physician if any parameters designated by the physician are exceeded. The technician enters findings into the physician's database and validates function by assessing if the lead data and arrhythmia events are normal or abnormal. After data is entered and evaluated, the technician generates a comprehensive report of all evaluated parameters, which is then delivered to the physician. All evaluations received within a 90-day period are included in this service.

Clinical Example (0580T)

A 60-year-old male with a substernal implantable cardioverter-defibrillator system implanted four months ago develops a pocket infection requiring removal of the generator. Once the infection is resolved, a new generator will be placed.

Description of Procedure (0580T)

Prepare the lateral left chest and administer anesthesia (local or general). Make an incision over the fifth-sixth ribs just below the left inframammary crease and carry down to the level of the capsule surrounding the generator. Perform subcutaneous dissection of the pulse generator. Disconnect the lead from the generator. Dissect the existing generator free from fibrous scar tissue. Often extensive removal of scar tissue or capsule is required. During the procedure, maintain adequate hemostasis and sterility. Close the pocket and dress the wound.

Category III Codes

● **0581T** Ablation, malignant breast tumor(s), percutaneous, cryotherapy, including imaging guidance when performed, unilateral

▶(Report 0581T only once per breast treated)◀

▶(Do not report 0581T in conjunction with 76641, 76642, 76940, 76942)◀

▶(For cryoablation of breast fibroadenoma[s], use 19105)◀

Rationale

In the Category III code section, code 0581T has been added to report ablation, malignant breast tumor(s), percutaneous, cryotherapy including imaging guidance when performed, unilateral. In addition, three parenthetical notes have been added to direct users to report the appropriate codes. Currently codes exist in the CPT code set that describe percutaneous cryoablation procedures of malignant tumors and refer to the procedures performed on a specific lesion. However, because no code exists that specifically describes cryoablation of a cancerous tumor in the breast, a new code was established. Instructional, exclusionary, and cross-reference parenthetical notes have been added following code 0581T to guide and instruct the user on appropriate reporting of the new code. An instructional parenthetical note has been added directing users to report code 0581T only once per breast treated. This is further clarified by the addition of "(s)" to "tumor" in the code descriptor. In addition, an exclusionary parenthetical note has also been added to restrict reporting of imaging in conjunction with this code because the descriptor includes imaging. Finally, this code is not intended for reporting cryoablation of breast fibroadenoma(s). As a result, a cross-reference parenthetical note has been added to direct users to report code 19105 for this procedure. In addition, a cross-reference parenthetical note has been added following code 19105 to direct users to report code 0581T for cryoablation of malignant breast tumor(s).

Clinical Example (0581T)

A 70-year-old female presented with stage IA (T1N0M0), estrogen and progesterone receptor (ER/PR) positive, HER2 negative, small, unifocal primary invasive ductal breast carcinoma, located at the union of the outer quadrants of her right breast. The physician offers surgical excision or cryoablation. The patient chooses to undergo percutaneous cryoablation of the tumor.

Description of Procedure (0581T)

Position, prepare, and drape the patient. Using ultrasound guidance, confirm the location of the breast tumor. Under local anesthesia, make a small incision with a scalpel. Introduce the cryoprobe through the incision under ultrasound guidance. Center the sharp cryoprobe tip in the breast tumor. Initiate the treatment cycle (based on tumor size) according to a programmed algorithm in the cryoablation system. If necessary, inject sterile saline between the tumor and skin surface to increase separation and prevent skin injury from the cold probe. Monitor the ice ball formation using ultrasound throughout the treatment cycle. Two complete freeze-thaw cycles are required to complete a single tissue ablation process. If needed, insert an external auxiliary temperature probe into the tissue to monitor temperature in the ice ball. At the end of the procedure, ensure that the warm phase is complete before the cryoprobe is safely removed from the patient's breast. After removal of cryoprobe, compress the puncture entry, clean and cover with sterile adhesive dressings, and transfer the patient to a recovery area.

● **0582T** Transurethral ablation of malignant prostate tissue by high-energy water vapor thermotherapy, including intraoperative imaging and needle guidance

▶(Do not report 0582T in conjunction with 52000, 72195, 72196, 72197, 76376, 76377, 76872, 76940, 76942, 77021, 77022)◀

▶(For transurethral destruction of prostate tissue by radiofrequency-generated water vapor thermotherapy for benign prostatic hypertrophy [BPH], use 53854)◀

Rationale

A new Category III code 0582T has been established for reporting transurethral ablation of malignant prostate tissue by high-energy water vapor thermotherapy, including intraoperative imaging and needle guidance. Parenthetical notes have been added to provide guidance on the appropriate reporting of code 0582T.

Clinical Example (0582T)

A 72-year-old male with an elevated PSA after prior negative prostate biopsy undergoes MRI, which reveals two suspicious lesions, one in the right apical peripheral zone and one in the left anterior transitional zone of his prostate. MRI/ultrasound (US) fusion biopsy of each lesion confirms Gleason 7 adenocarcinoma. The patient elects focal ablation of the lesions by high-energy water vapor thermotherapy with intraoperative imaging and needle guidance.

Description of Procedure (0582T)

The patient receives general anesthesia and is placed in the lithotomy position. Mount a transrectal US probe onto a stepper unit and position in the rectum to visualize the prostate. Complete a thorough US examination of the prostate (including volumetric and treatment measurements) as well as anterior rectal wall and periprostatic space. Under real-time US guidance, advance an 18-g needle just anterior to the rectum into the periprostatic space. Inject 1 to 2 cc of normal saline to assist identifying the proper location of the needle and then connect to a saline pump to be used later during the water vapor treatment cycle. Using a standard vapor cartridge, pass the disposable cystoscopic device into the prostatic urethra and localize by real-time US tracking. Using the MRI guidance system and uploaded MRI images, complete the MRI/US fusion process and identify the left anterior transitional zone target. Guide the vapor needle to the center of the target utilizing US and the needle tracking guidance system. As the needle is deployed, monitor the bio-capacitance safety system to avoid breach of the prostatic capsule. When the vapor needle location is confirmed, initiate the periprostatic saline infusion followed by vapor delivery into the target at the standard setting of 400 calories per vapor treatment. After each treatment, the needle may be slightly advanced or retracted and vapor treatment repeated if additional ablation is needed, until the target lesion is completely ablated. After confirming complete ablation of the left transitional zone lesion, retract the needle and replace into the right apical peripheral zone lesion. Repeat the water vapor treatment cycle(s) until that lesion is completely ablated. Retract the needle and remove the device. Place a Foley catheter and send the patient to the recovery room.

● **0583T** Tympanostomy (requiring insertion of ventilating tube), using an automated tube delivery system, iontophoresis local anesthesia

▶(Do not report 0583T in conjunction with 69209, 69210, 69420, 69421, 69433, 69436, 69990, 92504, 97033)◀

▶(For bilateral procedure, report 0583T with modifier 50)◀

Rationale

A new Category III code 0583T has been established to report tympanostomy with iontophoresis. In accordance with the addition of the new code, two parenthetical notes have been added to provide instruction regarding the intended use of this code. Code 0583T is a new procedure that describes different work for performing tympanostomy with an automated delivery system for tube placement using iontophoresis local anesthesia into the ear canal. This new procedure may be performed in an office setting and involves work by a physician that includes binocular microscopic cleaning of the ear canal, earset sizing and positioning for the insertion into the ear, introduction of anesthetic solution, followed by the iontophoresis and automated tube delivery. In addition, an exclusionary parenthetical note has been added to restrict reporting of certain procedures with code 0583T. An instructional parenthetical note has been added to further provide clarification when reporting modifier 50 for bilateral procedures.

Clinical Example (0583T)

A 2-year-old female presents with three episodes of acute otitis media within the past six months. Middle ear effusion is present on examination despite several courses of antibiotic therapy. Under iontophoresis local anesthesia, a tympanostomy tube is inserted using an automated tube delivery system.

Description of Procedure (0583T)

Position the patient sitting on the parent or guardian's lap, in a reclining procedure chair. Perform a surgical time-out. Perform an otoscopic examination using the operating microscope. Perform binocular microscopy for ear canal cleaning. Size the ear canal and fit the iontophoresis earset earplug into the ear canal. Place the return electrode. Introduce anesthetic solution into the ear canal and initiate iontophoresis. At the end of iontophoresis, the earset and return electrode are removed and the anesthetic solution is drained from the ear canal. Repeat binocular microscopy to clean material mobilized in the ear canal. The patient and parent or guardian are reclined into a near-supine position. Visualize the ear canal and tympanic membrane using the operating microscope. Assess adequacy of anesthesia of the tympanic membrane. Position the tube delivery device in contact with the tympanic membrane and deploy. Inspect the operative site and perform adjustments of tube position and/or suctioning as needed. Instill eardrops in the ear canal.

Category III Codes

- **0584T** Islet cell transplant, includes portal vein catheterization and infusion, including all imaging, including guidance, and radiological supervision and interpretation, when performed; percutaneous
- **0585T** laparoscopic
- **0586T** open

> ### Rationale
>
> Three new Category III codes (0584T, 0585T, 0586T) have been established to report islet cell transplantation including portal vein catheterization and infusion including all imaging, guidance, and radiological supervision and interpretation. The codes are differentiated by the approach with individual codes created for percutaneous (0584T), laparoscopic (0585T), and open (0586T) approach.
>
> In accordance with the addition of codes 0584T, 0585T, and 0586T, a parenthetical note has been added following code 48160, *Pancreatectomy, total or subtotal, with autologous transplantation of pancreas or pancreatic islet cells*, to direct users to these new codes to report pancreatic islet cell transplantation.

Clinical Example (0584T)

A 46-year-old female at the time of islet transplantation had a 26-year history of type 1 diabetes complicated by hypoglycemic unawareness and severe hypoglycemic events requiring intervention by others. After evaluation, the patient is placed on the United Network for Organ Sharing (UNOS) waitlist for islet cell transplantation.

Description of Procedure (0584T)

Before the procedure, take medical history, perform a physical examination, and review pre-transplant laboratory testing. Initiate induction immunosuppression to prevent graft rejection and recurrence of autoimmune diabetes. Ensure intensive peritransplant glucose monitoring. The islet transplant occurs by intraportal infusion by a QHP trained in percutaneous, transhepatic access of the portal vein. Apply local anesthesia at infusion site identified by ultrasound, access a peripheral portal vein branch with a fine needle, and confirm intraportal location with contrast. Pass guidewire into main portal vein and upsize percutaneous access to accept a 6Fr introducer. Advance a 6Fr arrow sheath into main portal vein and perform portal venogram. Infuse islet preparation following the manufacturer's instruction under intermittent portal vein pressure monitoring. After completion of islet cell infusion, retract sheath into the hepatic parenchymal tract under fluoroscopic and sonographic guidance. Embolize the tract with hemostatic agent. Perform postprocedure ultrasound to monitor for perihepatic hematoma and evaluate the patency of the portal system. Repeat after 24 hours, or before discharge. Dictate report of procedure for medical records. When bacteriology results of islet preparation or any new pertinent pancreas donor information is received, dictate an addendum to the report. If test results require change in treatment plan, call physician following the recipient and provide report. After the procedure, a QHP will monitor the patient. Depending on the islet graft function and treatment response in the recipient, additional islet infusions may be needed to achieve normoglycemia in the recipient.

Clinical Example (0585T)

A 50-year-old female patient at the time of islet transplantation had a 40-year history of type 1 diabetes complicated by hypoglycemic unawareness and severe hypoglycemic events. After evaluation, the patient is placed on the UNOS waitlist for islet cell transplantation. The patient also has a history of coronary artery disease with stent placement and a requirement for dual antiplatelet therapy, posing a relative contraindication for a percutaneous approach.

Description of Procedure (0585T)

Follow pre-transplant procedures and initiate induction of immunosuppression to prevent graft rejection and recurrence of autoimmune diabetes. Ensure intensive peritransplant glucose monitoring. A transplant surgeon trained in laparoscopy performs the procedure. The islet transplant occurs by intraportal infusion via a mesenteric vein in the operating room suite under general anesthesia with a short hospital or 24-hour observation stay. Position and prep patient aseptically for the intervention. Perform a small supraumbilical incision, and install a pneumoperitoneum with CO_2 insufflation. Place two 5-mm trocars in the right and left upper quadrants and a camera trocar supraumbilically. Identify a mesenteric vein. Insert and secure an angiocath connected to an infusion tubing. Infuse islet cell preparation under intermittent monitoring of portal pressure. After completion of infusion, remove the angiocath and ensure hemostasis. Remove trocars and close skin. Perform postprocedure ultrasound to monitor the patency of the portal system. Repeat after 24 hours, or before discharge. Dictate report of procedure for the medical record and posttransplant follow-up. When bacteriology results of the islet preparation or any new pertinent pancreas donor information is received, dictate addendum to the report. If test results require change in treatment plan, call physician following the recipient and provide the report.

Clinical Example (0586T)

A 62-year-old female patient at the time of islet transplantation had a 45-year history of type 1 diabetes complicated by severe hypoglycemic unawareness and peripheral vascular disease with previous stent placement and a requirement for dual antiplatelet therapy and previous abdominal surgery, rendering a minimally invasive laparoscopic approach more difficult. After evaluation, the patient is placed on the UNOS waitlist for islet cell transplantation.

Description of Procedure (0586T)

Follow pre-transplant procedures and initiate induction of immunosuppression to prevent graft rejection and recurrence of autoimmune diabetes. Ensure intensive peritransplant glucose monitoring. A transplant surgeon performs the procedure. The islet transplant occurs by intraportal infusion via a mesenteric vein in the operating room suite under general anesthesia. Position and prepare patient aseptically for the intervention. After induction of general anesthesia, perform periumbilical minilaparotomy. Insert and secure an angiocath linked to an infusion line into a large mesenteric vein. Infuse islet cell preparation under intermittent monitoring of portal pressure. After completion of infusion, remove the angiocath and ensure hemostasis. Close the minilaparotomy. Perform postprocedure ultrasound to monitor the patency of the portal system. Repeat after 24 hours, or before discharge. Dictate report of procedure for the medical record and posttransplant follow-up. When bacteriology results of the islet preparation or any new pertinent pancreas donor information is received, dictate an addendum to the report. If test results require change in treatment plan, call physician following the recipient and provide the report.

● **0587T** Percutaneous implantation or replacement of integrated single device neurostimulation system including electrode array and receiver or pulse generator, including analysis, programming, and imaging guidance when performed, posterior tibial nerve

▶(Do not report 0587T in conjunction with 64555, 64566, 64575, 64590, 95970, 95971, 95972, 0588T, 0589T, 0590T)◀

● **0588T** Revision or removal of integrated single device neurostimulation system including electrode array and receiver or pulse generator, including analysis, programming, and imaging guidance when performed, posterior tibial nerve

▶(Do not report 0588T in conjunction with 64555, 64566, 64575, 64590, 95970, 95971, 95972, 0587T, 0589T, 0590T)◀

● **0589T** Electronic analysis with simple programming of implanted integrated neurostimulation system (eg, electrode array and receiver), including contact group(s), amplitude, pulse width, frequency (Hz), on/off cycling, burst, dose lockout, patient-selectable parameters, responsive neurostimulation, detection algorithms, closed-loop parameters, and passive parameters, when performed by physician or other qualified health care professional, posterior tibial nerve, 1-3 parameters

▶(Do not report 0589T in conjunction with 43647, 43648, 43881, 43882, 61850-61888, 63650, 63655, 63661, 63662, 63663, 63664, 63685, 63688, 64553-64595, 95970, 95971, 95972, 95976, 95977, 95983, 95984, 0587T, 0588T, 0590T)◀

● **0590T** Electronic analysis with complex programming of implanted integrated neurostimulation system (eg, electrode array and receiver), including contact group(s), amplitude, pulse width, frequency (Hz), on/off cycling, burst, dose lockout, patient-selectable parameters, responsive neurostimulation, detection algorithms, closed-loop parameters, and passive parameters, when performed by physician or other qualified health care professional, posterior tibial nerve, 4 or more parameters

▶(Do not report 0590T in conjunction with 43647, 43648, 43881, 43882, 61850-61888, 63650, 63655, 63661, 63662, 63663, 63664, 63685, 63688, 64553-64595, 95970, 95971, 95972, 95976, 95977, 95983, 95984, 0587T, 0588T, 0589T)◀

Rationale

New Category III codes 0587T, 0588T, 0589T, and 0590T have been added to report percutaneous implantation or replacement and revision or removal of integrated single-device neurostimulation systems and separate electronic analysis with simple or complex programming of the implanted integrated neurostimulator system devices. In addition, parenthetical notes have been added within the Surgery/Neurostimulator and Medicine/Neurostimulators subsections and Category III code section to provide additional instruction regarding reporting of other neurostimulator electrode or generator implantation, removal, replacement, revision, imaging for placement, and programming for these integrated devices.

Codes 0587T and 0588T have been established to report percutaneous implantation or replacement and revision or removal of integrated single-device neurostimulators with analysis and programming. These codes have been added to identify the efforts of implanting or replacing (0587T) or revising or removing (0588T) an integrated, single-device neurostimulator. These neurostimulation devices are comprised of an electrode array and integrated receiver or pulse generator in a single unit/device and are used at the posterior tibial nerve (lower leg) to treat conditions such as overactive bladder and refractory urge incontinence.

Imaging guidance, programming, and analysis have been included as part of the placement procedure. Therefore, these services are inherently included as part of the procedures and not separately reported.

Separate codes have been established to identify electronic analysis with simple (0589T) and complex (0590T) programming. These codes are intended to be used when programming services are performed independent of placement and revision/removal services. Guidance for this has been included within the exclusionary parenthetical note that follows each code.

Other parenthetical notes within the Category III section for these codes and in other sections of the code set provide additional direction regarding the intended use for the new codes. These include exclusionary parenthetical notes that restrict reporting of placement and programming services and cross-references that direct users to the new codes for placement/replacement, revision/removal, and programming services for percutaneous implantation or replacement of integrated neurostimulation system for the posterior tibial nerve.

Clinical Example (0587T)

A 47-year-old female has a long history of debilitating urge incontinence and is voiding more than 20 times every 24 hours. She had been evaluated and found to have an overactive bladder. All available conservative remedies have been unsuccessful and she now elects percutaneous implantation of a posterior tibial nerve wirelessly powered neurostimulation system.

Description of Procedure (0587T)

Patient is placed in supine modified lateral position, so the medial leg is accessible on table. Prepare leg bilaterally and drape with sterile technique. Have integrated neurostimulation external unit available. Then, remove small sleeve from introducer. Palpate medial malleolus on ankle and the Achilles tendon. Place a mark one-third of the way between medial malleolus and Achilles tendon, approximately 2 to 3 cm from the medial malleolus, and draw a parallel line along the tibia. Use local anesthesia at the insertion point and make a small nick at the insertion mark with a #11 blade. Hold the lead introducer vertically to penetrate the fascia, drop the needle, and advance from the insertion point retrograde to the hub of the introducer parallel to tibia. Stimulate with J-hook cable through the small sleeve cut into the introducer needle and increase stimulator slowly until patient feels tingling stimulation. Movement of toes confirms tibial nerve stimulation. Advance stimulator through the lead introducer. Withdraw introducer to the mark on the lead with electrodes exposed and tines still within the introducer. Remove the stylet and stimulate with integrated neurostimulation unit in sterile bag. Note motor and sensory response. Remove the introducer needle and deploy tines. Suture through the stimulator tubing to connective tissue. Suture to dermis to avoid skin irritation and erosion of the suture and trim lead beyond the 7-cm marker. Bury under the dermis and create a small subcutaneous space below the dermis, 1-cm distal to insertion point, with a hemostat. Close skin nick with absorbable suture, skin glue, or steri-strip. Final X rays (anteroposterior and lateral) confirm device placement.

Clinical Example (0588T)

A 65-year-old female had undergone previous percutaneous implantation of a posterior tibial nerve neurostimulation system three years ago. The device had worked well until two months ago when she no longer noted adequate control of her urge incontinence. Imaging studies revealed migration of the device away from the posterior tibial nerve. She has elected to undergo revision of the wirelessly powered neurostimulation system.

Description of Procedure (0588T)

Make an incision over the previous lead insertion site. Isolate and externalize the lead. Remove the lead by wrapping it around a curved hemostat and turning it under tension. If the lead breaks, extend the incision and carry the dissection down to the tibial to remove all fragments. After removal of the integrated neurostimulation system, close the wound in standard fashion.

Clinical Example (0589T)

A 55-year-old female with severe urgency incontinence recently underwent percutaneous implantation of an integrated single device neurostimulation system including electrode array and receiver adjacent to the posterior tibial nerve. During the procedure, initial electronic analysis and programming were performed.

Description of Procedure (0589T)

Physician performs electronic analysis and programming of the integrated system. Tests three separate implant parameters while assessing the degree of response and side effect improvement or worsening after each programming change.

Clinical Example (0590T)

A 57-year-old female with refractory overactive bladder symptoms recently underwent percutaneous implantation of an integrated single device neurostimulation system including electrode array and receiver adjacent to the posterior tibial nerve. During the procedure, initial electronic analysis and programming were performed.

Description of Procedure (0590T)

Physician performs electronic analysis and programming of the integrated system. Tests over four combinations of the implant parameters while assessing the degree of response and side effect improvement or worsening after each programming change.

►Health and Well-Being Coaching◄

►Health and well-being coaching is a patient-centered approach wherein patients determine their goals, use self-discovery or active learning processes together with content education to work toward their goals, and self-monitor behaviors to increase accountability, all within the context of an interpersonal relationship with a coach. The coach is a nonphysician health care professional certified by the National Board for Health and Wellness Coaching or National Commission for Health Education Credentialing, Inc. Coaches' training includes behavioral change theory, motivational strategies, communication techniques, health education and promotion theories, which are used to assist patients to develop intrinsic motivation and obtain skills to create sustainable change for improved health and well-being.◄

- ● **0591T** Health and well-being coaching face-to-face; individual, initial assessment
- ● **0592T** individual, follow-up session, at least 30 minutes

  ►(Do not report 0592T in conjunction with 96156, 96158, 96159, 98960, 0488T, 0591T)◄

  ►(For medical nutrition therapy, see 97802, 97803, 97804)◄

- ● **0593T** group (2 or more individuals), at least 30 minutes

  ►(Do not report 0593T in conjunction with 96164, 96165, 97150, 98961, 98962, 0403T)◄

Rationale

In the Category III section, three Category III codes (0591T, 0592T, 0593T) have been added to report health coaching services. A new heading "Health and Well-Being Coaching" has been added along with introductory guidelines to address the intended use for these services. In addition, three parenthetical notes have been added following the new codes to guide users in the appropriate reporting of these services in conjunction with other services in the CPT code set.

Category III codes 0591T, 0592T, and 0593T are intended to describe health and well-being coaching. These codes represent a new approach geared toward patients such as those who experience chronic pain and any other forms of chronic disorders and provide opportunities for patients to develop knowledge, skill, and self-confidence to participate in decision making and to implement long-term behavior changes that prevent the trajectory of lifestyle-related disease (eg, chronic low back pain, obesity, hypertension, and many others). Health coaching also provides guidance to patients by aiding in creating visions for optimal health and exploration of long-term goals to align with the patient's visions. These codes have been established to specifically describe a patient-centered approach wherein patients determine their goals, use self-discovery, or active learning processes together with content education to work toward their goals, and self-monitor behaviors to increase accountability. The new Category III codes include codes for health and well-being coaching face-to-face (0591T), follow-up individual session (0592T), and group session (0593T). It is important to note that the new Category III guidelines define health and well-being coaching and who performs these services. In addition, exclusionary and instructional parenthetical notes have been added following codes 0592T and 0593T to guide and instruct the user on appropriate reporting of these new services in conjunction with related or similar services. The exclusionary parenthetical note added following code 0592T restricts reporting of certain procedures that are inherently included as part of the service. The restricted services are health and behavior assessment and intervention (96156, 96158, 96159); education and training for patient self-management (98960); preventive behavior change (0488T); and face-to-face health and well-being coaching (0591T). An additional instructional parenthetical note has been added to direct users to the codes for medical nutrition therapy (97802, 97803, 97804). Finally, an exclusionary parenthetical note has been added following code 0593T to restrict reporting health behavior intervention, group procedures (96164, 96165); therapeutic procedure[s] (97150); education and training (98961, 98962); and preventive behavior change (0403T).

Clinical Example (0591T)

A 48-year-old female with chronic disease is referred to a health coach to set realistic health and well-being goals centered around her health and well-being priorities and values.

Description of Procedure (0591T)

Health coaching is provided by a trained health coach. Initial coaching sessions occur between a health coach and individual. These services are typically provided in outpatient clinical settings but may also include inpatient settings. The initial session is 60 to 90 minutes.

It can be done either physically face-to-face or via real-time synchronous audio-visual communication. Introduce the concepts of health coaching, as well as learn what is most important in the patient's life, their support structure, and awareness of impact of social determinants of health on their well-being. Guide patients in creating a vision of their optimal health, and explore long-term goals that align with that vision. Although patients will have chronic illness, the focus of health coaching visits and subsequent goal-setting is set by the patient. Help patients create specific, realistic goals in the context of moving toward their optimal health vision, with these goals further broken down into small, realistic action steps. Utilize motivational interviewing, reflective listening, and behavior change theory. Help the patient learn to anticipate obstacles that may arise and leverage the patient's own unique problem-solving skills to work the desired behavior change into daily life. Document all visits in the medical record.

Clinical Example (0592T)

A 48-year-old female with chronic disease has a follow-up visit with a trained health coach to continue work centered around her health and well-being goals, priorities, and values.

Description of Procedure (0592T)

Health coaching is provided by a trained health coach. Follow-up coaching sessions occur between a health coach and individual. These services are typically provided in outpatient clinical settings but may also include inpatient settings. The follow-up sessions are typically 30 to 60 minutes. Coaching typically occurs weekly at the start of coaching to establish effective communication between the health coach and the patient, and with a minimal frequency of biweekly. After three months, coaching is tapered to monthly for most patients. The coaching sessions occur physically face-to-face or via real-time synchronous audio-visual communication. During follow-up sessions, ask patients what is important to them about their health and how well they think they manage their health. Guide the patient in creating a vision of optimal health, and explore long-term goals that align with that vision. Help the patient create specific, realistic goals in the context of moving toward their optimal health vision, with these goals further broken down into small, realistic action steps. Health coaches utilize motivational interviewing, reflective listening, and behavior change theory. At each subsequent session, the coach and patient discuss what was successful, what challenges arose, and most importantly what the patient learned about themselves in the process of implementing the prior session's action steps. Each session's action steps build on each other until the goal is consistently met. In addition, the health coach helps the patient learn to anticipate obstacles week to week, and leverages the patient's own unique problem-solving skills to implement the desired behavior change into daily life. During the coaching sessions, the coach continuously helps the patient link their individual values and personal sense of meaning with the behavioral goals to elicit intrinsic motivation that assists patients to sustain the behavior change far beyond the coaching period. All visits are documented in the medical record.

Clinical Example (0593T)

A 50-year-old male veteran with chronic disease is referred to a group health coaching session to set realistic health and well-being goals centered around his health and well-being priorities and values.

Description of Procedure (0593T)

Health coaching is provided by a trained health coach. Group health coaching sessions occur between a health coach and group of patients. These services are typically offered in outpatient clinical settings but may also include inpatient settings. Group health coaching sessions are typically 60 minutes. Group health coaching typically occurs weekly at the start of coaching to establish effective communication between the health coach and the patients with a minimal frequency of biweekly. After three months, it can be tapered to monthly in most situations. It can be done face-to-face or via real-time synchronous audio-visual communication. During sessions, guide patients in creating a vision of their optimal health, and explore long-term goals that align with that vision. Help patients create specific, realistic goals in the context of moving toward their optimal health vision, with these goals further broken down into small, realistic action steps. Utilize motivational interviewing, reflective listening, and behavior change theory. At each subsequent session, discuss with the patients what was successful, what challenges arose, and most importantly what the patients learned about themselves in the process of implementing the prior session's action steps. Each session's action steps build on each other until the goal is consistently met. Help the patients learn to anticipate obstacles week to week, and leverage the patients' own unique problem-solving skills to work the desired behavior change into daily life. During the coaching sessions, continuously help the patients link their individual values and personal sense of meaning with the behavioral goals to elicit intrinsic motivation that assists patients to sustain the behavior change far beyond the coaching period. Health coaches are trained to facilitate group sessions to allow for shared experiences and group learning, as well as develop a support system for fellow participants. Document all visits in the medical record.

Appendix A

Summary of Additions, Deletions, and Revisions

The summary of changes shows the actual changes that have been made to the code descriptors.

New codes appear with a bullet (●) and are indicated as "Code added." Revised codes are preceded with a triangle (▲). Within revised codes, or if a code symbol has been deleted, the deleted language and code symbol appear with a strikethrough (⊖), while new text appears underlined.

The ⁄ symbol is used to identify codes for vaccines that are pending FDA approval. The # symbol is used to identify codes that have been resequenced. CPT add-on codes are annotated by the + symbol. The ⊘ symbol is used to identify codes that are exempt from the use of modifier 51. The ★ symbol is used to identify codes that may be used for reporting telemedicine services. The ⋈ is used to identify proprietary laboratory analyses (PLA) test that has an identical descriptor as another PLA test. A PLA code that satisfies Category I code criteria and has been accepted by the CPT Editorial Panel is annotated with the ↕ symbol.

Modifier	Modifier Descriptor
50	▶**Bilateral Procedure:** Unless otherwise identified in the listings, bilateral procedures that are performed at the same session, should be identified by adding modifier 50 to the appropriate 5 digit code. **Note:** This modifier should not be appended to designated "add-on" codes (see Appendix D).◀
63	▶**Procedure Performed on Infants less than 4 kg:** Procedures performed on neonates and infants up to a present body weight of 4 kg may involve significantly increased complexity and physician or other qualified health care professional work commonly associated with these patients. This circumstance may be reported by adding modifier 63 to the procedure number. **Note:** Unless otherwise designated, this modifier may only be appended to procedures/services listed in the 20100-69990 code series and 92920, 92928, 92953, 92960, 92986, 92987, 92990, 92997, 92998, 93312, 93313, 93314, 93315, 93316, 93317, 93318, 93452, 93505, 93530, 93531, 93532, 93533, 93561, 93562, 93563, 93564, 93568, 93580, 93582, 93590, 93591, 93592, 93615, 93616 from the Medicine/Cardiovascular section. Modifier 63 should not be appended to any CPT codes listed in the **Evaluation and Management Services, Anesthesia, Radiology, Pathology/Laboratory,** or **Medicine** sections (other than those identified above from the Medicine/Cardiovascular section).◀

Appendix A

Modifiers

50 ▶**Bilateral Procedure:** Unless otherwise identified in the listings, bilateral procedures that are performed at the same session, should be identified by adding modifier 50 to the appropriate 5 digit code. **Note:** This modifier should not be appended to designated "add-on" codes (see Appendix D).◀

Rationale

The guidelines for modifier 50, *Bilateral Procedure,* have been revised with instructions for reporting add-on procedures that are performed bilaterally. Previously, the instructions for reporting add-on procedures when performed bilaterally varied throughout the code set whereby some add-on codes were reported twice, while others were reported with modifier 50, *Bilateral Procedure,* appended.

For 2020, the instruction for reporting add-on procedures when performed bilaterally has been standardized to indicate that add-on codes should be reported twice, instead of reporting modifier 50.

63 ▶**Procedure Performed on Infants less than 4 kg:** Procedures performed on neonates and infants up to a present body weight of 4 kg may involve significantly increased complexity and physician or other qualified health care professional work commonly associated with these patients. This circumstance may be reported by adding modifier 63 to the procedure number. **Note:** Unless otherwise designated, this modifier may only be appended to procedures/services listed in the 20100-69990 code series and 92920, 92928, 92953, 92960, 92986, 92987, 92990, 92997, 92998, 93312, 93313, 93314, 93315, 93316, 93317, 93318, 93452, 93505, 93530, 93531, 93532, 93533, 93561, 93562, 93563, 93564, 93568, 93580, 93582, 93590, 93591, 93592, 93615, 93616 from the Medicine/Cardiovascular section. Modifier 63 should not be appended to any CPT codes listed in the **Evaluation and Management Services, Anesthesia, Radiology, Pathology/Laboratory,** or **Medicine** sections (other than those identified above from the Medicine/Cardiovascular section).◀

Rationale

The codes in the definition of modifier 63 have been revised to include services from the Medicine/Cardiovascular section.

The codes now listed in the description of modifier 63 represent invasive cardiovascular procedures that may be used to treat infants less than 4 kg. As with the procedures/services listed in the 20100-69990 code series, when an invasive cardiovascular procedure is performed on an infant less than 4 kg, it represents significantly more physician or other qualified health care professional work.

The revised descriptor now includes codes 92920, 92928, 92953, 92960, 92986, 92987, 92990, 92997, 92998, 93312, 93313, 93314, 93315, 93316, 93317, 93318, 93452, 93505, 93530, 93531, 93532, 93533, 93561, 93562, 93563, 93564, 93568, 93580, 93582, 93590, 93591, 93592, 93615, and 93616 from the Medicine/Cardiovascular section.

Modifiers Approved for Ambulatory Surgery Center (ASC) Hospital Outpatient Use

CPT Level I Modifiers

50 ▶**Bilateral Procedure:** Unless otherwise identified in the listings, bilateral procedures that are performed at the same session, should be identified by adding modifier 50 to the appropriate 5 digit code. **Note:** This modifier should not be appended to designated "add-on" codes (see Appendix D).◀

Rationale

In the Modifiers Approved for Ambulatory Surgery Center (ASC) Hospital Outpatient Use subsection of Appendix A, the guidelines for modifier 50, *Bilateral Procedure,* have been revised with instructions for reporting add-on procedures that are performed bilaterally. Previously, the instructions for reporting add-on procedures when performed bilaterally varied throughout the code set whereby some add-on codes were reported twice, while others were reported with modifier 50, *Bilateral Procedure,* appended.

For 2020, the instruction for reporting add-on procedures when performed bilaterally has been standardized to indicate that add-on codes should be reported twice instead of reporting modifier 50.

Appendix E

Summary of Additions, Deletions, and Revisions

The summary of changes shows the actual changes that have been made to the code descriptors.

New codes appear with a bullet (●) and are indicated as "Code added." Revised codes are preceded with a triangle (▲). Within revised codes, or if a code symbol has been deleted, the deleted language and code symbol appear with a strikethrough (⊖), while new text appears underlined.

The ⁄ symbol is used to identify codes for vaccines that are pending FDA approval. The # symbol is used to identify codes that have been resequenced. CPT add-on codes are annotated by the + symbol. The ⊘ symbol is used to identify codes that are exempt from the use of modifier 51. The ★ symbol is used to identify codes that may be used for reporting telemedicine services. The ⋈ is used to identify proprietary laboratory analyses (PLA) test that has an identical descriptor as another PLA test. A PLA code that satisfies Category I code criteria and has been accepted by the CPT Editorial Panel is annotated with the ↑↓ symbol.

Code
17004
31500
36620
93451
93456
93503
93631
95992

Appendix E

Summary of CPT Codes Exempt from Modifier 51

This listing is a summary of CPT codes that are exempt from the use of modifier 51. Procedures on this list are typically performed with another procedure but may be a stand-alone procedure and not always performed with other specified procedures. For add-on codes, see Appendix D. This is not an exhaustive list of procedures that are typically exempt from multiple procedure reductions. The codes listed below are identified in CPT 2020 with a ⊘ symbol.

20697	93602	93618
20974	93603	94610
20975	93610	95905
44500	93612	99151
61107	93615	99152
93600	93616	

Rationale

Appendix E has been updated by deleting eight codes from its listing. Codes 17004, 31500, 36620, 93451, 93456, 93503, 93631, and 95992 were reviewed because of a survey requested by the AMA/Specialty Relative Value Scale (RVS) Update Committee (RUC) Relativity Assessment Workgroup (RAW), which identified that there was duplication on pre- and post-work related to the services with which these codes are typically reported.

To ensure that there is no duplication in work, codes 17004, 31500, 36620, 93451, 93456, 93503, 93631, and 95992 have been removed from the Appendix E listing and the ⊘ symbol has been removed from these codes.

Appendix O

Summary of Additions, Deletions, and Revisions

The summary of changes shows the actual changes that have been made to the code descriptors.

New codes appear with a bullet (●) and are indicated as "Code added." Revised codes are preceded with a triangle (▲). Within revised codes, or if a code symbol has been deleted, the deleted language and code symbol appear with a ~~strikethrough~~ (⊖), while new text appears underlined.

The ⁄ symbol is used to identify codes for vaccines that are pending FDA approval. The # symbol is used to identify codes that have been resequenced. CPT add-on codes are annotated by the + symbol. The ⊘ symbol is used to identify codes that are exempt from the use of modifier 51. The ★ symbol is used to identify codes that may be used for reporting telemedicine services. The ✣ is used to identify proprietary laboratory analyses (PLA) test that has an identical descriptor as another PLA test. A PLA code that satisfies Category I code criteria and has been accepted by the CPT Editorial Panel is annotated with the ↿⇂ symbol.

Proprietary Name and Clinical Laboratory or Manufacturer	Alpha-Numeric Code	Code Descriptor
Administrative Codes for Multianalyte Assays with Algorithmic Analyses (MAAA)		
ASH FibroSURE™, ▶BioPredictive S.A.S◀	0002M	Liver disease, ten biochemical assays (ALT, A2-macroglobulin, apolipoprotein A-1, total bilirubin, GGT, haptoglobin, AST, glucose, total cholesterol and triglycerides) utilizing serum, prognostic algorithm reported as quantitative scores for fibrosis, steatosis and alcoholic steatohepatitis (ASH)
NASH FibroSURE™, ▶BioPredictive S.A.S◀	0003M	Liver disease, ten biochemical assays (ALT, A2-macroglobulin, apolipoprotein A-1, total bilirubin, GGT, haptoglobin, AST, glucose, total cholesterol and triglycerides) utilizing serum, prognostic algorithm reported as quantitative scores for fibrosis, steatosis and nonalcoholic steatohepatitis (NASH)

~~VisibiliT test, Sequenom Center for Molecular Medicine, LLC~~	▶(0009M has been deleted)◀	~~Fetal aneuploidy (trisomy 21, and 18) DNA sequence analysis of selected regions using maternal plasma, algorithm reported as a risk score for each trisomy~~
NeoLAB™ Prostate Liquid Biopsy, NeoGenomics Laboratories	▲0011M	▶Oncology, prostate cancer, mRNA expression assay of 12 genes (10 content and 2 housekeeping), RT-PCR test utilizing blood plasma and urine, algorithms to predict high-grade prostate cancer risk◀
▶EndoPredict®, Myriad Genetic Laboratories, Inc◀	●81522	▶Oncology (breast), mRNA, gene expression profiling by RT-PCR of 12 genes (8 content and 4 housekeeping), utilizing formalin-fixed paraffin-embedded tissue, algorithm reported as recurrence risk score◀

(Continued on page 238)

▲=Revised code   ●=New code   ▶◀=Contains new or revised text   ✣=Duplicate PLA test   ↿⇂=Category I PLA

Appendix O

Proprietary Name and Clinical Laboratory or Manufacturer	Alpha-Numeric Code	Code Descriptor
▶Decipher® Prostate, Decipher® Biosciences◀	●81542	▶Oncology (prostate) mRNA, microarray gene expression profiling of 22 content genes, utilizing formalin-fixed paraffin-embedded tissue, algorithm reported as metastasis risk score◀
▶DecisionDx®-UM test, Castle Biosciences, Inc◀	●81552	▶Oncology (uveal melanoma), mRNA, gene expression profiling by real-time RT-PCR of 15 genes (12 content and 3 housekeeping), utilizing fine needle aspirate or formalin-fixed paraffin-embedded tissue, algorithm reported as risk of metastasis◀
▶ ~~AmHPR Helicobacter pylori~~ AmHPR® H. pylori Antibiotic Resistance ~~Next Generation Sequencing~~ Panel, American Molecular Laboratories, Inc◀	▲0008U	▶Helicobacter pylori detection and antibiotic resistance, DNA, 16S and 23S rRNA, gyrA, pbp1, rdxA and rpoB, next generation sequencing, formalin-fixed paraffin-embedded or fresh tissue <u>or fecal sample</u>, predictive, reported as positive or negative for resistance to clarithromycin, fluoroquinolones, metronidazole, amoxicillin, tetracycline, and rifabutin◀
~~ToxLok, InSource Diagnostics, InSource Diagnostics~~	▶(0020U has been deleted)◀	~~Drug test(s), presumptive, with definitive confirmation of positive results, any number of drug classes, urine, with specimen verification including DNA authentication in comparison to buccal DNA, per date of service~~ ~~(For additional PLA code with identical clinical descriptor, see 0007U. See Appendix O to determine appropriate code assignment)~~
~~CYP2D6 Genotype Cascade, Mayo Clinic, Mayo Clinic~~	▶(0028U has been deleted)◀	~~CYP2D6 (cytochrome P450, family 2, subfamily D, polypeptide 6) (eg, drug metabolism) gene analysis, copy number variants, common variants with reflex to targeted sequence~~
~~RNA Sequencing by NGS, OmniSeq, Inc, Life Technologies Corporation~~	▶(0057U has been deleted)◀	~~Oncology (solid organ neoplasia), mRNA, gene expression profiling by massively parallel sequencing for analysis of 51 genes, utilizing formalin-fixed paraffin-embedded tissue, algorithm reported as a normalized percentile rank~~
▶SLE-key® Rule Out, Veracis Inc Veracis Inc◀	●0062U	▶Autoimmune (systemic lupus erythematosus), IgG and IgM analysis of 80 biomarkers, utilizing serum, algorithm reported with a risk score◀
▶NPDX ASD ADM Panel I, Stemina Biomarker Discovery, Inc, Stemina Biomarker Discovery, Inc d/b/a NeuroPointDX◀	●0063U	▶Neurology (autism), 32 amines by LC-MS/MS, using plasma, algorithm reported as metabolic signature associated with autism spectrum disorder◀
▶BioPlex 2200 Syphilis Total & RPR Assay, Bio-Rad Laboratories, Bio-Rad Laboratories◀	●0064U	▶Antibody, Treponema pallidum, total and rapid plasma reagin (RPR), immunoassay, qualitative◀
▶BioPlex 2200 RPR Assay, Bio-Rad Laboratories, Bio-Rad Laboratories◀	●0065U	▶Syphilis test, non-treponemal antibody, immunoassay, qualitative (RPR)◀

Appendix O

Proprietary Name and Clinical Laboratory or Manufacturer	Alpha-Numeric Code	Code Descriptor
▶PartoSure™ Test, Parsagen Diagnostics, Inc, Parsagen Diagnostics, Inc, a QIAGEN Company◀	●0066U	▶Placental alpha-micro globulin-1 (PAMG-1), immunoassay with direct optical observation, cervico-vaginal fluid, each specimen◀
▶BBDRisk Dx™, Silbiotech, Inc, Silbiotech, Inc◀	●0067U	▶Oncology (breast), immunohistochemistry, protein expression profiling of 4 biomarkers (matrix metalloproteinase-1 [MMP-1], carcinoembryonic antigen-related cell adhesion molecule 6 [CEACAM6], hyaluronoglucosaminidase [HYAL1], highly expressed in cancer protein [HEC1]), formalin-fixed paraffin-embedded precancerous breast tissue, algorithm reported as carcinoma risk score◀
▶MYCODART Dual Amplification Real Time PCR Panel for 6 Candida species, RealTime Laboratories, Inc, RealTime Laboratories, Inc◀	●0068U	▶Candida species panel (*C. albicans, C. glabrata, C. parapsilosis, C. kruseii, C. tropicalis,* and *C. auris*), amplified probe technique with qualitative report of the presence or absence of each species◀
▶miR-31now™, GoPath Laboratories, GoPath Laboratories◀	●0069U	▶Oncology (colorectal), microRNA, RT-PCR expression profiling of miR-31-3p, formalin-fixed paraffin-embedded tissue, algorithm reported as an expression score◀
▶*CYP2D6* Common Variants and Copy Number, Mayo Clinic, Laboratory Developed Test◀	●0070U	▶*CYP2D6 (cytochrome P450, family 2, subfamily D, polypeptide 6)* (eg, drug metabolism) gene analysis, common and select rare variants (ie, *2, *3, *4, *4N, *5, *6, *7, *8, *9, *10, *11, *12, *13, *14A, *14B, *15, *17, *29, *35, *36, *41, *57, *61, *63, *68, *83, *xN)◀
▶*CYP2D6* Full Gene Sequencing, Mayo Clinic, Laboratory Developed Test◀	+●0071U	▶*CYP2D6 (cytochrome P450, family 2, subfamily D, polypeptide 6)* (eg, drug metabolism) gene analysis, full gene sequence (List separately in addition to code for primary procedure)◀ ▶(Use 0071U in conjunction with 0070U)◀
▶*CYP2D6-2D7* Hybrid Gene Targeted Sequence Analysis, Mayo Clinic, Laboratory Developed Test◀	+●0072U	▶*CYP2D6 (cytochrome P450, family 2, subfamily D, polypeptide 6)* (eg, drug metabolism) gene analysis, targeted sequence analysis (ie, CYP2D6-2D7 hybrid gene) (List separately in addition to code for primary procedure)◀ ▶(Use 0072U in conjunction with 0070U)◀
▶*CYP2D7-2D6* Hybrid Gene Targeted Sequence Analysis, Mayo Clinic, Laboratory Developed Test◀	+●0073U	▶*CYP2D6 (cytochrome P450, family 2, subfamily D, polypeptide 6)* (eg, drug metabolism) gene analysis, targeted sequence analysis (ie, CYP2D7-2D6 hybrid gene) (List separately in addition to code for primary procedure)◀ ▶(Use 0073U in conjunction with 0070U)◀

(Continued on page 240)

▲=Revised code   ●=New code   ▶◀=Contains new or revised text   ⋈=Duplicate PLA test   ↑↓=Category I PLA

Proprietary Name and Clinical Laboratory or Manufacturer	Alpha-Numeric Code	Code Descriptor
▶CYP2D6 trans-duplication/multiplication non-duplicated gene targeted sequence analysis, Mayo Clinic, Laboratory Developed Test◀	+●0074U	▶CYP2D6 (cytochrome P450, family 2, subfamily D, polypeptide 6) (eg, drug metabolism) gene analysis, targeted sequence analysis (ie, non-duplicated gene when duplication/multiplication is trans) (List separately in addition to code for primary procedure)◀ ▶(Use 0074U in conjunction with 0070U)◀
▶CYP2D6 5' gene duplication/multiplication targeted sequence analysis, Mayo Clinic, Laboratory Developed Test◀	+●0075U	▶CYP2D6 (cytochrome P450, family 2, subfamily D, polypeptide 6) (eg, drug metabolism) gene analysis, targeted sequence analysis (ie, 5' gene duplication/multiplication) (List separately in addition to code for primary procedure)◀ ▶(Use 0075U in conjunction with 0070U)◀
▶CYP2D6 3' gene duplication/multiplication targeted sequence analysis, Mayo Clinic, Laboratory Developed Test◀	+●0076U	▶CYP2D6 (cytochrome P450, family 2, subfamily D, polypeptide 6) (eg, drug metabolism) gene analysis, targeted sequence analysis (ie, 3' gene duplication/multiplication) (List separately in addition to code for primary procedure)◀ ▶(Use 0076U in conjunction with 0070U)◀
▶M-Protein Detection and Isotyping by MALDI-TOF Mass Spectrometry, Mayo Clinic, Laboratory Developed Test◀	●0077U	▶Immunoglobulin paraprotein (M-protein), qualitative, immunoprecipitation and mass spectrometry, blood or urine, including isotype◀
▶INFINITI® Neural Response Panel, PersonalizeDx Labs, AutoGenomics Inc◀	●0078U	▶Pain management (opioid-use disorder) genotyping panel, 16 common variants (ie, ABCB1, COMT, DAT1, DBH, DOR, DRD1, DRD2, DRD4, GABA, GAL, HTR2A, HTTLPR, MTHFR, MUOR, OPRK1, OPRM1), buccal swab or other germline tissue sample, algorithm reported as positive or negative risk of opioid-use disorder◀
▶ToxLok™, InSource Diagnostics, InSource Diagnostics◀	●0079U	▶Comparative DNA analysis using multiple selected single-nucleotide polymorphisms (SNPs), urine and buccal DNA, for specimen identity verification◀
▶BDX-XL2, Biodesix®, Inc, Biodesix®, Inc◀	●0080U	▶Oncology (lung), mass spectrometric analysis of galectin-3-binding protein and scavenger receptor cysteine-rich type 1 protein M130, with five clinical risk factors (age, smoking status, nodule diameter, nodule-spiculation status and nodule location), utilizing plasma, algorithm reported as a categorical probability of malignancy◀
DecisionDx®-UM, Castle Biosciences, Inc	▶(0081U has been deleted. To report, use 81552)◀	Oncology (uveal melanoma), mRNA, gene expression profiling by real-time RT-PCR of 15 genes (12 content and 3 housekeeping genes), utilizing fine needle aspirate or formalin-fixed paraffin-embedded tissue, algorithm reported as risk of metastasis

CPT Changes 2020 — Appendix O

Proprietary Name and Clinical Laboratory or Manufacturer	Alpha-Numeric Code	Code Descriptor
▶NextGen Precision™ Testing, Precision Diagnostics, Precision Diagnostics LBN Precision Toxicology, LLC◀	●0082U	▶Drug test(s), definitive, 90 or more drugs or substances, definitive chromatography with mass spectrometry, and presumptive, any number of drug classes, by instrument chemistry analyzer (utilizing immunoassay), urine, report of presence or absence of each drug, drug metabolite or substance with description and severity of significant interactions per date of service◀
▶Onco4D™, Animated Dynamics, Inc, Animated Dynamics, Inc◀	●0083U	▶Oncology, response to chemotherapy drugs using motility contrast tomography, fresh or frozen tissue, reported as likelihood of sensitivity or resistance to drugs or drug combinations◀
▶BLOODchip® ID CORE XT™, Grifols Diagnostic Solutions Inc◀	●0084U	▶Red blood cell antigen typing, DNA, genotyping of 10 blood groups with phenotype prediction of 37 red blood cell antigens◀
▶IB*Schek*™, Commonwealth Diagnostics International, Inc◀	●0085U	▶Cytolethal distending toxin B (CdtB) and vinculin IgG antibodies by immunoassay (ie, ELISA)◀
▶Accelerate PhenoTest™ BC kit, Accelerate Diagnostics, Inc◀	●0086U	▶Infectious disease (bacterial and fungal), organism identification, blood culture, using rRNA FISH, 6 or more organism targets, reported as positive or negative with phenotypic minimum inhibitory concentration (MIC)-based antimicrobial susceptibility◀
▶Molecular Microscope® MMDx—Heart, Kashi Clinical Laboratories◀	●0087U	▶Cardiology (heart transplant), mRNA gene expression profiling by microarray of 1283 genes, transplant biopsy tissue, allograft rejection and injury algorithm reported as a probability score◀
▶Molecular Microscope® MMDx—Kidney, Kashi Clinical Laboratories◀	●0088U	▶Transplantation medicine (kidney allograft rejection), microarray gene expression profiling of 1494 genes, utilizing transplant biopsy tissue, algorithm reported as a probability score for rejection◀
▶Pigmented Lesion Assay (PLA), DermTech◀	●0089U	▶Oncology (melanoma), gene expression profiling by RTqPCR, *PRAME* and *LINC00518*, superficial collection using adhesive patch(es)◀
▶myPath® Melanoma, Myriad Genetic Laboratories◀	●0090U	▶Oncology (cutaneous melanoma), mRNA gene expression profiling by RT-PCR of 23 genes (14 content and 9 housekeeping), utilizing formalin-fixed paraffin-embedded tissue, algorithm reported as a categorical result (ie, benign, indeterminate, malignant)◀
▶FirstSight^CRC, CellMax Life◀	●0091U	▶Oncology (colorectal) screening, cell enumeration of circulating tumor cells, utilizing whole blood, algorithm, for the presence of adenoma or cancer, reported as a positive or negative result◀
▶REVEAL Lung Nodule Characterization, MagArray, Inc◀	●0092U	▶Oncology (lung), three protein biomarkers, immunoassay using magnetic nanosensor technology, plasma, algorithm reported as risk score for likelihood of malignancy◀

(Continued on page 242)

▲=Revised code ●=New code ▶◀=Contains new or revised text ✣=Duplicate PLA test ↑↓=Category I PLA

Proprietary Name and Clinical Laboratory or Manufacturer	Alpha-Numeric Code	Code Descriptor
▶ComplyRX, Claro Labs◀	●0093U	▶Prescription drug monitoring, evaluation of 65 common drugs by LC-MS/MS, urine, each drug reported detected or not detected◀
▶RCIGM Rapid Whole Genome Sequencing, Rady Children's Institute for Genomic Medicine (RCIGM)◀	●0094U	▶Genome (eg, unexplained constitutional or heritable disorder or syndrome), rapid sequence analysis◀
▶Esophageal String Test™ (EST), Cambridge Biomedical, Inc◀	●0095U	▶Inflammation (eosinophilic esophagitis), ELISA analysis of eotaxin-3 *(CCL26 [C-C motif chemokine ligand 26])* and major basic protein *(PRG2 [proteoglycan 2, pro eosinophil major basic protein])*, specimen obtained by swallowed nylon string, algorithm reported as predictive probability index for active eosinophilic esophagitis◀
▶HPV, High-Risk, Male Urine, Molecular Testing Labs◀	●0096U	▶Human papillomavirus (HPV), high-risk types (ie, 16, 18, 31, 33, 35, 39, 45, 51, 52, 56, 58, 59, 66, 68), male urine◀
▶BioFire® FilmArray® Gastrointestinal (GI) Panel, BioFire® Diagnostics◀	●0097U	▶Gastrointestinal pathogen, multiplex reverse transcription and multiplex amplified probe technique, multiple types or subtypes, 22 targets (Campylobacter [C. jejuni/C. coli/C. upsaliensis], Clostridium difficile [C. difficile] toxin A/B, Plesiomonas shigelloides, Salmonella, Vibrio [V. parahaemolyticus/V. vulnificus/V. cholerae], including specific identification of Vibrio cholerae, Yersinia enterocolitica, Enteroaggregative Escherichia coli [EAEC], Enteropathogenic Escherichia coli [EPEC], Enterotoxigenic Escherichia coli [ETEC] lt/st, Shiga-like toxin-producing Escherichia coli [STEC] stx1/stx2 [including specific identification of the E. coli O157 serogroup within STEC], Shigella/Enteroinvasive Escherichia coli [EIEC], Cryptosporidium, Cyclospora cayetanensis, Entamoeba histolytica, Giardia lamblia [also known as G. intestinalis and G. duodenalis], adenovirus F 40/41, astrovirus, norovirus GI/GII, rotavirus A, sapovirus [Genogroups I, II, IV, and V])◀
▶BioFire® FilmArray® Respiratory Panel (RP) EZ, BioFire® Diagnostics◀	●0098U	▶Respiratory pathogen, multiplex reverse transcription and multiplex amplified probe technique, multiple types or subtypes, 14 targets (adenovirus, coronavirus, human metapneumovirus, influenza A, influenza A subtype H1, influenza A subtype H3, influenza A subtype H1-2009, influenza B, parainfluenza virus, human rhinovirus/enterovirus, respiratory syncytial virus, Bordetella pertussis, Chlamydophila pneumoniae, Mycoplasma pneumoniae)◀

Proprietary Name and Clinical Laboratory or Manufacturer	Alpha-Numeric Code	Code Descriptor
▶BioFire® FilmArray® Respiratory Panel (RP), BioFire® Diagnostics◀	●0099U	▶Respiratory pathogen, multiplex reverse transcription and multiplex amplified probe technique, multiple types or subtypes, 20 targets (adenovirus, coronavirus 229E, coronavirus HKU1, coronavirus, coronavirus OC43, human metapneumovirus, influenza A, influenza A subtype, influenza A subtype H3, influenza A subtype H1-2009, influenza, parainfluenza virus, parainfluenza virus 2, parainfluenza virus 3, parainfluenza virus 4, human rhinovirus/enterovirus, respiratory syncytial virus, Bordetella pertussis, Chlamydophila pneumonia, Mycoplasma pneumoniae)◀
▶BioFire® FilmArray® Respiratory Panel 2 (RP2), BioFire® Diagnostics◀	●0100U	▶Respiratory pathogen, multiplex reverse transcription and multiplex amplified probe technique, multiple types or subtypes, 21 targets (adenovirus, coronavirus 229E, coronavirus HKU1, coronavirus NL63, coronavirus OC43, human metapneumovirus, human rhinovirus/enterovirus, influenza A, including subtypes H1, H1-2009, and H3, influenza B, parainfluenza virus 1, parainfluenza virus 2, parainfluenza virus 3, parainfluenza virus 4, respiratory syncytial virus, Bordetella parapertussis [IS1001], Bordetella pertussis [ptxP], Chlamydia pneumoniae, Mycoplasma pneumoniae)◀
▶ColoNext®, Ambry Genetics®, Ambry Genetics®◀	●0101U	▶Hereditary colon cancer disorders (eg, Lynch syndrome, PTEN hamartoma syndrome, Cowden syndrome, familial adenomatosis polyposis), genomic sequence analysis panel utilizing a combination of NGS, Sanger, MLPA, and array CGH, with mRNA analytics to resolve variants of unknown significance when indicated (15 genes [sequencing and deletion/duplication], *EPCAM* and *GREM1* [deletion/duplication only])◀
▶BreastNext®, Ambry Genetics®, Ambry Genetics®◀	●0102U	▶Hereditary breast cancer-related disorders (eg, hereditary breast cancer, hereditary ovarian cancer, hereditary endometrial cancer), genomic sequence analysis panel utilizing a combination of NGS, Sanger, MLPA, and array CGH, with mRNA analytics to resolve variants of unknown significance when indicated (17 genes [sequencing and deletion/duplication])◀
▶OvaNext®, Ambry Genetics®, Ambry Genetics®◀	●0103U	▶Hereditary ovarian cancer (eg, hereditary ovarian cancer, hereditary endometrial cancer), genomic sequence analysis panel utilizing a combination of NGS, Sanger, MLPA, and array CGH, with mRNA analytics to resolve variants of unknown significance when indicated (24 genes [sequencing and deletion/duplication], *EPCAM* [deletion/duplication only])◀

(Continued on page 244)

Appendix O   CPT Changes 2020

Proprietary Name and Clinical Laboratory or Manufacturer	Alpha-Numeric Code	Code Descriptor
~~CancerNext®, Ambry Genetics®, Ambry Genetics®~~	▶(0104U has been deleted)◀	~~Hereditary pan cancer (eg, hereditary breast and ovarian cancer, hereditary endometrial cancer, hereditary colorectal cancer), genomic sequence analysis panel utilizing a combination of NGS, Sanger, MLPA, and array CGH, with mRNA analytics to resolve variants of unknown significance when indicated (32 genes)~~
▶KidneyIntelX™, RenalytixAI, RenalytixAI◀	●0105U	▶Nephrology (chronic kidney disease), multiplex electrochemiluminescent immunoassay (ECLIA) of tumor necrosis factor receptor 1A, receptor superfamily 2 *(TNFR1, TNFR2)*, and kidney injury molecule-1 (KIM-1) combined with longitudinal clinical data, including *APOL1* genotype if available, and plasma (isolated fresh or frozen), algorithm reported as probability score for rapid kidney function decline (RKFD)◀
▶13C-Spirulina Gastric Emptying Breath Test (GEBT), Cairn Diagnostics d/b/a Advanced Breath Diagnostics, LLC, Cairn Diagnostics d/b/a Advanced Breath Diagnostics, LLC◀	●0106U	▶Gastric emptying, serial collection of 7 timed breath specimens, non-radioisotope carbon-13 (^{13}C) spirulina substrate, analysis of each specimen by gas isotope ratio mass spectrometry, reported as rate of $^{13}CO_2$ excretion◀
▶Singulex Clarity C.diff toxins A/B Assay, Singulex◀	●0107U	▶Clostridium difficile toxin(s) antigen detection by immunoassay technique, stool, qualitative, multiple-step method◀
▶TissueCypher® Barrett's Esophagus Assay, Cernostics, Cernostics◀	●0108U	▶Gastroenterology (Barrett's esophagus), whole slide–digital imaging, including morphometric analysis, computer-assisted quantitative immunolabeling of 9 protein biomarkers (p16, AMACR, p53, CD68, COX-2, CD45RO, HIF1a, HER-2, K20) and morphology, formalin-fixed paraffin-embedded tissue, algorithm reported as risk of progression to high-grade dysplasia or cancer◀
▶MYCODART Dual Amplification Real Time PCR Panel for 4 Aspergillus species, RealTime Laboratories, Inc/MycoDART, Inc◀	●0109U	▶Infectious disease (Aspergillus species), real-time PCR for detection of DNA from 4 species *(A. fumigatus, A. terreus, A. niger,* and *A. flavus)*, blood, lavage fluid, or tissue, qualitative reporting of presence or absence of each species◀
▶Oral OncolyticAssuranceRX, Firstox Laboratories, LLC, Firstox Laboratories, LLC◀	●0110U	▶Prescription drug monitoring, one or more oral oncology drug(s) and substances, definitive tandem mass spectrometry with chromatography, serum or plasma from capillary blood or venous blood, quantitative report with steady-state range for the prescribed drug(s) when detected◀
▶Praxis(TM) Extended RAS Panel, Illumina, Illumina◀	●0111U	▶Oncology (colon cancer), targeted *KRAS* (codons 12, 13, and 61) and *NRAS* (codons 12, 13, and 61) gene analysis, utilizing formalin-fixed paraffin-embedded tissue◀
▶MicroGenDX qPCR & NGS For Infection, MicroGenDX, MicroGenDX◀	●0112U	▶Infectious agent detection and identification, targeted sequence analysis (16S and 18S rRNA genes) with drug-resistance gene◀

Proprietary Name and Clinical Laboratory or Manufacturer	Alpha-Numeric Code	Code Descriptor
▶MiPS (Mi-Prostate Score), MLabs, MLabs◀	●0113U	▶Oncology (prostate), measurement of *PCA3* and *TMPRSS2-ERG* in urine and PSA in serum following prostatic massage, by RNA amplification and fluorescence-based detection, algorithm reported as risk score◀
▶EsoGuard™, Lucid Diagnostics, Lucid Diagnostics◀	●0114U	▶Gastroenterology (Barrett's esophagus), *VIM* and *CCNA1* methylation analysis, esophageal cells, algorithm reported as likelihood for Barrett's esophagus◀
▶ePlex Respiratory Pathogen (RP) Panel, GenMark Diagnostics, Inc, GenMark Diagnostics, Inc◀	●0115U	▶Respiratory infectious agent detection by nucleic acid (DNA and RNA), 18 viral types and subtypes and 2 bacterial targets, amplified probe technique, including multiplex reverse transcription for RNA targets, each analyte reported as detected or not detected◀
▶Snapshot Oral Fluid Compliance, Ethos Laboratories◀	●0116U	▶Prescription drug monitoring, enzyme immunoassay of 35 or more drugs confirmed with LC-MS/MS, oral fluid, algorithm results reported as a patient-compliance measurement with risk of drug to drug interactions for prescribed medications◀
▶Foundation PI^{SM}, Ethos Laboratories◀	●0117U	▶Pain management, analysis of 11 endogenous analytes (methylmalonic acid, xanthurenic acid, homocysteine, pyroglutamic acid, vanilmandelate, 5-hydroxyindoleacetic acid, hydroxymethylglutarate, ethylmalonate, 3-hydroxypropyl mercapturic acid (3-HPMA), quinolinic acid, kynurenic acid), LC-MS/MS, urine, algorithm reported as a pain-index score with likelihood of atypical biochemical function associated with pain◀
▶Viracor TRAC™ dd-cfDNA, Viracor Eurofins, Viracor Eurofins◀	●0118U	▶Transplantation medicine, quantification of donor-derived cell-free DNA using whole genome next-generation sequencing, plasma, reported as percentage of donor-derived cell-free DNA in the total cell-free DNA◀
▶MI-HEART Ceramides, Plasma, Mayo Clinic, Laboratory Developed Test◀	●0119U	▶Cardiology, ceramides by liquid chromatography–tandem mass spectrometry, plasma, quantitative report with risk score for major cardiovascular events◀
▶Lymph3Cx Lymphoma Molecular Subtyping Assay, Mayo Clinic, Laboratory Developed Test◀	●0120U	▶Oncology (B-cell lymphoma classification), mRNA, gene expression profiling by fluorescent probe hybridization of 58 genes (45 content and 13 housekeeping genes), formalin-fixed paraffin-embedded tissue, algorithm reported as likelihood for primary mediastinal B-cell lymphoma (PMBCL) and diffuse large B-cell lymphoma (DLBCL) with cell of origin subtyping in the latter◀

(Continued on page 246)

Proprietary Name and Clinical Laboratory or Manufacturer	Alpha-Numeric Code	Code Descriptor
▶Flow Adhesion of Whole Blood on VCAM-1 (FAB-V), Functional Fluidics, Functional Fluidics◀	●0121U	▶Sickle cell disease, microfluidic flow adhesion (VCAM-1), whole blood◀
▶Flow Adhesion of Whole Blood to P-SELECTIN (WB-PSEL), Functional Fluidics, Functional Fluidics◀	●0122U	▶Sickle cell disease, microfluidic flow adhesion (P-Selectin), whole blood◀
▶Mechanical Fragility, RBC by shear stress profiling and spectral analysis, Functional Fluidics, Functional Fluidics◀	●0123U	▶Mechanical fragility, RBC, shear stress and spectral analysis profiling◀
▶First Trimester Screen	Fß^{SM}, Eurofins NTD, LLC, Eurofins NTD, LLC◀	●0124U	▶Fetal congenital abnormalities, biochemical assays of 3 analytes (free beta-hCG, PAPP-A, AFP), time-resolved fluorescence immunoassay, maternal dried-blood spot, algorithm reported as risk scores for fetal trisomies 13/18 and 21◀
▶Maternal Fetal Screen	T1^{SM}, Eurofins NTD, LLC, Eurofins NTD, LLC◀	●0125U	▶Fetal congenital abnormalities and perinatal complications, biochemical assays of 5 analytes (free beta-hCG, PAPP-A, AFP, placental growth factor, and inhibin-A), time-resolved fluorescence immunoassay, maternal serum, algorithm reported as risk scores for fetal trisomies 13/18, 21, and preeclampsia◀
▶Maternal Fetal Screen	T1 + Y Chromosome^{SM}, Eurofins NTD, LLC, Eurofins NTD, LLC◀	●0126U	▶Fetal congenital abnormalities and perinatal complications, biochemical assays of 5 analytes (free beta-hCG, PAPP-A, AFP, placental growth factor, and inhibin-A), time-resolved fluorescence immunoassay, includes qualitative assessment of Y chromosome in cell-free fetal DNA, maternal serum and plasma, predictive algorithm reported as risk scores for fetal trisomies 13/18, 21, and preeclampsia◀
▶Preeclampsia Screen	T1^{SM}, Eurofins NTD, LLC, Eurofins NTD, LLC◀	●0127U	▶Obstetrics (preeclampsia), biochemical assays of 3 analytes (PAPP-A, AFP, and placental growth factor), time-resolved fluorescence immunoassay, maternal serum, predictive algorithm reported as a risk score for preeclampsia◀
▶Preeclampsia Screen	T1 + Y Chromosome^{SM}, Eurofins NTD, LLC, Eurofins NTD, LLC◀	●0128U	▶Obstetrics (preeclampsia), biochemical assays of 3 analytes (PAPP-A, AFP, and placental growth factor), time-resolved fluorescence immunoassay, includes qualitative assessment of Y chromosome in cell-free fetal DNA, maternal serum and plasma, predictive algorithm reported as a risk score for preeclampsia◀

Proprietary Name and Clinical Laboratory or Manufacturer	Alpha-Numeric Code	Code Descriptor
▶BRCAplus, Ambry Genetics◀	●0129U	▶Hereditary breast cancer–related disorders (eg, hereditary breast cancer, hereditary ovarian cancer, hereditary endometrial cancer), genomic sequence analysis and deletion/duplication analysis panel *(ATM, BRCA1, BRCA2, CDH1, CHEK2, PALB2, PTEN,* and *TP53)*◀
▶+RNAinsight™ for ColoNext®, Ambry Genetics◀	+●0130U	▶Hereditary colon cancer disorders (eg, Lynch syndrome, PTEN hamartoma syndrome, Cowden syndrome, familial adenomatosis polyposis), targeted mRNA sequence analysis panel *(APC, CDH1, CHEK2, MLH1, MSH2, MSH6, MUTYH, PMS2, PTEN,* and *TP53)* (List separately in addition to code for primary procedure)◀ ▶ (Use 0130U in conjunction with 81435, 0101U)◀
▶+RNAinsight™ for BreastNext®, Ambry Genetics◀	+●0131U	▶Hereditary breast cancer–related disorders (eg, hereditary breast cancer, hereditary ovarian cancer, hereditary endometrial cancer), targeted mRNA sequence analysis panel (13 genes) (List separately in addition to code for primary procedure)◀ ▶(Use 0131U in conjunction with 81162, 81432, 0102U)◀
▶+RNAinsight™ for OvaNext®, Ambry Genetics◀	+●0132U	▶Hereditary ovarian cancer–related disorders (eg, hereditary breast cancer, hereditary ovarian cancer, hereditary endometrial cancer), targeted mRNA sequence analysis panel (17 genes) (List separately in addition to code for primary procedure)◀ ▶(Use 0132U in conjunction with 81162, 81432, 0103U)◀
▶+RNAinsight™ for ProstateNext®, Ambry Genetics◀	+●0133U	▶Hereditary prostate cancer–related disorders, targeted mRNA sequence analysis panel (11 genes) (List separately in addition to code for primary procedure)◀ ▶(Use 0133U in conjunction with 81162)◀
▶+RNAinsight™ for CancerNext®, Ambry Genetics◀	+●0134U	▶Hereditary pan cancer (eg, hereditary breast and ovarian cancer, hereditary endometrial cancer, hereditary colorectal cancer), targeted mRNA sequence analysis panel (18 genes) (List separately in addition to code for primary procedure)◀ ▶(Use 0134U in conjunction with 81162, 81432, 81435)◀
▶+RNAinsight™ for GYNPlus®, Ambry Genetics◀	+●0135U	▶Hereditary gynecological cancer (eg, hereditary breast and ovarian cancer, hereditary endometrial cancer, hereditary colorectal cancer), targeted mRNA sequence analysis panel (12 genes) (List separately in addition to code for primary procedure)◀ ▶(Use 0135U in conjunction with 81162)◀

(Continued on page 248)

Proprietary Name and Clinical Laboratory or Manufacturer	Alpha-Numeric Code	Code Descriptor
►+RNAinsight™ for *ATM*, Ambry Genetics◄	+●0136U	►*ATM (ataxia telangiectasia mutated)* (eg, ataxia telangiectasia) mRNA sequence analysis (List separately in addition to code for primary procedure)◄ ►(Use 0136U in conjunction with 81408)◄
►+RNAinsight™ for *PALB2*, Ambry Genetics◄	+●0137U	►*PALB2 (partner and localizer of BRCA2)* (eg, breast and pancreatic cancer) mRNA sequence analysis (List separately in addition to code for primary procedure)◄ ►(Use 0137U in conjunction with 81307)◄
►+RNAinsight™ for *BRCA1/2*, Ambry Genetics◄	+●0138U	►*BRCA1 (BRCA1, DNA repair associated), BRCA2 (BRCA2, DNA repair associated)* (eg, hereditary breast and ovarian cancer) mRNA sequence analysis (List separately in addition to code for primary procedure)◄ ►(Use 0138U in conjunction with 81162)◄

Appendix O

Multianalyte Assays with Algorithmic Analyses and Proprietary Laboratory Analyses

The following list includes three types of CPT codes:

1. Multianalyte assays with algorithmic analyses (MAAA) administrative codes
2. Category I MAAA codes
3. Proprietary laboratory analyses (PLA) codes

1. Multianalyte assays with algorithmic analyses (MAAAs) are procedures that utilize multiple results derived from assays of various types, including molecular pathology assays, fluorescent in situ hybridization assays and non-nucleic acid based assays (eg, proteins, polypeptides, lipids, carbohydrates). Algorithmic analysis using the results of these assays as well as other patient information (if used) is then performed and reported typically as a numeric score(s) or as a probability. MAAAs are typically unique to a single clinical laboratory or manufacturer. The results of individual component procedure(s) that are inputs to the MAAAs may be provided on the associated laboratory report, however these assays are not reported separately using additional codes. MAAAs, by nature, are typically unique to a single clinical laboratory or manufacturer.

The list includes a proprietary name and clinical laboratory or manufacturer in the first column, an alpha-numeric code in the second column and code descriptor in the third column. The format for the code descriptor usually includes (in order):

- Disease type (eg, oncology, autoimmune, tissue rejection),
- Chemical(s) analyzed (eg, DNA, RNA, protein, antibody),
- Number of markers (eg, number of genes, number of proteins),
- Methodology(s) (eg, microarray, real-time [RT]-PCR, in situ hybridization [ISH], enzyme linked immunosorbent assays [ELISA]),
- Number of functional domains (if indicated),
- Specimen type (eg, blood, fresh tissue, formalin-fixed paraffin-embedded),
- Algorithm result type (eg, prognostic, diagnostic),
- Report (eg, probability index, risk score).

MAAA procedures that have been assigned a Category I code are noted in the list below and additionally listed in the Category I MAAA section (81500-81599). The Category I MAAA section introductory language and associated parenthetical instruction(s) should be used to govern the appropriate use for Category I MAAA codes. If a specific MAAA procedure has not been assigned a Category I code, it is indicated as a four-digit number followed by the letter M.

When a specific MAAA procedure is not included in either the list below or in the Category I MAAA section, report the analysis using the Category I MAAA unlisted code (81599). The codes below are specific to the assays identified in Appendix O by proprietary name. In order to report an MAAA code, the analysis performed must fulfill the code descriptor and, if proprietary, must be the test represented by the proprietary name listed in Appendix O. When an analysis is performed that may potentially fall within a specific descriptor, however the proprietary name is not included in the list below, the MAAA unlisted code (81599) should be used.

Additions in this section may be released tri-annually (or quarterly for PLA codes) via the AMA CPT website to expedite dissemination for reporting. The list will be published annually in the CPT codebook. Go to www.ama-assn.org/go/cpt for the most current listing.

These administrative codes encompass all analytical services required for the algorithmic analysis (eg, cell lysis, nucleic acid stabilization, extraction, digestion, amplification, hybridization and detection) in addition to the algorithmic analysis itself, when applicable. Procedures that are required prior to cell lysis (eg, microdissection, codes 88380 and 88381) should be reported separately.

Appendix O

The codes in this list are provided as an administrative coding set to facilitate accurate reporting of MAAA services. The minimum standard for inclusion in this list is that an analysis is generally available for patient care. The AMA has not reviewed procedures in the administrative coding set for clinical utility. The list is not a complete list of all MAAA procedures.

2. Category I MAAA codes are included below along with their proprietary names. These codes are also listed in the Pathology and Laboratory section of the CPT code set (81490-81599).

3. PLA codes created in response to the Protecting Access to Medicare Act (PAMA) of 2014 are listed along with their proprietary names. These codes are also located at the end of the Pathology and Laboratory section of the CPT code set. In some instances, the descriptor language of PLA codes may be identical, which are differentiated only by the listed propriety names.

Proprietary Name and Clinical Laboratory or Manufacturer	Alpha-Numeric Code	Code Descriptor
Administrative Codes for Multianalyte Assays with Algorithmic Analyses (MAAA)		
—	0001M has been deleted, use 81596)	—
ASH FibroSURE™, ▶BioPredictive S.A.S◀	0002M	Liver disease, ten biochemical assays (ALT, A2-macroglobulin, apolipoprotein A-1, total bilirubin, GGT, haptoglobin, AST, glucose, total cholesterol and triglycerides) utilizing serum, prognostic algorithm reported as quantitative scores for fibrosis, steatosis and alcoholic steatohepatitis (ASH)
NASH FibroSURE™, ▶BioPredictive S.A.S◀	0003M	Liver disease, ten biochemical assays (ALT, A2-macroglobulin, apolipoprotein A-1, total bilirubin, GGT, haptoglobin, AST, glucose, total cholesterol and triglycerides) utilizing serum, prognostic algorithm reported as quantitative scores for fibrosis, steatosis and nonalcoholic steatohepatitis (NASH)
ScoliScore™ Transgenomic	0004M	Scoliosis, DNA analysis of 53 single nucleotide polymorphisms (SNPs), using saliva, prognostic algorithm reported as a risk score
HeproDX™, GoPath Laboratories, LLC	0006M	Oncology (hepatic), mRNA expression levels of 161 genes, utilizing fresh hepatocellular carcinoma tumor tissue, with alpha-fetoprotein level, algorithm reported as a risk classifier
NETest, Wren Laboratories, LLC	0007M	Oncology (gastrointestinal neuroendocrine tumors), real-time PCR expression analysis of 51 genes, utilizing whole peripheral blood, algorithm reported as a nomogram of tumor disease index
—	(0008M has been deleted, use 81520)	—
—	▶(0009M has been deleted)◀	—
NeoLAB™ Prostate Liquid Biopsy, NeoGenomics Laboratories	▲0011M	▶Oncology, prostate cancer, mRNA expression assay of 12 genes (10 content and 2 housekeeping), RT-PCR test utilizing blood plasma and urine, algorithms to predict high-grade prostate cancer risk◀

Proprietary Name and Clinical Laboratory or Manufacturer	Alpha-Numeric Code	Code Descriptor
Cxbladder™ Detect, Pacific Edge Diagnostics USA, Ltd	0012M	Oncology (urothelial), mRNA, gene expression profiling by real-time quantitative PCR of five genes (MDK, HOXA13, CDC2 [CDK1], IGFBP5, and CXCR2), utilizing urine, algorithm reported as a risk score for having urothelial carcinoma
Cxbladder™ Monitor, Pacific Edge Diagnostics USA, Ltd	0013M	Oncology (urothelial), mRNA, gene expression profiling by real-time quantitative PCR of five genes (MDK, HOXA13, CDC2 [CDK1], IGFBP5, and CXCR2), utilizing urine, algorithm reported as a risk score for having recurrent urothelial carcinoma
Category I Codes for Multianalyte Assays with Algorithmic Analyses (MAAA)		
Vectra® DA, Crescendo Bioscience, Inc	81490	Autoimmune (rheumatoid arthritis), analysis of 12 biomarkers using immunoassays, utilizing serum, prognostic algorithm reported as a disease activity score (Do not report 81490 in conjunction with 86140)
Corus® CAD, CardioDx, Inc	81493	Coronary artery disease, mRNA, gene expression profiling by real-time RT-PCR of 23 genes, utilizing whole peripheral blood, algorithm reported as a risk score
AlloMap®, CareDx, Inc	81595	Cardiology (heart transplant), mRNA, gene expression profiling by real-time quantitative PCR of 20 genes (11 content and 9 housekeeping), utilizing subfraction of peripheral blood, algorithm reported as a rejection risk score
Risk of Ovarian Malignancy Algorithm (ROMA)™, Fujirebio Diagnostics	81500	Oncology (ovarian), biochemical assays of two proteins (CA-125 and HE4), utilizing serum, with menopausal status, algorithm reported as a risk score
OVA1™, Vermillion, Inc	81503	Oncology (ovarian), biochemical assays of five proteins (CA-125, apolipoprotein A1, beta-2 microglobulin, transferrin, and pre-albumin), utilizing serum, algorithm reported as a risk score
Tissue of Origin Test Kit-FFPE, Cancer Genetics, Inc	81504	Oncology (tissue of origin), microarray gene expression profiling of >2000 genes, utilizing formalin-fixed paraffin-embedded tissue, algorithm reported as tissue similarity scores
PreDx Diabetes Risk Score™, Tethys Clinical Laboratory	81506	Endocrinology (type 2 diabetes), biochemical assays of seven analytes (glucose, HbA1c, insulin, hs-CRP, adiponectin, ferritin, interleukin 2-receptor alpha), utilizing serum or plasma, algorithm reporting a risk score
Harmony™ Prenatal Test, Ariosa Diagnostics	81507	Fetal aneuploidy (trisomy 21, 18, and 13) DNA sequence analysis of selected regions using maternal plasma, algorithm reported as a risk score for each trisomy

(*Continued on page 252*)

Proprietary Name and Clinical Laboratory or Manufacturer	Alpha-Numeric Code	Code Descriptor
No proprietary name and clinical laboratory or manufacturer. Maternal serum screening procedures are well-established procedures and are performed by many laboratories throughout the country. The concept of prenatal screens has existed and evolved for over 10 years and is not exclusive to any one facility.	81508	Fetal congenital abnormalities, biochemical assays of two proteins (PAPP-A, hCG [any form]), utilizing maternal serum, algorithm reported as a risk score
	81509	Fetal congenital abnormalities, biochemical assays of three proteins (PAPP-A, hCG [any form], DIA), utilizing maternal serum, algorithm reported as a risk score
	81510	Fetal congenital abnormalities, biochemical assays of three analytes (AFP, uE3, hCG [any form]), utilizing maternal serum, algorithm reported as a risk score
	81511	Fetal congenital abnormalities, biochemical assays of four analytes (AFP, uE3, hCG [any form], DIA) utilizing maternal serum, algorithm reported as a risk score (may include additional results from previous biochemical testing)
	81512	Fetal congenital abnormalities, biochemical assays of five analytes (AFP, uE3, total hCG, hyperglycosylated hCG, DIA) utilizing maternal serum, algorithm reported as a risk score
Breast Cancer Index, Biotheranostics, Inc	81518	Oncology (breast), mRNA, gene expression profiling by real-time RT-PCR of 11 genes (7 content and 4 housekeeping), utilizing formalin-fixed paraffin-embedded tissue, algorithms reported as percentage risk for metastatic recurrence and likelihood of benefit from extended endocrine therapy
►EndoPredict®, Myriad Genetic Laboratories, Inc◄	#●81522	►Oncology (breast), mRNA, gene expression profiling by RT-PCR of 12 genes (8 content and 4 housekeeping), utilizing formalin-fixed paraffin-embedded tissue, algorithm reported as recurrence risk score◄
Oncotype DX®, Genomic Health	81519	Oncology (breast), mRNA, gene expression profiling by real-time RT-PCR of 21 genes, utilizing formalin-fixed paraffin-embedded tissue, algorithm reported as recurrence score
Prosigna® Breast Cancer Assay, NanoString Technologies, Inc	81520	Oncology (breast), mRNA gene expression profiling by hybrid capture of 58 genes (50 content and 8 housekeeping), utilizing formalin-fixed paraffin-embedded tissue, algorithm reported as a recurrence risk score
MammaPrint®, Agendia, Inc	81521	Oncology (breast), mRNA, microarray gene expression profiling of 70 content genes and 465 housekeeping genes, utilizing fresh frozen or formalin-fixed paraffin-embedded tissue, algorithm reported as index related to risk of distant metastasis
Oncotype DX® Colon Cancer Assay, Genomic Health	81525	Oncology (colon), mRNA, gene expression profiling by real-time RT-PCR of 12 genes (7 content and 5 housekeeping), utilizing formalin-fixed paraffin-embedded tissue, algorithm reported as a recurrence score

Proprietary Name and Clinical Laboratory or Manufacturer	Alpha-Numeric Code	Code Descriptor
Cologuard™, Exact Sciences, Inc	81528	Oncology (colorectal) screening, quantitative real-time target and signal amplification of 10 DNA markers (KRAS mutations, promoter methylation of NDRG4 and BMP3) and fecal hemoglobin, utilizing stool, algorithm reported as a positive or negative result (Do not report 81528 in conjunction with 81275, 82274)
ChemoFX®, Helomics, Corp	81535 +81536	Oncology (gynecologic), live tumor cell culture and chemotherapeutic response by DAPI stain and morphology, predictive algorithm reported as a drug response score; first single drug or drug combination each additional single drug or drug combination (List separately in addition to code for primary procedure) (Use 81536 in conjunction with 81535)
VeriStrat, Biodesix, Inc	81538	Oncology (lung), mass spectrometric 8-protein signature, including amyloid A, utilizing serum, prognostic and predictive algorithm reported as good versus poor overall survival
4Kscore test, OPKO Health, Inc	81539	Oncology (high-grade prostate cancer), biochemical assay of four proteins (Total PSA, Free PSA, Intact PSA and human kallikrein-2 [hK2]), utilizing plasma or serum, prognostic algorithm reported as a probability score
CancerTYPE ID, bioTheranostics, Inc	81540	Oncology (tumor of unknown origin), mRNA, gene expression profiling by real-time RT-PCR of 92 genes (87 content and 5 housekeeping) to classify tumor into main cancer type and subtype, utilizing formalin-fixed paraffin-embedded tissue, algorithm reported as a probability of a predicted main cancer type and subtype
Prolaris®, Myriad Genetic Laboratories, Inc	81541	Oncology (prostate), mRNA gene expression profiling by real-time RT-PCR of 46 genes (31 content and 15 housekeeping), utilizing formalin-fixed paraffin-embedded tissue, algorithm reported as a disease-specific mortality risk score
▶Decipher® Prostate, Decipher® Biosciences◀	●81542	▶Oncology (prostate) mRNA, microarray gene expression profiling of 22 content genes, utilizing formalin-fixed paraffin-embedded tissue, algorithm reported as metastasis risk score◀
Afirma® Gene Expression Classifier, Veracyte, Inc	81545	Oncology (thyroid), gene expression analysis of 142 genes, utilizing fine needle aspirate, algorithm reported as a categorical result (eg, benign or suspicious)
ConfirmMDx® for Prostate Cancer, MDxHealth, Inc	81551	Oncology (prostate), promoter methylation profiling by real-time PCR of 3 genes (GSTP1, APC, RASSF1), utilizing formalin-fixed paraffin-embedded tissue, algorithm reported as a likelihood of prostate cancer detection on repeat biopsy

(Continued on page 254)

Appendix O

CPT Changes 2020

Proprietary Name and Clinical Laboratory or Manufacturer	Alpha-Numeric Code	Code Descriptor
▶DecisionDx®-UM test, Castle Biosciences, Inc◀	●81552	▶Oncology (uveal melanoma), mRNA, gene expression profiling by real-time RT-PCR of 15 genes (12 content and 3 housekeeping), utilizing fine needle aspirate or formalin-fixed paraffin-embedded tissue, algorithm reported as risk of metastasis◀
HCV FibroSURE™, FibroTest™, BioPredictive S.A.S.	81596	Infectious disease, chronic hepatitis C virus (HCV) infection, six biochemical assays (ALT, A2-macroglobulin, apolipoprotein A-1, total bilirubin, GGT, and haptoglobin) utilizing serum, prognostic algorithm reported as scores for fibrosis and necroinflammatory activity in liver
—	81599	Unlisted multianalyte assay with algorithmic analysis
Proprietary Laboratory Analyses (PLA)		
PreciseType® HEA Test, Immucor, Inc	0001U	Red blood cell antigen typing, DNA, human erythrocyte antigen gene analysis of 35 antigens from 11 blood groups, utilizing whole blood, common RBC alleles reported
PolypDX™, Atlantic Diagnostic Laboratories, LLC, Metabolomic Technologies, Inc	0002U	Oncology (colorectal), quantitative assessment of three urine metabolites (ascorbic acid, succinic acid and carnitine) by liquid chromatography with tandem mass spectrometry (LC-MS/MS) using multiple reaction monitoring acquisition, algorithm reported as likelihood of adenomatous polyps
Overa (OVA1 Next Generation), Asprira Labs, Inc, Vermillion, Inc	0003U	Oncology (ovarian) biochemical assays of five proteins (apolipoprotein A-1, CA 125 II, follicle stimulating hormone, human epididymis protein 4, transferrin), utilizing serum, algorithm reported as a likelihood score
—	(0004U has been deleted)	—
ExosomeDx® Prostate (IntelliScore), Exosome Diagnostics, Inc, Exosome Diagnostics, Inc	0005U	Oncology (prostate) gene expression profile by real-time RT-PCR of 3 genes (*ERG, PCA3,* and *SPDEF*), urine, algorithm reported as risk score
Drug-drug, Drug-substance Identification and Interaction, Aegis Sciences Corporation	0006U	Detection of interacting medications, substances, supplements and foods, 120 or more analytes, definitive chromatography with mass spectrometry, urine, description and severity of each interaction identified, per date of service
ToxProtect, Genotox Laboratories Ltd	0007U	Drug test(s), presumptive, with definitive confirmation of positive results, any number of drug classes, urine, includes specimen verification including DNA authentication in comparison to buccal DNA, per date of service

★=Telemedicine   +=Add-on code   ⁄=FDA approval pending   #=Resequenced code   ⊘=Modifier 51 exempt

CPT Changes 2020 — Appendix O

Proprietary Name and Clinical Laboratory or Manufacturer	Alpha-Numeric Code	Code Descriptor
▶AmHPR® H. pylori Antibiotic Resistance Panel, American Molecular Laboratories, Inc◀	▲0008U	▶Helicobacter pylori detection and antibiotic resistance, DNA, 16S and 23S rRNA, gyrA, pbp1, rdxA and rpoB, next generation sequencing, formalin-fixed paraffin-embedded or fresh tissue or fecal sample, predictive, reported as positive or negative for resistance to clarithromycin, fluoroquinolones, metronidazole, amoxicillin, tetracycline, and rifabutin◀
DEPArray™ HER2, PacificDx	0009U	Oncology (breast cancer), *ERBB2* (HER2) copy number by FISH, tumor cells from formalin-fixed paraffin-embedded tissue isolated using image-based dielectrophoresis (DEP) sorting, reported as *ERBB2* gene amplified or non-amplified
Bacterial Typing by Whole Genome Sequencing, Mayo Clinic	0010U	Infectious disease (bacterial), strain typing by whole genome sequencing, phylogenetic-based report of strain relatedness, per submitted isolate
Cordant CORE™, Cordant Health Solutions	0011U	Prescription drug monitoring, evaluation of drugs present by LC-MS/MS, using oral fluid, reported as a comparison to an estimated steady-state range, per date of service including all drug compounds and metabolites
MatePair Targeted Rearrangements, Congenital, Mayo Clinic	0012U	Germline disorders, gene rearrangement detection by whole genome next-generation sequencing, DNA, whole blood, report of specific gene rearrangement(s)
MatePair Targeted Rearrangements, Oncology, Mayo Clinic	0013U	Oncology (solid organ neoplasia), gene rearrangement detection by whole genome next-generation sequencing, DNA, fresh or frozen tissue or cells, report of specific gene rearrangement(s)
MatePair Targeted Rearrangements, Hematologic, Mayo Clinic	0014U	Hematology (hematolymphoid neoplasia), gene rearrangement detection by whole genome next-generation sequencing, DNA, whole blood or bone marrow, report of specific gene rearrangement(s)
—	(0015U has been deleted)	—
BCR-ABL1 major and minor breakpoint fusion transcripts, University of Iowa, Department of Pathology, Asuragen	0016U	Oncology (hematolymphoid neoplasia), RNA, *BCR/ABL1* major and minor breakpoint fusion transcripts, quantitative PCR amplification, blood or bone marrow, report of fusion not detected or detected with quantitation
JAK2 Mutation, University of Iowa, Department of Pathology	0017U	Oncology (hematolymphoid neoplasia), *JAK2* mutation, DNA, PCR amplification of exons 12-14 and sequence analysis, blood or bone marrow, report of *JAK2* mutation not detected or detected
ThyraMIR™, Interpace Diagnostics	0018U	Oncology (thyroid), microRNA profiling by RT-PCR of 10 microRNA sequences, utilizing fine needle aspirate, algorithm reported as a positive or negative result for moderate to high risk of malignancy

(Continued on page 256)

▲ = Revised code   ● = New code   ▶◀ = Contains new or revised text   ✄ = Duplicate PLA test   ↕ = Category I PLA

Proprietary Name and Clinical Laboratory or Manufacturer	Alpha-Numeric Code	Code Descriptor
OncoTarget/OncoTreat, Columbia University Department of Pathology and Cell Biology, Darwin Health	0019U	Oncology, RNA, gene expression by whole transcriptome sequencing, formalin-fixed paraffin-embedded tissue or fresh frozen tissue, predictive algorithm reported as potential targets for therapeutic agents
—	▶(0020U has been deleted)◀	—
Apifiny®, Armune BioScience, Inc	0021U	Oncology (prostate), detection of 8 autoantibodies (ARF 6, NKX3-1, 5'-UTR-BMI1, CEP 164, 3'-UTR-Ropporin, Desmocollin, AURKAIP-1, CSNK2A2), multiplexed immunoassay and flow cytometry serum, algorithm reported as risk score
Oncomine™ Dx Target Test, Thermo Fisher Scientific	0022U	Targeted genomic sequence analysis panel, non-small cell lung neoplasia, DNA and RNA analysis, 23 genes, interrogation for sequence variants and rearrangements, reported as presence/absence of variants and associated therapy(ies) to consider
LeukoStrat® CDx *FLT3* Mutation Assay, LabPMM LLC, an Invivoscribe Technologies, Inc Company, Invivoscribe Technologies, Inc	0023U	Oncology (acute myelogenous leukemia), DNA, genotyping of internal tandem duplication, p.D835, p.I836, using mononuclear cells, reported as detection or non-detection of *FLT3* mutation and indication for or against the use of midostaurin
GlycA, Laboratory Corporation of America, Laboratory Corporation of America	0024U	Glycosylated acute phase proteins (GlycA), nuclear magnetic resonance spectroscopy, quantitative
UrSure Tenofovir Quantification Test, Synergy Medical Laboratories, UrSure Inc	0025U	Tenofovir, by liquid chromatography with tandem mass spectrometry (LC-MS/MS), urine, quantitative
Thyroseq Genomic Classifier, CBLPath, Inc, University of Pittsburgh Medical Center	0026U	Oncology (thyroid), DNA and mRNA of 112 genes, next-generation sequencing, fine needle aspirate of thyroid nodule, algorithmic analysis reported as a categorical result ("Positive, high probability of malignancy" or "Negative, low probability of malignancy")
JAK2 Exons 12 to 15 Sequencing, Mayo Clinic, Mayo Clinic	0027U	*JAK2 (Janus kinase 2)* (eg, myeloproliferative disorder) gene analysis, targeted sequence analysis exons 12-15
—	▶(0028U has been deleted)◀	—
Focused Pharmacogenomics Panel, Mayo Clinic, Mayo Clinic	0029U	Drug metabolism (adverse drug reactions and drug response), targeted sequence analysis (ie, *CYP1A2, CYP2C19, CYP2C9, CYP2D6, CYP3A4, CYP3A5, CYP4F2, SLCO1B1, VKORC1* and rs12777823)
Warfarin Response Genotype, Mayo Clinic, Mayo Clinic	0030U	Drug metabolism (warfarin drug response), targeted sequence analysis (ie, *CYP2C9, CYP4F2, VKORC1,* rs12777823)
Cytochrome P450 1A2 Genotype, Mayo Clinic, Mayo Clinic	0031U	*CYP1A2 (cytochrome P450 family 1, subfamily A, member 2)* (eg, drug metabolism) gene analysis, common variants (ie, *1F, *1K, *6, *7)

Proprietary Name and Clinical Laboratory or Manufacturer	Alpha-Numeric Code	Code Descriptor
Catechol-O-Methyltransferase (COMT) Genotype, Mayo Clinic, Mayo Clinic	0032U	*COMT (catechol-O-methyltransferase)* (eg, drug metabolism) gene analysis, c.472G>A (rs4680) variant
Serotonin Receptor Genotype (*HTR2A* and *HTR2C*), Mayo Clinic, Mayo Clinic	0033U	*HTR2A (5-hydroxytryptamine receptor 2A), HTR2C (5-hydroxytryptamine receptor 2C)* (eg, citalopram metabolism) gene analysis, common variants (ie, *HTR2A* rs7997012 [c.614-2211T>C], *HTR2C* rs3813929 [c.-759C>T] and rs1414334 [c.551-3008C>G])
Thiopurine Methyltransferase (*TPMT*) and Nudix Hydrolase (*NUDT15*) Genotyping, Mayo Clinic, Mayo Clinic	0034U	*TPMT (thiopurine S-methyltransferase), NUDT15 (nudix hydroxylase 15)* (eg, thiopurine metabolism) gene analysis, common variants (ie, *TPMT* *2, *3A, *3B, *3C, *4, *5, *6, *8, *12; *NUDT15* *3, *4, *5)
Real-time quaking-induced conversion for prion detection (RT-QuIC), National Prion Disease Pathology Surveillance Center	0035U	Neurology (prion disease), cerebrospinal fluid, detection of prion protein by quaking-induced conformational conversion, qualitative
EXaCT-1 Whole Exome Testing, Lab of Oncology-Molecular Detection, Weill Cornell Medicine-Clinical Genomics Laboratory	0036U	Exome (ie, somatic mutations), paired formalin-fixed paraffin-embedded tumor tissue and normal specimen, sequence analyses
FoundationOne CDx™ (F1CDx), Foundation Medicine, Inc, Foundation Medicine, Inc	0037U	Targeted genomic sequence analysis, solid organ neoplasm, DNA analysis of 324 genes, interrogation for sequence variants, gene copy number amplifications, gene rearrangements, microsatellite instability and tumor mutational burden
Sensieva™ Droplet 25OH Vitamin D2/D3 Microvolume LC/MS Assay, InSource Diagnostics, InSource Diagnostics	0038U	Vitamin D, 25 hydroxy D2 and D3, by LC-MS/MS, serum microsample, quantitative
Anti-dsDNA, High Salt/Avidity, University of Washington, Department of Laboratory Medicine, Bio-Rad	0039U	Deoxyribonucleic acid (DNA) antibody, double stranded, high avidity
MRDx BCR-ABL Test, MolecularMD, MolecularMD	0040U	*BCR/ABL1 (t(9;22))* (eg, chronic myelogenous leukemia) translocation analysis, major breakpoint, quantitative
Lyme ImmunoBlot IgM, IGeneX Inc, ID-FISH Technology Inc (ASR) (Lyme ImmunoBlot IgM Strips Only)	0041U	Borrelia burgdorferi, antibody detection of 5 recombinant protein groups, by immunoblot, IgM
Lyme ImmunoBlot IgG, IGeneX Inc, ID-FISH Technology Inc (ASR) (Lyme ImmunoBlot IgG Strips Only)	0042U	Borrelia burgdorferi, antibody detection of 12 recombinant protein groups, by immunoblot, IgG
Tick-Borne Relapsing Fever (TBRF) Borrelia ImmunoBlots IgM Test, IGeneX Inc, ID-FISH Technology (Provides TBRF ImmunoBlot IgM Strips)	0043U	Tick-borne relapsing fever Borrelia group, antibody detection to 4 recombinant protein groups, by immunoblot, IgM

(Continued on page 258)

Proprietary Name and Clinical Laboratory or Manufacturer	Alpha-Numeric Code	Code Descriptor
Tick-Borne Relapsing Fever (TBRF) Borrelia ImmunoBlots IgG Test, IGeneX Inc, ID-FISH Technology Inc (Provides TBRF ImmunoBlot IgG Strips)	0044U	Tick-borne relapsing fever Borrelia group, antibody detection to 4 recombinant protein groups, by immunoblot, IgG
The Oncotype DX® Breast DCIS Score™ Test, Genomic Health, Inc, Genomic Health, Inc	0045U	Oncology (breast ductal carcinoma in situ), mRNA, gene expression profiling by real-time RT-PCR of 12 genes (7 content and 5 housekeeping), utilizing formalin-fixed paraffin-embedded tissue, algorithm reported as recurrence score
FLT3 ITD MRD by NGS, LabPMM LLC, an Invivoscribe Technologies, Inc Company	0046U	FLT3 (fms-related tyrosine kinase 3) (eg, acute myeloid leukemia) internal tandem duplication (ITD) variants, quantitative
Oncotype DX Genomic Prostate Score, Genomic Health, Inc, Genomic Health, Inc	0047U	Oncology (prostate), mRNA, gene expression profiling by real-time RT-PCR of 17 genes (12 content and 5 housekeeping), utilizing formalin-fixed paraffin-embedded tissue, algorithm reported as a risk score
MSK-IMPACT (Integrated Mutation Profiling of Actionable Cancer Targets), Memorial Sloan Kettering Cancer Center	0048U	Oncology (solid organ neoplasia), DNA, targeted sequencing of protein-coding exons of 468 cancer-associated genes, including interrogation for somatic mutations and microsatellite instability, matched with normal specimens, utilizing formalin-fixed paraffin-embedded tumor tissue, report of clinically significant mutation(s)
NPM1 MRD by NGS, LabPMM LLC, an Invivoscribe Technologies, Inc Company	0049U	NPM1 (nucleophosmin) (eg, acute myeloid leukemia) gene analysis, quantitative
MyAML NGS Panel, LabPMM LLC, an Invivoscribe Technologies, Inc Company	0050U	Targeted genomic sequence analysis panel, acute myelogenous leukemia, DNA analysis, 194 genes, interrogation for sequence variants, copy number variants or rearrangements
UCompliDx, Elite Medical Laboratory Solutions, LLC, Elite Medical Laboratory Solutions, LLC (LDT)	0051U	Prescription drug monitoring, evaluation of drugs present by LC-MS/MS, urine, 31 drug panel, reported as quantitative results, detected or not detected, per date of service
VAP Cholesterol Test, VAP Diagnostics Laboratory, Inc, VAP Diagnostics Laboratory, Inc	0052U	Lipoprotein, blood, high resolution fractionation and quantitation of lipoproteins including all five major lipoprotein classes and the subclasses of HDL, LDL, and VLDL by vertical auto profile ultracentrifugation
Prostate Cancer Risk Panel, Mayo Clinic, Laboratory Developed Test	0053U	Oncology (prostate cancer), FISH analysis of 4 genes (ASAP1, HDAC9, CHD1 and PTEN), needle biopsy specimen, algorithm reported as probability of higher tumor grade
AssuranceRx Micro Serum, Firstox Laboratories, LLC, Firstox Laboratories, LLC	0054U	Prescription drug monitoring, 14 or more classes of drugs and substances, definitive tandem mass spectrometry with chromatography, capillary blood, quantitative report with therapeutic and toxic ranges, including steady-state range for the prescribed dose when detected, per date of service

Proprietary Name and Clinical Laboratory or Manufacturer	Alpha-Numeric Code	Code Descriptor
myTAIHEART, TAI Diagnostics, Inc, TAI Diagnostics, Inc	0055U	Cardiology (heart transplant), cell-free DNA, PCR assay of 96 DNA target sequences (94 single nucleotide polymorphism targets and two control targets), plasma
MatePair Acute Myeloid Leukemia Panel, Mayo Clinic, Laboratory Developed Test	0056U	Hematology (acute myelogenous leukemia), DNA, whole genome next-generation sequencing to detect gene rearrangement(s), blood or bone marrow, report of specific gene rearrangement(s)
—	▶(0057U has been deleted)◀	—
Merkel SmT Oncoprotein Antibody Titer, University of Washington, Department of Laboratory Medicine	0058U	Oncology (Merkel cell carcinoma), detection of antibodies to the Merkel cell polyoma virus oncoprotein (small T antigen), serum, quantitative
Merkel Virus VP1 Capsid Antibody, University of Washington, Department of Laboratory Medicine	0059U	Oncology (Merkel cell carcinoma), detection of antibodies to the Merkel cell polyoma virus capsid protein (VP1), serum, reported as positive or negative
Twins Zygosity PLA, Natera, Inc, Natera, Inc	0060U	Twin zygosity, genomic-targeted sequence analysis of chromosome 2, using circulating cell-free fetal DNA in maternal blood
Transcutaneous multispectral measurement of tissue oxygenation and hemoglobin using spatial frequency domain imaging (SFDI), Modulated Imaging, Inc, Modulated Imaging, Inc	0061U	Transcutaneous measurement of five biomarkers (tissue oxygenation [StO_2], oxyhemoglobin [$ctHbO_2$], deoxyhemoglobin [ctHbR], papillary and reticular dermal hemoglobin concentrations [ctHb1 and ctHb2]), using spatial frequency domain imaging (SFDI) and multi-spectral analysis
▶SLE-key® Rule Out, Veracis Inc Veracis Inc◀	●0062U	▶Autoimmune (systemic lupus erythematosus), IgG and IgM analysis of 80 biomarkers, utilizing serum, algorithm reported with a risk score◀
▶NPDX ASD ADM Panel I, Stemina Biomarker Discovery, Inc, Stemina Biomarker Discovery, Inc d/b/a NeuroPointDX◀	●0063U	▶Neurology (autism), 32 amines by LC-MS/MS, using plasma, algorithm reported as metabolic signature associated with autism spectrum disorder◀
▶BioPlex 2200 Syphilis Total & RPR Assay, Bio-Rad Laboratories, Bio-Rad Laboratories◀	●0064U	▶Antibody, Treponema pallidum, total and rapid plasma reagin (RPR), immunoassay, qualitative◀
▶BioPlex 2200 RPR Assay, Bio-Rad Laboratories, Bio-Rad Laboratories◀	●0065U	▶Syphilis test, non-treponemal antibody, immunoassay, qualitative (RPR)◀
▶PartoSure™ Test, Parsagen Diagnostics, Inc, Parsagen Diagnostics, Inc, a QIAGEN Company◀	●0066U	▶Placental alpha-micro globulin-1 (PAMG-1), immunoassay with direct optical observation, cervico-vaginal fluid, each specimen◀

(Continued on page 260)

Proprietary Name and Clinical Laboratory or Manufacturer	Alpha-Numeric Code	Code Descriptor
▶BBDRisk Dx™, Silbiotech, Inc, Silbiotech, Inc◀	●0067U	▶Oncology (breast), immunohistochemistry, protein expression profiling of 4 biomarkers (matrix metalloproteinase-1 [MMP-1], carcinoembryonic antigen-related cell adhesion molecule 6 [CEACAM6], hyaluronoglucosaminidase [HYAL1], highly expressed in cancer protein [HEC1]), formalin-fixed paraffin-embedded precancerous breast tissue, algorithm reported as carcinoma risk score◀
▶MYCODART Dual Amplification Real Time PCR Panel for 6 Candida species, RealTime Laboratories, Inc, RealTime Laboratories, Inc◀	●0068U	▶Candida species panel (*C. albicans, C. glabrata, C. parapsilosis, C. kruseii, C. tropicalis,* and *C. auris*), amplified probe technique with qualitative report of the presence or absence of each species◀
▶miR-31now™, GoPath Laboratories, GoPath Laboratories◀	●0069U	▶Oncology (colorectal), microRNA, RT-PCR expression profiling of miR-31-3p, formalin-fixed paraffin-embedded tissue, algorithm reported as an expression score◀
▶*CYP2D6* Common Variants and Copy Number, Mayo Clinic, Laboratory Developed Test◀	●0070U	▶*CYP2D6 (cytochrome P450, family 2, subfamily D, polypeptide 6)* (eg, drug metabolism) gene analysis, common and select rare variants (ie, *2, *3, *4, *4N, *5, *6, *7, *8, *9, *10, *11, *12, *13, *14A, *14B, *15, *17, *29, *35, *36, *41, *57, *61, *63, *68, *83, *xN)◀
▶*CYP2D6* Full Gene Sequencing, Mayo Clinic, Laboratory Developed Test◀	+●0071U	▶*CYP2D6 (cytochrome P450, family 2, subfamily D, polypeptide 6)* (eg, drug metabolism) gene analysis, full gene sequence (List separately in addition to code for primary procedure)◀
		▶(Use 0071U in conjunction with 0070U)◀
▶*CYP2D6-2D7* Hybrid Gene Targeted Sequence Analysis, Mayo Clinic, Laboratory Developed Test◀	+●0072U	▶*CYP2D6 (cytochrome P450, family 2, subfamily D, polypeptide 6)* (eg, drug metabolism) gene analysis, targeted sequence analysis (ie, CYP2D6-2D7 hybrid gene) (List separately in addition to code for primary procedure)◀
		▶(Use 0072U in conjunction with 0070U)◀
▶*CYP2D7-2D6* Hybrid Gene Targeted Sequence Analysis, Mayo Clinic, Laboratory Developed Test◀	+●0073U	▶*CYP2D6 (cytochrome P450, family 2, subfamily D, polypeptide 6)* (eg, drug metabolism) gene analysis, targeted sequence analysis (ie, CYP2D7-2D6 hybrid gene) (List separately in addition to code for primary procedure)◀
		▶(Use 0073U in conjunction with 0070U)◀
▶*CYP2D6* trans-duplication/multiplication non-duplicated gene targeted sequence analysis, Mayo Clinic, Laboratory Developed Test◀	+●0074U	▶*CYP2D6 (cytochrome P450, family 2, subfamily D, polypeptide 6)* (eg, drug metabolism) gene analysis, targeted sequence analysis (ie, non-duplicated gene when duplication/multiplication is trans) (List separately in addition to code for primary procedure)◀
		▶(Use 0074U in conjunction with 0070U)◀

Proprietary Name and Clinical Laboratory or Manufacturer	Alpha-Numeric Code	Code Descriptor
►CYP2D6 5' gene duplication/multiplication targeted sequence analysis, Mayo Clinic, Laboratory Developed Test◄	+●0075U	►CYP2D6 (cytochrome P450, family 2, subfamily D, polypeptide 6) (eg, drug metabolism) gene analysis, targeted sequence analysis (ie, 5' gene duplication/multiplication) (List separately in addition to code for primary procedure)◄ ►(Use 0075U in conjunction with 0070U)◄
►CYP2D6 3' gene duplication/multiplication targeted sequence analysis, Mayo Clinic, Laboratory Developed Test◄	+●0076U	►CYP2D6 (cytochrome P450, family 2, subfamily D, polypeptide 6) (eg, drug metabolism) gene analysis, targeted sequence analysis (ie, 3' gene duplication/multiplication) (List separately in addition to code for primary procedure)◄ ►(Use 0076U in conjunction with 0070U)◄
►M-Protein Detection and Isotyping by MALDI-TOF Mass Spectrometry, Mayo Clinic, Laboratory Developed Test◄	●0077U	►Immunoglobulin paraprotein (M-protein), qualitative, immunoprecipitation and mass spectrometry, blood or urine, including isotype◄
►INFINITI® Neural Response Panel, PersonalizeDx Labs, AutoGenomics Inc◄	●0078U	►Pain management (opioid-use disorder) genotyping panel, 16 common variants (ie, ABCB1, COMT, DAT1, DBH, DOR, DRD1, DRD2, DRD4, GABA, GAL, HTR2A, HTTLPR, MTHFR, MUOR, OPRK1, OPRM1), buccal swab or other germline tissue sample, algorithm reported as positive or negative risk of opioid-use disorder◄
►ToxLok™, InSource Diagnostics, InSource Diagnostics◄	●0079U	►Comparative DNA analysis using multiple selected single-nucleotide polymorphisms (SNPs), urine and buccal DNA, for specimen identity verification◄
►BDX-XL2, Biodesix®, Inc, Biodesix®, Inc◄	●0080U	►Oncology (lung), mass spectrometric analysis of galectin-3-binding protein and scavenger receptor cysteine-rich type 1 protein M130, with five clinical risk factors (age, smoking status, nodule diameter, nodule-spiculation status and nodule location), utilizing plasma, algorithm reported as a categorical probability of malignancy◄
—	►(0081U has been deleted. To report, use 81552)◄	—
►NextGen Precision™ Testing, Precision Diagnostics, Precision Diagnostics LBN Precision Toxicology, LLC◄	●0082U	►Drug test(s), definitive, 90 or more drugs or substances, definitive chromatography with mass spectrometry, and presumptive, any number of drug classes, by instrument chemistry analyzer (utilizing immunoassay), urine, report of presence or absence of each drug, drug metabolite or substance with description and severity of significant interactions per date of service◄
►Onco4D™, Animated Dynamics, Inc, Animated Dynamics, Inc◄	●0083U	►Oncology, response to chemotherapy drugs using motility contrast tomography, fresh or frozen tissue, reported as likelihood of sensitivity or resistance to drugs or drug combinations◄

(Continued on page 262)

Proprietary Name and Clinical Laboratory or Manufacturer	Alpha-Numeric Code	Code Descriptor
▶BLOODchip® ID CORE XT™, Grifols Diagnostic Solutions Inc◀	●0084U	▶Red blood cell antigen typing, DNA, genotyping of 10 blood groups with phenotype prediction of 37 red blood cell antigens◀
▶IB*Schek*™, Commonwealth Diagnostics International, Inc◀	●0085U	▶Cytolethal distending toxin B (CdtB) and vinculin IgG antibodies by immunoassay (ie, ELISA)◀
▶Accelerate PhenoTest™ BC kit, Accelerate Diagnostics, Inc◀	●0086U	▶Infectious disease (bacterial and fungal), organism identification, blood culture, using rRNA FISH, 6 or more organism targets, reported as positive or negative with phenotypic minimum inhibitory concentration (MIC)-based antimicrobial susceptibility◀
▶Molecular Microscope® MMDx—Heart, Kashi Clinical Laboratories◀	●0087U	▶Cardiology (heart transplant), mRNA gene expression profiling by microarray of 1283 genes, transplant biopsy tissue, allograft rejection and injury algorithm reported as a probability score◀
▶Molecular Microscope® MMDx—Kidney, Kashi Clinical Laboratories◀	●0088U	▶Transplantation medicine (kidney allograft rejection), microarray gene expression profiling of 1494 genes, utilizing transplant biopsy tissue, algorithm reported as a probability score for rejection◀
▶Pigmented Lesion Assay (PLA), DermTech◀	●0089U	▶Oncology (melanoma), gene expression profiling by RTqPCR, *PRAME* and *LINC00518*, superficial collection using adhesive patch(es)◀
▶myPath® Melanoma, Myriad Genetic Laboratories◀	●0090U	▶Oncology (cutaneous melanoma), mRNA gene expression profiling by RT-PCR of 23 genes (14 content and 9 housekeeping), utilizing formalin-fixed paraffin-embedded tissue, algorithm reported as a categorical result (ie, benign, indeterminate, malignant)◀
▶FirstSight^CRC, CellMax Life◀	●0091U	▶Oncology (colorectal) screening, cell enumeration of circulating tumor cells, utilizing whole blood, algorithm, for the presence of adenoma or cancer, reported as a positive or negative result◀
▶REVEAL Lung Nodule Characterization, MagArray, Inc◀	●0092U	▶Oncology (lung), three protein biomarkers, immunoassay using magnetic nanosensor technology, plasma, algorithm reported as risk score for likelihood of malignancy◀
▶ComplyRX, Claro Labs◀	●0093U	▶Prescription drug monitoring, evaluation of 65 common drugs by LC-MS/MS, urine, each drug reported detected or not detected◀
▶RCIGM Rapid Whole Genome Sequencing, Rady Children's Institute for Genomic Medicine (RCIGM)◀	●0094U	▶Genome (eg, unexplained constitutional or heritable disorder or syndrome), rapid sequence analysis◀

Proprietary Name and Clinical Laboratory or Manufacturer	Alpha-Numeric Code	Code Descriptor
▶Esophageal String Test™ (EST), Cambridge Biomedical, Inc◀	●0095U	▶Inflammation (eosinophilic esophagitis), ELISA analysis of eotaxin-3 *(CCL26 [C-C motif chemokine ligand 26])* and major basic protein *(PRG2 [proteoglycan 2, pro eosinophil major basic protein])*, specimen obtained by swallowed nylon string, algorithm reported as predictive probability index for active eosinophilic esophagitis◀
▶HPV, High-Risk, Male Urine, Molecular Testing Labs◀	●0096U	▶Human papillomavirus (HPV), high-risk types (ie, 16, 18, 31, 33, 35, 39, 45, 51, 52, 56, 58, 59, 66, 68), male urine◀
▶BioFire® FilmArray® Gastrointestinal (GI) Panel, BioFire® Diagnostics◀	●0097U	▶Gastrointestinal pathogen, multiplex reverse transcription and multiplex amplified probe technique, multiple types or subtypes, 22 targets (Campylobacter [C. jejuni/C. coli/C. upsaliensis], Clostridium difficile [C. difficile] toxin A/B, Plesiomonas shigelloides, Salmonella, Vibrio [V. parahaemolyticus/V. vulnificus/V. cholerae], including specific identification of Vibrio cholerae, Yersinia enterocolitica, Enteroaggregative Escherichia coli [EAEC], Enteropathogenic Escherichia coli [EPEC], Enterotoxigenic Escherichia coli [ETEC] lt/st, Shiga-like toxin-producing Escherichia coli [STEC] stx1/stx2 [including specific identification of the E. coli O157 serogroup within STEC], Shigella/Enteroinvasive Escherichia coli [EIEC], Cryptosporidium, Cyclospora cayetanensis, Entamoeba histolytica, Giardia lamblia [also known as G. intestinalis and G. duodenalis], adenovirus F 40/41, astrovirus, norovirus GI/GII, rotavirus A, sapovirus [Genogroups I, II, IV, and V])◀
▶BioFire® FilmArray® Respiratory Panel (RP) EZ, BioFire® Diagnostics◀	●0098U	▶Respiratory pathogen, multiplex reverse transcription and multiplex amplified probe technique, multiple types or subtypes, 14 targets (adenovirus, coronavirus, human metapneumovirus, influenza A, influenza A subtype H1, influenza A subtype H3, influenza A subtype H1-2009, influenza B, parainfluenza virus, human rhinovirus/enterovirus, respiratory syncytial virus, Bordetella pertussis, Chlamydophila pneumoniae, Mycoplasma pneumoniae)◀

(Continued on page 264)

Appendix O

Proprietary Name and Clinical Laboratory or Manufacturer	Alpha-Numeric Code	Code Descriptor
▶BioFire® FilmArray® Respiratory Panel (RP), BioFire® Diagnostics◀	●0099U	▶Respiratory pathogen, multiplex reverse transcription and multiplex amplified probe technique, multiple types or subtypes, 20 targets (adenovirus, coronavirus 229E, coronavirus HKU1, coronavirus, coronavirus OC43, human metapneumovirus, influenza A, influenza A subtype, influenza A subtype H3, influenza A subtype H1-2009, influenza, parainfluenza virus, parainfluenza virus 2, parainfluenza virus 3, parainfluenza virus 4, human rhinovirus/enterovirus, respiratory syncytial virus, Bordetella pertussis, Chlamydophila pneumonia, Mycoplasma pneumoniae)◀
▶BioFire® FilmArray® Respiratory Panel 2 (RP2), BioFire® Diagnostics◀	●0100U	▶Respiratory pathogen, multiplex reverse transcription and multiplex amplified probe technique, multiple types or subtypes, 21 targets (adenovirus, coronavirus 229E, coronavirus HKU1, coronavirus NL63, coronavirus OC43, human metapneumovirus, human rhinovirus/enterovirus, influenza A, including subtypes H1, H1-2009, and H3, influenza B, parainfluenza virus 1, parainfluenza virus 2, parainfluenza virus 3, parainfluenza virus 4, respiratory syncytial virus, Bordetella parapertussis [IS1001], Bordetella pertussis [ptxP], Chlamydia pneumoniae, Mycoplasma pneumoniae)◀
▶ColoNext®, Ambry Genetics®, Ambry Genetics®◀	●0101U	▶Hereditary colon cancer disorders (eg, Lynch syndrome, PTEN hamartoma syndrome, Cowden syndrome, familial adenomatosis polyposis), genomic sequence analysis panel utilizing a combination of NGS, Sanger, MLPA, and array CGH, with mRNA analytics to resolve variants of unknown significance when indicated (15 genes [sequencing and deletion/duplication], *EPCAM* and *GREM1* [deletion/duplication only])◀
▶BreastNext®, Ambry Genetics®, Ambry Genetics®◀	●0102U	▶Hereditary breast cancer-related disorders (eg, hereditary breast cancer, hereditary ovarian cancer, hereditary endometrial cancer), genomic sequence analysis panel utilizing a combination of NGS, Sanger, MLPA, and array CGH, with mRNA analytics to resolve variants of unknown significance when indicated (17 genes [sequencing and deletion/duplication])◀
▶OvaNext®, Ambry Genetics®, Ambry Genetics®◀	●0103U	▶Hereditary ovarian cancer (eg, hereditary ovarian cancer, hereditary endometrial cancer), genomic sequence analysis panel utilizing a combination of NGS, Sanger, MLPA, and array CGH, with mRNA analytics to resolve variants of unknown significance when indicated (24 genes [sequencing and deletion/duplication], *EPCAM* [deletion/duplication only])◀

CPT Changes 2020 — Appendix O

Proprietary Name and Clinical Laboratory or Manufacturer	Alpha-Numeric Code	Code Descriptor
—	▶(0104U has been deleted)◀	—
▶KidneyIntelX™, RenalytixAI, RenalytixAI◀	●0105U	▶Nephrology (chronic kidney disease), multiplex electrochemiluminescent immunoassay (ECLIA) of tumor necrosis factor receptor 1A, receptor superfamily 2 *(TNFR1, TNFR2)*, and kidney injury molecule-1 (KIM-1) combined with longitudinal clinical data, including *APOL1* genotype if available, and plasma (isolated fresh or frozen), algorithm reported as probability score for rapid kidney function decline (RKFD)◀
▶13C-Spirulina Gastric Emptying Breath Test (GEBT), Cairn Diagnostics d/b/a Advanced Breath Diagnostics, LLC, Cairn Diagnostics d/b/a Advanced Breath Diagnostics, LLC◀	●0106U	▶Gastric emptying, serial collection of 7 timed breath specimens, non-radioisotope carbon-13 (^{13}C) spirulina substrate, analysis of each specimen by gas isotope ratio mass spectrometry, reported as rate of $^{13}CO_2$ excretion◀
▶Singulex Clarity C.diff toxins A/B Assay, Singulex◀	●0107U	▶Clostridium difficile toxin(s) antigen detection by immunoassay technique, stool, qualitative, multiple-step method◀
▶TissueCypher® Barrett's Esophagus Assay, Cernostics, Cernostics◀	●0108U	▶Gastroenterology (Barrett's esophagus), whole slide–digital imaging, including morphometric analysis, computer-assisted quantitative immunolabeling of 9 protein biomarkers (p16, AMACR, p53, CD68, COX-2, CD45RO, HIF1a, HER-2, K20) and morphology, formalin-fixed paraffin-embedded tissue, algorithm reported as risk of progression to high-grade dysplasia or cancer◀
▶MYCODART Dual Amplification Real Time PCR Panel for 4 Aspergillus species, RealTime Laboratories, Inc/MycoDART, Inc◀	●0109U	▶Infectious disease (Aspergillus species), real-time PCR for detection of DNA from 4 species *(A. fumigatus, A. terreus, A. niger,* and *A. flavus)*, blood, lavage fluid, or tissue, qualitative reporting of presence or absence of each species◀
▶Oral OncolyticAssuranceRX, Firstox Laboratories, LLC, Firstox Laboratories, LLC◀	●0110U	▶Prescription drug monitoring, one or more oral oncology drug(s) and substances, definitive tandem mass spectrometry with chromatography, serum or plasma from capillary blood or venous blood, quantitative report with steady-state range for the prescribed drug(s) when detected◀
▶Praxis™ Extended RAS Panel, Illumina, Illumina◀	●0111U	▶Oncology (colon cancer), targeted *KRAS* (codons 12, 13, and 61) and *NRAS* (codons 12, 13, and 61) gene analysis, utilizing formalin-fixed paraffin-embedded tissue◀
▶MicroGenDX qPCR & NGS For Infection, MicroGenDX, MicroGenDX◀	●0112U	▶Infectious agent detection and identification, targeted sequence analysis (16S and 18S rRNA genes) with drug-resistance gene◀
▶MiPS (Mi-Prostate Score), MLabs, MLabs◀	●0113U	▶Oncology (prostate), measurement of *PCA3* and *TMPRSS2-ERG* in urine and PSA in serum following prostatic massage, by RNA amplification and fluorescence-based detection, algorithm reported as risk score◀

(Continued on page 266)

▲ = Revised code   ● = New code   ▶◀ = Contains new or revised text   ✕ = Duplicate PLA test   ↕ = Category I PLA

Appendix O

Proprietary Name and Clinical Laboratory or Manufacturer	Alpha-Numeric Code	Code Descriptor
▶EsoGuard™, Lucid Diagnostics, Lucid Diagnostics◀	●0114U	▶Gastroenterology (Barrett's esophagus), *VIM* and *CCNA1* methylation analysis, esophageal cells, algorithm reported as likelihood for Barrett's esophagus◀
▶ePlex Respiratory Pathogen (RP) Panel, GenMark Diagnostics, Inc, GenMark Diagnostics, Inc◀	●0115U	▶Respiratory infectious agent detection by nucleic acid (DNA and RNA), 18 viral types and subtypes and 2 bacterial targets, amplified probe technique, including multiplex reverse transcription for RNA targets, each analyte reported as detected or not detected◀
▶Snapshot Oral Fluid Compliance, Ethos Laboratories◀	●0116U	▶Prescription drug monitoring, enzyme immunoassay of 35 or more drugs confirmed with LC-MS/MS, oral fluid, algorithm results reported as a patient-compliance measurement with risk of drug to drug interactions for prescribed medications◀
▶Foundation PI^{SM}, Ethos Laboratories◀	●0117U	▶Pain management, analysis of 11 endogenous analytes (methylmalonic acid, xanthurenic acid, homocysteine, pyroglutamic acid, vanilmandelate, 5-hydroxyindoleacetic acid, hydroxymethylglutarate, ethylmalonate, 3-hydroxypropyl mercapturic acid (3-HPMA), quinolinic acid, kynurenic acid), LC-MS/MS, urine, algorithm reported as a pain-index score with likelihood of atypical biochemical function associated with pain◀
▶Viracor TRAC™ dd-cfDNA, Viracor Eurofins, Viracor Eurofins◀	●0118U	▶Transplantation medicine, quantification of donor-derived cell-free DNA using whole genome next-generation sequencing, plasma, reported as percentage of donor-derived cell-free DNA in the total cell-free DNA◀
▶MI-HEART Ceramides, Plasma, Mayo Clinic, Laboratory Developed Test◀	●0119U	▶Cardiology, ceramides by liquid chromatography–tandem mass spectrometry, plasma, quantitative report with risk score for major cardiovascular events◀
▶Lymph3Cx Lymphoma Molecular Subtyping Assay, Mayo Clinic, Laboratory Developed Test◀	●0120U	▶Oncology (B-cell lymphoma classification), mRNA, gene expression profiling by fluorescent probe hybridization of 58 genes (45 content and 13 housekeeping genes), formalin-fixed paraffin-embedded tissue, algorithm reported as likelihood for primary mediastinal B-cell lymphoma (PMBCL) and diffuse large B-cell lymphoma (DLBCL) with cell of origin subtyping in the latter◀
▶Flow Adhesion of Whole Blood on VCAM-1 (FAB-V), Functional Fluidics, Functional Fluidics◀	●0121U	▶Sickle cell disease, microfluidic flow adhesion (VCAM-1), whole blood◀
▶Flow Adhesion of Whole Blood to P-SELECTIN (WB-PSEL), Functional Fluidics, Functional Fluidics◀	●0122U	▶Sickle cell disease, microfluidic flow adhesion (P-Selectin), whole blood◀

CPT Changes 2020 — Appendix O

Proprietary Name and Clinical Laboratory or Manufacturer	Alpha-Numeric Code	Code Descriptor
▶Mechanical Fragility, RBC by shear stress profiling and spectral analysis, Functional Fluidics, Functional Fluidics◀	●0123U	▶Mechanical fragility, RBC, shear stress and spectral analysis profiling◀
▶First Trimester Screen	Fß^{SM}, Eurofins NTD, LLC, Eurofins NTD, LLC◀	●0124U	▶Fetal congenital abnormalities, biochemical assays of 3 analytes (free beta-hCG, PAPP-A, AFP), time-resolved fluorescence immunoassay, maternal dried-blood spot, algorithm reported as risk scores for fetal trisomies 13/18 and 21◀
▶Maternal Fetal Screen	T1^{SM}, Eurofins NTD, LLC, Eurofins NTD, LLC◀	●0125U	▶Fetal congenital abnormalities and perinatal complications, biochemical assays of 5 analytes (free beta-hCG, PAPP-A, AFP, placental growth factor, and inhibin-A), time-resolved fluorescence immunoassay, maternal serum, algorithm reported as risk scores for fetal trisomies 13/18, 21, and preeclampsia◀
▶Maternal Fetal Screen	T1 + Y Chromosome^{SM}, Eurofins NTD, LLC, Eurofins NTD, LLC◀	●0126U	▶Fetal congenital abnormalities and perinatal complications, biochemical assays of 5 analytes (free beta-hCG, PAPP-A, AFP, placental growth factor, and inhibin-A), time-resolved fluorescence immunoassay, includes qualitative assessment of Y chromosome in cell-free fetal DNA, maternal serum and plasma, predictive algorithm reported as risk scores for fetal trisomies 13/18, 21, and preeclampsia◀
▶Preeclampsia Screen	T1^{SM}, Eurofins NTD, LLC, Eurofins NTD, LLC◀	●0127U	▶Obstetrics (preeclampsia), biochemical assays of 3 analytes (PAPP-A, AFP, and placental growth factor), time-resolved fluorescence immunoassay, maternal serum, predictive algorithm reported as a risk score for preeclampsia◀
▶Preeclampsia Screen	T1 + Y Chromosome^{SM}, Eurofins NTD, LLC, Eurofins NTD, LLC◀	●0128U	▶Obstetrics (preeclampsia), biochemical assays of 3 analytes (PAPP-A, AFP, and placental growth factor), time-resolved fluorescence immunoassay, includes qualitative assessment of Y chromosome in cell-free fetal DNA, maternal serum and plasma, predictive algorithm reported as a risk score for preeclampsia◀
▶BRCAplus, Ambry Genetics◀	●0129U	▶Hereditary breast cancer–related disorders (eg, hereditary breast cancer, hereditary ovarian cancer, hereditary endometrial cancer), genomic sequence analysis and deletion/duplication analysis panel *(ATM, BRCA1, BRCA2, CDH1, CHEK2, PALB2, PTEN,* and *TP53)*◀
▶+RNAinsight™ for ColoNext®, Ambry Genetics◀	+●0130U	▶Hereditary colon cancer disorders (eg, Lynch syndrome, PTEN hamartoma syndrome, Cowden syndrome, familial adenomatosis polyposis), targeted mRNA sequence analysis panel *(APC, CDH1, CHEK2, MLH1, MSH2, MSH6, MUTYH, PMS2, PTEN,* and *TP53)* (List separately in addition to code for primary procedure)◀
		▶ (Use 0130U in conjunction with 81435, 0101U)◀

(Continued on page 268)

▲ = Revised code   ● = New code   ▶◀ = Contains new or revised text   ✕ = Duplicate PLA test   ↕ = Category I PLA

Appendix O

Proprietary Name and Clinical Laboratory or Manufacturer	Alpha-Numeric Code	Code Descriptor
▶+RNAinsight™ for BreastNext®, Ambry Genetics◀	+●0131U	▶Hereditary breast cancer–related disorders (eg, hereditary breast cancer, hereditary ovarian cancer, hereditary endometrial cancer), targeted mRNA sequence analysis panel (13 genes) (List separately in addition to code for primary procedure)◀ ▶(Use 0131U in conjunction with 81162, 81432, 0102U)◀
▶+RNAinsight™ for OvaNext®, Ambry Genetics◀	+●0132U	▶Hereditary ovarian cancer–related disorders (eg, hereditary breast cancer, hereditary ovarian cancer, hereditary endometrial cancer), targeted mRNA sequence analysis panel (17 genes) (List separately in addition to code for primary procedure)◀ ▶(Use 0132U in conjunction with 81162, 81432, 0103U)◀
▶+RNAinsight™ for ProstateNext®, Ambry Genetics◀	+●0133U	▶Hereditary prostate cancer–related disorders, targeted mRNA sequence analysis panel (11 genes) (List separately in addition to code for primary procedure)◀ ▶(Use 0133U in conjunction with 81162)◀
▶+RNAinsight™ for CancerNext®, Ambry Genetics◀	+●0134U	▶Hereditary pan cancer (eg, hereditary breast and ovarian cancer, hereditary endometrial cancer, hereditary colorectal cancer), targeted mRNA sequence analysis panel (18 genes) (List separately in addition to code for primary procedure)◀ ▶(Use 0134U in conjunction with 81162, 81432, 81435)◀
▶+RNAinsight™ for GYNPlus®, Ambry Genetics◀	+●0135U	▶Hereditary gynecological cancer (eg, hereditary breast and ovarian cancer, hereditary endometrial cancer, hereditary colorectal cancer), targeted mRNA sequence analysis panel (12 genes) (List separately in addition to code for primary procedure)◀ ▶(Use 0135U in conjunction with 81162)◀
▶+RNAinsight™ for *ATM*, Ambry Genetics◀	+●0136U	▶*ATM (ataxia telangiectasia mutated)* (eg, ataxia telangiectasia) mRNA sequence analysis (List separately in addition to code for primary procedure)◀ ▶(Use 0136U in conjunction with 81408)◀
▶+RNAinsight™ for *PALB2*, Ambry Genetics◀	+●0137U	▶*PALB2 (partner and localizer of BRCA2)* (eg, breast and pancreatic cancer) mRNA sequence analysis (List separately in addition to code for primary procedure)◀ ▶(Use 0137U in conjunction with 81307)◀
▶+RNAinsight™ for *BRCA1/2*, Ambry Genetics◀	+●0138U	▶*BRCA1 (BRCA1, DNA repair associated), BRCA2 (BRCA2, DNA repair associated)* (eg, hereditary breast and ovarian cancer) mRNA sequence analysis (List separately in addition to code for primary procedure)◀ ▶(Use 0138U in conjunction with 81162)◀

Rationale

In accordance with the changes (addition of new codes, including the PLA codes) in the Pathology and Laboratory section, Appendix O has been revised to reflect these changes. One administrative MAAA code (0009M) has been deleted and one administrative MAAA code (0011M) has been revised to remove the term "/or" from "and/or" in the descriptor. Three new Category I MAAA codes (81522, 81542, 81552) have been added. In addition, five PLA codes (0020U, 0028U, 0057U, 0081U, 0104U) have been deleted, one PLA code (0008U) has been revised, and 75 PLA codes (0062U-0080U, 0082U-0103U, 0105U-0138U) have been added.

Refer to the codebook and Rationale for codes 81522, 81542, and 81552 and PLA codes in the Pathology and Laboratory section for a full discussion of these changes.

Notes

Indexes

Instructions for the Use of the Changes Indexes

The Changes Indexes are **not** a substitute for the main text of *CPT Changes 2020* or the main text of the CPT codebook. The changes indexes consist of two types of content—coding changes and modifiers—all of which are intended to assist users in searching and locating information quickly within *CPT Changes 2020*.

Index of Coding Changes

The Index of Coding Changes list new, revised, and deleted codes, and/or some codes that may be affected by revised and/or new guidelines and parenthetical notes. This index enables users to quickly search and locate the codes within a page(s), in addition to discerning the status of a code (new, revised, deleted, or textually changed) because the status of each new, revised, or deleted code is noted in parentheses next to the code number:

99444 (deleted) 5, 6, 7, 10, 14, 16
99423 (new) 3, 5-9, 10

Index of Modifiers

The Index of Modifiers does not list all modifiers unless they are new, revised, or deleted, and/or if the modifier may be affected by revised and/or new guidelines and parenthetical notes. A limited Index of Modifiers, ie, limited to only those modifiers that appear in the Rationales, is provided to help users quickly locate these modifiers and to know where in the book these modifiers are listed or mentioned in the Rationales.

52, Reduced Services 72, 78
59, Distinct Procedural Service 98

Indexes

Index of Coding Changes

Code	Pages
0002M (revised)	250
0003M (revised)	250
0009M (deleted)	269
0011M (revised)	269
0008U (revised)	127, 131, 256, 269
0020U (deleted)	127, 131, 238, 256, 269
0028U (deleted)	127, 131, 256, 269
0057U (deleted)	127, 131, 259, 269
0062U (new)	127, 131, 259, 269
0063U (new)	127, 131, 259
0064U (new)	127, 131, 259
0065U (new)	127, 131, 259
0066U (new)	127, 131, 132, 239, 259
0067U (new)	127, 132, 239, 260
0068U (new)	127, 132, 239, 260
0069U (new)	127, 132, 239, 260
0070U (new)	127, 132, 239, 260
0071U (new)	127, 132, 239, 260
0072U (new)	127, 132, 239, 260
0073U (new)	127, 133, 239, 260
0074U (new)	127, 133, 240, 260
0075U (new)	127, 133, 240, 261
0076U (new)	128, 133, 240, 261
0077U (new)	128, 133, 240, 261
0078U (new)	128, 133, 134, 240, 261
0079U (new)	128, 134, 240, 261
0080U (new)	128, 134, 240, 261, 269
0062U-0080U	269
0081U (deleted)	128, 240, 261, 269
0082U (new)	128, 134, 241, 261, 269
0083U (new)	128, 134, 241, 261
0084U (new)	128, 134, 241, 262
0085U (new)	128, 134, 135, 241, 262
0086U (new)	128, 135, 241, 262
0087U (new)	128, 135, 241, 262
0088U (new)	128, 135, 241, 262
0089U (new)	128, 135, 241, 262
0090U (new)	128, 135, 241, 262
0091U (new)	128, 135, 241, 262
0092U (new)	128, 136, 241, 262
0093U (new)	128, 136, 242, 262
0094U (new)	128, 136, 242, 262
0095U (new)	128, 136, 242, 263
0096U (new)	128, 136, 242, 263
0097U (new)	128, 136, 242, 263
0098U (new)	129, 136-137, 242, 263
0099U (new)	129, 137, 243, 264
0100U (new)	129, 137, 243, 264
0101U (new)	129, 137, 243, 264
0102U (new)	129, 137, 243, 264
0103U (new)	129, 137-138, 243, 264
0082U-0103U	269
0104U (deleted)	129, 131, 265, 269
0105U (new)	129, 138, 265, 269
0106U (new)	129, 138, 265
0107U (new)	129, 138, 244, 265
0108U (new)	129, 138, 244, 265
0109U (new)	129, 138, 244, 265
0110U (new)	129, 138, 244, 265
0111U (new)	129, 139, 244, 265
0112U (new)	129, 139, 244, 265
0113U (new)	129, 139, 245, 265
0114U (new)	129, 139, 245, 266
0115U (new)	129, 139, 245, 266
0116U (new)	130, 139, 245, 266
0117U (new)	130, 139, 140, 245, 266
0118U (new)	130, 140, 245, 266
0119U (new)	130, 140, 245, 266
0120U (new)	130, 140, 245, 266
0121U (new)	130, 140, 246, 266
0122U (new)	130, 140, 246, 266
0123U (new)	130, 140, 246, 267
0124U (new)	130, 140, 141, 246, 267
0125U (new)	130, 141, 246, 267
0126U (new)	130, 141, 246, 267
0127U (new)	130, 141, 246, 267
0128U (new)	130, 141, 246, 267
0129U (new)	130, 141, 247, 267
0130U (new)	130, 141, 247, 267
0131U (new)	130, 142, 247, 268
0132U (new)	130, 142, 247, 268
0133U (new)	130, 142, 247, 268
0134U (new)	130, 142, 247, 268
0135U (new)	130, 142, 247, 268
0136U (new)	131, 142, 143, 248, 268
0137U (new)	131, 143, 248, 268
0138U (new)	131, 143, 248, 268
0105U-0138U	269
0205T (deleted)	198
0206T (deleted)	198
0249T (deleted)	63-65, 94, 95, 200
0254T (deleted)	56, 58, 61, 62, 93, 200
0341T (deleted)	200
0345T	46, 158-160, 200, 201, 204, 206
0357T (deleted)	126, 198
0375T (deleted)	35, 202
0377T (deleted)	63, 65, 202
0380T (deleted)	202
0399T (deleted)	158, 202
0402T (revised)	203
0482T (deleted)	98, 203
0543T (new)	204, 205
0544T (new)	46, 47, 158-160, 201, 204-207
0545T (new)	46, 47, 158-160, 201, 204-207

Index of Coding Changes

Code	Pages
0546T (new)	28, 208
0547T (new)	208
0548T (new)	209
0549T (new)	209
0550T (new)	200, 203, 209, 210
0551T (new)	209, 210
0552T (new)	210
0553T (new)	211
0554T (new)	211, 212
0555T (new)	211, 212
0556T (new)	211, 212
0557T (new)	211, 212
0558T (new)	211-213
0559T (new)	94, 213, 214
0560T (new)	94, 213, 214
0561T (new)	94, 213-215
0562T (new)	94, 213-215
0559T-0562T	94
0564T (new)	215, 216
0565T (new)	216
0566T (new)	216, 217
0567T (new)	217
0568T (new)	217
0569T (new)	46, 162, 218, 219
0570T (new)	46, 162, 218, 219, 220
0571T (new)	42, 44, 220, 221-223
0572T (new)	42, 44, 220, 221-223
0573T (new)	42, 44, 220, 221-223
0574T (new)	42, 44, 220-222, 224
0575T (new)	42, 44, 220-224
0576T (new)	42, 44, 220-224
0577T (new)	42, 44, 162, 220-225
0578T (new)	42, 44, 156, 157, 221-222, 225
0579T (new)	42, 44, 156, 157, 221-222, 225
0580T (new)	42, 44, 220-223, 225
0571T-0580T	42, 44
0581T (new)	27, 226
0582T (new)	67, 94, 95, 226, 227
0583T (new)	84, 85, 227
0584T (new)	65, 228
0585T (new)	65, 228
0586T (new)	65, 228, 229
0587T (new)	78, 179, 229, 230
0588T (new)	179, 229, 230
0589T (new)	178, 179, 229, 230
0590T (new)	178, 179, 229, 230
0591T (new)	231
0592T (new)	231, 232
0593T (new)	231, 232
2022F (revised)	192
2023F (new)	192
2024F (revised)	192
2025F (new)	192
2026F (revised)	192
2033F (new)	192
3045F (deleted)	192, 193
3051F (new)	192, 193
3052F (new)	192, 193
15769 (new)	22, 23, 33-35, 37, 84, 200, 203, 204, 216
15771 (new)	22, 23, 25, 33-35, 37, 200, 203, 204, 216
15772 (new)	22-25, 33-35, 37, 200, 203, 204, 216
15773 (new)	22-25, 33-35, 37, 84, 200, 203, 204, 216
15774 (new)	22-25, 33-35, 37, 84, 200, 203, 204, 216
15876-15879	25
19260 (deleted)	26, 27, 34, 38, 39, 62
19271 (deleted)	26, 27, 34, 38, 39
19272 (deleted)	26, 27, 34, 38, 39
20560 (new)	29, 185, 186
20561 (new)	29, 30, 185, 186
20700 (new)	21, 30, 31
20701 (new)	21, 30-32
20702 (new)	21, 30-32
20703 (new)	21, 30-32
20704 (new)	21, 30-32
20705 (new)	21, 30, 31, 33
20700-20705	31
20926 (deleted)	23, 33, 35, 37, 84, 200, 203, 204
21601 (new)	26, 27, 34, 37-39, 62
21602 (new)	26, 27, 34, 37, 38
21603 (new)	26, 27, 34, 37, 38
21601-21603	27
31233 (revised)	35-37
31235 (revised)	35-37
31292 (revised)	36, 37
31293 (revised)	36, 37
31294 (revised)	36, 37
31295 (revised)	36, 37
31296 (revised)	36, 37
31297 (revised)	36, 37
31298 (revised)	35-37
31295-31298	37
33010 (deleted)	39
33011 (deleted)	39
33015 (deleted)	39, 40
33016 (new)	36, 37, 94
33017 (new)	36, 37, 93, 94
33018 (new)	39-41, 93, 94
33019 (new)	39-41, 93, 94
33016-33019	39
33275 (revised)	42-45, 220, 222
33858 (new)	45, 47, 48, 55, 56, 58
33859 (new)	45, 47, 49, 55, 56, 58
33860 (deleted)	45, 47, 56, 58
33858-33864	48
33870 (deleted)	47, 56, 58
33871 (new)	47-49, 55, 56, 58
34717 (new)	50-54, 56-58, 61, 62, 93, 200
34718 (new)	50-58, 61, 62, 93, 200
35701 (revised)	58, 59
35702 (new)	59, 60
35703 (new)	59, 60
35721 (deleted)	59
35741 (deleted)	59
35761 (deleted)	59

Index of Coding Changes

Code	Pages
43401 (deleted)	62, 63
46945 (revised)	63, 64
46946 (revised)	63, 64
46948 (new)	63-65, 94, 95, 200
49013 (new)	65
49014 (new)	65, 66
54640 (revised)	67
62270 (revised)	68, 69, 95, 104
62272 (revised)	68, 69, 95
62328 (new)	68, 69, 95
62329 (new)	68, 69, 95
64400 (revised)	70-73, 78
64402 (deleted)	71, 72
64405 (revised)	70, 71
64408 (revised)	70, 71, 73
64410 (deleted)	71, 72
64413 (deleted)	71, 72
64415 (revised)	70, 71
64416 (revised)	70, 71, 73
64417 (revised)	70, 71, 73
64418 (revised)	70, 71
64420 (revised)	70, 72, 73
64421 (revised)	70, 72, 73
64425 (revised)	70, 72, 74
64430 (revised)	72, 74
64435 (revised)	72, 74
64445 (revised)	72, 74, 75
64446 (revised)	72, 75
64447 (revised)	72, 75
64448 (revised)	72, 75
64449 (revised)	72, 76
64450 (revised)	70-72
64400-64450	72
64451 (new)	71, 72, 76, 77, 167
64454 (new)	70-72, 76, 78
64479-64484	77
64624 (new)	70-72, 78, 79
64625 (new)	79, 167
66711 (revised)	80, 81
66982 (revised)	80, 81
66984 (revised)	80-82
66987 (new)	80-82
66988 (new)	80, 81, 83
74022 (revised)	89
74210 (revised)	89, 90
74220 (revised)	89-91
74221 (new)	89-91
74230 (revised)	89, 90
74240 (revised)	89-91
74241 (deleted)	89, 90
74245 (deleted)	89, 90
74246 (revised)	89-92
74247 (deleted)	89, 90
74248 (new)	89, 90, 92
74249 (deleted)	89, 90
74250 (revised)	89-92
74251 (revised)	89-92
74260 (deleted)	90, 91
74270 (revised)	90, 91, 93
74280 (revised)	90, 91, 93
76930 (deleted)	39, 94
78205 (deleted)	96
78206 (deleted)	96
78320 (deleted)	96
78429 (new)	96-99, 101
78459 (revised)	97, 98, 101, 102
78430 (new)	96-99, 101
78431 (new)	96-98, 100
78432 (new)	96-98, 100
78433 (new)	96-98, 101
78434 (new)	96-98, 102, 203
78491 (revised)	96-98, 101, 103
78492 (revised)	96-98, 103
78607 (deleted)	104
78647 (deleted)	104
78710 (deleted)	104
78800 (revised)	96-98, 104-106
78801 (revised)	96, 97, 104-106
78802 (revised)	96, 97, 104-106
78803 (revised)	96-98, 104-106
78804 (revised)	96-98, 104-106
78800-78804	96-98, 104
78805 (deleted)	105
78806 (deleted)	105
78807 (deleted)	105
78830 (new)	96-98, 104, 105, 107
78831 (new)	96-98, 104, 105, 107
78832 (new)	96-98, 104, 105, 107
78835 (new)	96-98, 104, 105, 108
80145 (new)	113
80187 (new)	113
80230 (new)	113
80235 (new)	113, 114
80280 (new)	113, 114
80285 (new)	113, 114
81277 (new)	114, 115, 123
81307 (new)	114, 115, 123, 131, 248, 268
81308 (new)	114, 115, 123
81309 (new)	115, 116, 119
81350 (revised)	116
81404 (revised)	116, 119
81406 (revised)	114, 115, 119, 123
81407 (revised)	123, 124
81522 (new)	124, 237, 252, 269
81542 (new)	124, 125, 238, 253, 269
81552 (new)	125, 128, 240, 254, 261, 269
87563 (new)	125
87798	125
90460-90472	149
90619 (new)	149
90694 (new)	149
90734 (revised)	149, 150
90911 (deleted)	150, 151
90912 (new)	150, 151

Index of Coding Changes

Code	Pages
90913 (new)	150, 151
92201 (new)	7, 8, 12, 150, 151, 165, 184, 186
92202 (new)	7, 8, 12
92225 (deleted)	151
92226 (deleted)	151
92548 (revised)	152, 153
92549 (new)	152, 153
92626 (revised)	154
92627 (revised)	154
93299 (deleted)	44, 45, 155-157
93356 (new)	158, 202, 203
93784 (revised)	11, 162, 163
93786 (revised)	11, 162, 163
93788 (revised)	11, 162, 163
93790 (revised)	11, 162, 163
93985 (new)	164, 165
93986 (new)	164, 165
94728 (revised)	165, 166
95700-95726	67, 166, 167, 172
95705-95716	172
95717-95726	172, 173
95719-95720	173
95813 (revised)	166-168, 170
95827 (deleted)	167
95831 (deleted)	167, 184, 185
95832 (deleted)	167
95833 (deleted)	167
95834 (deleted)	167, 184, 185
95831-95834	167, 184, 185
95950 (deleted)	67, 166, 169, 172
95951 (deleted)	67, 166, 169, 172
95953 (deleted)	67, 166, 169, 172
95956 (deleted)	67, 166, 169, 171, 172
95715 (new)	169-173, 175
95716 (new)	168-173, 175
95717 (new)	166-173, 175
95718 (new)	166-173, 175, 176
95719 (new)	166, 168-173, 175, 176
95720 (new)	166, 168-173, 176
95721 (new)	166, 168-173, 176
95722 (new)	166, 168-173, 177
95723 (new)	166, 168-173, 177
95724 (new)	166, 168-173, 177
95725 (new)	166, 168-173, 178
95726 (new)	67, 166, 168-173, 178
96150 (deleted)	6, 179-182, 201, 202
96151 (deleted)	6, 179-182, 187, 201, 202
96152 (deleted)	6, 179-182, 187, 201, 202
96153 (deleted)	6, 179-182, 187, 201, 202
96154 (deleted)	6, 179-182, 187, 201, 202
96155 (deleted)	6, 179-182, 187, 201, 202
96156 (new)	6, 179-182, 186, 187, 201, 202, 231
96158 (new)	6, 179-182, 186, 187, 201, 202, 231
96159 (new)	6, 179-187, 201, 202, 231
96164 (new)	6, 179-183, 186, 187, 201, 202, 231
96165 (new)	6, 179-183, 187, 201, 202, 231
96167 (new)	6, 179-183, 186, 187, 201, 202, 231
96168 (new)	6, 179-183, 186, 187, 201, 202
96170 (new)	6, 179-183, 186, 187, 201, 202
96171 (new)	6, 179-182, 184, 186, 187, 201, 202
97127 (deleted)	180, 181, 184, 185
97129 (new)	180, 181, 184, 185
97130 (new)	184, 185
97161-97172	167
98969 (deleted)	4, 5, 10, 14-16, 163, 187, 188
98970 (new)	4, 5, 7, 10, 14, 16, 188
98971 (new)	4, 5, 7, 10, 14, 16, 188, 189
98972 (new)	4, 5, 7, 10, 14, 16, 188, 189
99421 (new)	4, 5-10, 14, 16, 163, 187, 188
99422 (new)	4, 5-10, 14, 16, 163, 187, 188
99423 (new)	4, 5-10, 14, 16, 163, 187, 188
99444 (deleted)	4, 5-8, 10, 14-16, 150, 163
99473 (new)	10-13, 162, 163
99474 (new)	10-13, 162, 163
99457 (revised)	10-13
99458 (new)	12, 13

Index of Modifiers

Modifier, Descriptor — Page Numbers

50, Bilateral Procedure 25, 34, 56, 58, 61, 66, 70, 72, 77, 79, 80, 199, 216, 227, 234, 270
51, Multiple Procedures 161
52, Reduced Services 72, 78
59, Distinct Procedural Service 98
63, Procedure Performed on Infants less than 4 kg 234

NOTES

NOTES

NOTES

NOTES

NOTES

NOTES

NOTES